Senior Acquisitions Editor: Sonya Seigafuse
Senior Product Manager: Kerry Barrett
Vendor Manager: Bridgett Dougherty
Senior Manufacturing Manager: Ben Rivera
Senior Marketing Manager: Kim Schonberger
Creative Director: Doug Smock
Production Service: Aptara, Inc.

Two Commerce Square
2001 Market Street
Philadelphia, PA 19103

Printed in China

Library of Congress Cataloging-in-Publication Data

Bridgeforth, George M.
Lippincott's primary care musculoskeletal radiology / George M. Bridgeforth, John Cherf ; associate editor, Mitesh Trivedi.
p. ; cm.
Other title: Primary care musculoskeletal radiology
Includes bibliographical references and index.
ISBN-13: 978-0-7817-9377-3 (alk. paper)
ISBN-10: 0-7817-9377-7 (alk. paper)
1. Musculoskeletal system—Radiography. 2. Musculoskeletal system—Diseases—Diagnosis. 3. Primary care (Medicine) I. Cherf, John. II. Trivedi, Mitesh. III. Title. IV. Title: Primary care musculoskeletal radiology.
[DNLM: 1. Musculoskeletal Diseases—radiography. 2. Diagnostic Imaging—methods. 3. Musculoskeletal System—radiography. WE 141]
RC925.7.B75 2011
616.7'0757—dc22 2010029762

Care has been taken to confirm the accuracy of the information presented and to describe generally accepted practices. However, the authors, editors, and publisher are not responsible for errors or omissions or for any consequences from application of the information in this book and make no warranty, expressed or implied, with respect to the currency, completeness, or accuracy of the contents of the publication. Application of the information in a particular situation remains the professional responsibility of the practitioner.

The authors, editors, and publisher have exerted every effort to ensure that drug selection and dosage set forth in this text are in accordance with current recommendations and practice at the time of publication. However, in view of ongoing research, changes in government regulations, and the constant flow of information relating to drug therapy and drug reactions, the reader is urged to check the package insert for each drug for any change in indications and dosage and for added warnings and precautions. This is particularly important when the recommended agent is a new or infrequently employed drug.

Some drugs and medical devices presented in the publication have Food and Drug Administration (FDA) clearance for limited use in restricted research settings. It is the responsibility of the health care provider to ascertain the FDA status of each drug or device planned for use in their clinical practice.

To purchase additional copies of this book, call our customer service department at (800) 638-3030 or fax orders to (301) 223-2320. International customers should call (301) 223-2300.

Visit Lippincott Williams & Wilkins on the Internet: at LWW.com. Lippincott Williams & Wilkins customer service representatives are available from 8:30 am to 6 pm, EST.

10 9 8 7 6 5 4 3 2 1

CCS0910

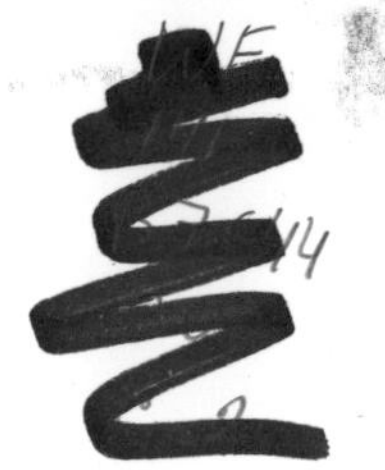

Lippincott's Primary

Musculosk

Radiology

George M

John Che

ASSOCIATE EDI

Mitesh T

Wolters Kluwer Health | Lippincott Williams & Wilkins

Dedication

This book is dedicated to my mother for her eternal sacrifices on my behalf and to my very special wife, Ewa for her eternal sacrifices on behalf of our two wonderful children—Courtny and Dylan.

-GB

This book is dedicated to my inspiring parents, Virginia and Frank; to my beautiful wife, Kelly; and to our extraordinary twin daughters, Elizabeth and Alexandra.

-JC

To my father and mother, Shashank and Smita Trivedi, whose dedication toward and sacrifice for their children is impossibly unparalleled and selfless. I love you both.

-MT

Contributors

Kris J. Alden, MD, PhD
Clinical Associate
Department of Surgery
University of Chicago Bone & Joint Center
Weiss Memorial Hospital
Chicago, Illinois

Kevin J. Bozic, MD, MBA
Associate Professor and Vice Chair
Department of Orthopaedic Surgery
University of California, San Francisco (UCSF) School of Medicine
Attending Surgeon
University of California, San Francisco (UCSF) Medical Center
San Francisco, California

George M. Bridgeforth, MD, MPH
Center Medical Director
Concentra Medical Centers
Chicago, Illinois

Charles Carroll IV, MD
Associate Professor of Clinical Orthopedic Surgery
Department of Orthopedic Surgery
Northwestern University Feinberg School of Medicine
Attending Surgeon
Northwestern Memorial Hospital
Chicago, Illinois

John Cherf, MD, MPH, MBA
President
The Chicago Institute of Orthopedics
Chicago, Illinois

Brian J. Cole, MD, MBA
Professor, Departments of Orthopedics & Anatomy and Cell Biology
Division of Sports Medicine
Section Head, Cartilage Restoration Center at Rush
Rush University Medical Center
Chicago, Illinois

Rachel M. Frank, BA, BS
Research Fellow
Department of Orthopedic Surgery
Rush University Medical Center
Chicago, Illinois

Thomas M. Hearty, MD, DPT
Resident Physician
Department of Orthopaedics
Northwestern University Feinberg School of Medicine
Northwestern Memorial Hospital
Chicago, Illinois

George B. Holmes, Jr., MD
Chief of Foot & Ankle Section
Assistant Professor
Department of Orthopaedic Surgery
Rush University Medical Center
Midwest Orthopaedics at Rush
Chicago, Illinois

Kathryn J. McCarthy, MD
Resident
Department of Orthopaedics
McGaw-Northwestern Memorial Hospital
Chicago, Illinois

Shane J. Nho, MD, MS
Assistant Professor
Division of Sports Medicine
Department of Orthopedic Surgery
Rush University Medical Center
Chicago, Illinois

Mark T. Nolden, MD
Clinical Instructor
Department of Orthopaedic Surgery
Northwestern University Feinberg School of Medicine
Attending Spine Surgeon
Northwestern Memorial Hospital
Chicago, Illinois

Jay J. Patel, MD, MS
Resident
Department of Orthopaedic Surgery
University of California, Irvine
Orange, California

Jessica H. Peelman, MD
Resident
Department of Orthopaedic Surgery
Northwestern University Feinberg School of Medicine
Northwestern Memorial Hospital
Chicago, Illinois

David W. Roberts, MD
Resident Physician
Department of Orthopaedic Surgery
Northwestern University Feinberg School of Medicine
Chicago, Illinois

Kimberly Shellcroft, PA-C
Physician Assistant
Department of Orthopedics
Chicago Orthopaedics and Sports Medicine
Chicago, Illinois

Mitesh Trivedi, MD
Chief Resident
Department of Radiology
Christiana Care Health System
Newark, Delaware

Brian M. Weatherford, MD
Resident
Department of Orthopaedic Surgery
Northwestern University Feinberg School of Medicine
Northwestern Memorial Hospital
Chicago, Illinois

David S. Wellman, MD
Resident
Department of Orthopaedic Surgery
Northwestern University Feinberg School of Medicine
Northwestern Memorial Hospital
Chicago, Illinois

Joan R. Williams, MD
Resident Physician
Department of Orthopaedic Surgery
Northwestern University Feinberg School of Medicine
Northwestern Memorial Hospital
Chicago, Illinois

Introduction to Lippincott's Primary Care Series

Welcome to Lippincott's Primary Care Series. The intended goal of this series is to help assist you in all of the use-case scenarios that you might encounter each day.

In this product, Primary Care Musculoskeletal Radiology, you will find:

1. **Book:** The book contains both bulleted points for quick look-up access when you need an answer right away, as well as longer text for the occasions when you need a little more information.

   Additionally we have included pedagogy to highlight certain aspects of the text. These elements include:

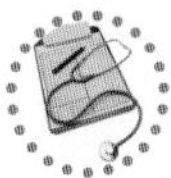 **Patient Assessment—Quick reference for the physical examination**

 **Not to Be Missed—Things to watch out for or possible diagnoses to keep in mind during the examination**

 **When to Refer—When to suggest further options to your patient**

2. **Website** that includes:
   - Fully searchable text of the book
   - Image bank that can be downloadable into PowerPoint for presentations
   - PDF downloadable Patient Information Sheets
3. **Anatomical Chart for Your Office**

We certainly hope this product is useful and meets your needs.

Please look for other titles in the Lippincott's Primary Care Series.

Preface

A musculoskeletal radiology course should be an integral part of the core curriculum of every physician's training with a basic course for upper level medical students followed by a more advanced course for all primary care residents. In addition, there should be an updated current concepts course for senior level physicians. This textbook was designed to fill that gap in the medical education of primary care residents and senior physicians. Primary care physicians who have a comprehensive understanding of musculoskeletal radiology are not only highly skilled clinicians but also are more effective in communicating with their radiology, orthopedic and neurosurgical colleagues. The end result is a higher standard of care.

Unlike many other radiology texts that focus mainly on the depiction of fractures, *Lippincott's Primary Care Musculoskeletal Radiology* adopts a more comprehensive approach. Each chapter integrates the functional anatomy, mechanism of injury, clinical presentation, differential diagnosis, radiological interpretation, and indications for referral and treatment. Because the majority of falls and acute trauma cases are seen initially by primary care physicians, this more comprehensive approach was designed to meet the needs of today's primary care providers. Instead of avoiding more challenging concepts and injuries (e.g., spinal cord injuries), we actually embraced these challenges. Moreover, there is a major focus on recognizing and avoiding many pitfalls that can lead to unintended but costly errors.

When evaluating musculoskeletal problems, it is critical to understand that good doctors understand what they are looking at, but better doctors understand what they are looking for. For example, certain types of fractures such as scaphoid fractures (which are the second most common fractures to the distal forearm and wrist following a fall on the outstretched hand) are commonly missed on standard radiographs. Over time, a misdiagnosis may lead to premature degenerative arthritis and permanent impairment. Our integrative approach discusses how to recognize and avoid this pitfall and many others like it. At the conclusion of the textbook, the physician should not only have a greater understanding of classic injuries but also a greater understanding of more subtle injuries which may confound even excellent physicians.

Contributing authors include some of the nation's leading specialists who provide a detailed but practical common sense approach to patient care. In addition, these leading specialists provide specific guidelines for both immediate and prompt referrals as well as discuss indications for an MRI versus a CT scan. Furthermore, nonsurgical and surgical treatments and prognosis are explored, so that the primary care physician can provide acutely injured patients with a higher standard of care. In addition to all of this, patient education handouts are provided online as a supplement, so patients will have a better idea what to expect on the road to recovery.

With today's technological developments, today's digital radiographs afford primary care physicians the unprecedented opportunity of viewing radiographs in the office setting. This technology will allow for a greater didactic interchange among colleagues which will result in improved patient assessment and better patient care. Within a five-year span, physicians will be able to review radiographs on mobile devices and at home as well. In the process of developing this textbook, we reviewed over 15,000 cases and selected those cases that we felt were most pertinent to the practice of medicine. This integrative didactic approach will not only improve the physician's comfort zone with evaluating radiographs but also provides many key clinical pearls for improving one's musculoskeletal clinical skills. The authors hope that the medical community will enjoy reading it as much as we did writing it.

Acknowledgments

I would like to extend a very special thank you to Kerry Barrett, Sonya Seigafuse, Martha Cushman and Sandhya Joshi at Aptara for their tremendous advice and support. In addition, I would like to extend my deepest appreciation to neurosurgeon, Leonard Cerullo and orthopedic surgeons, Craig Westin, Chris Giannoulias and James Cohen for their advice. Hand specialist, Nolan Lewis was very generous with his time as well. I am very grateful to Julia Salgado for pulling over 15,000 x-rays for me to review. Also, I would like to thank my support staff, Monique Thomas and orthopedic physician assistant, Erika Armstrong for their assistance. I would like to acknowledge Concentra executive physicians, John Anderson, Tom Fogarty and Jane Derebery. Finally, I would like to recognize my two mentors, Thomas Killup and Conal Wilmot for their counsel and their direction. – GB

I can't be more appreciative of the dedication, persistence and professionalism of Dr. George Bridgeforth to bring this book to print. – JC

I would like to acknowledge Vinay Gheyi, MD and Kedar Kulkarni, MD who had presented this wonderful opportunity to me. – MT

Contents

SECTION 1

Spine

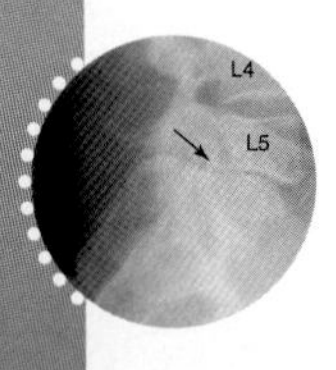

Chapter 1 Degenerative Disc Disease

George M. Bridgeforth and Mark Nolden

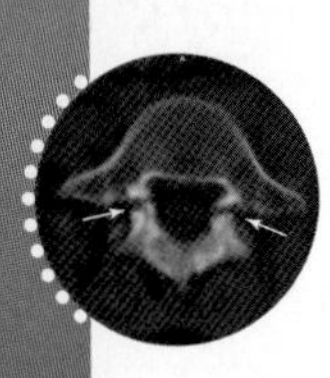

Chapter 2 Spondylolysis vs. Spondylolisthesis

George M. Bridgeforth and Mark Nolden

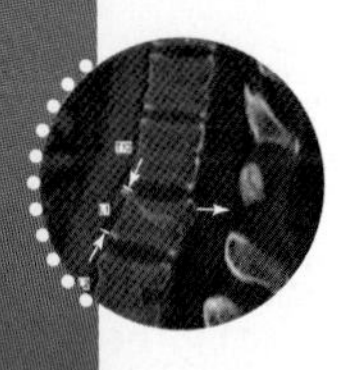

Chapter 3 Comminuted Vertebral Body Fractures

George M. Bridgeforth and Mark Nolden

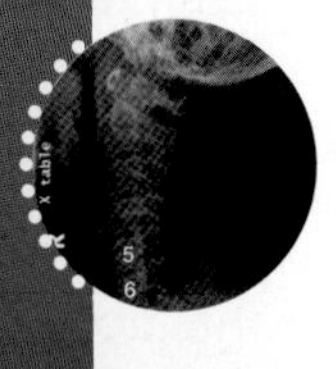

Chapter 4 Wedge Fractures

George M. Bridgeforth and Mark Nolden

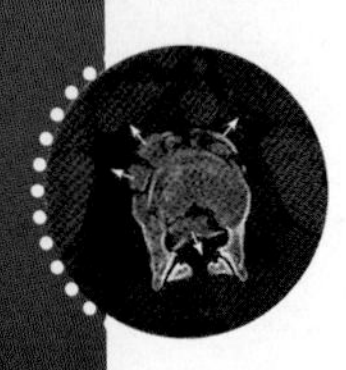

Chapter 5 Burst Fractures

George M. Bridgeforth and Mark Nolden

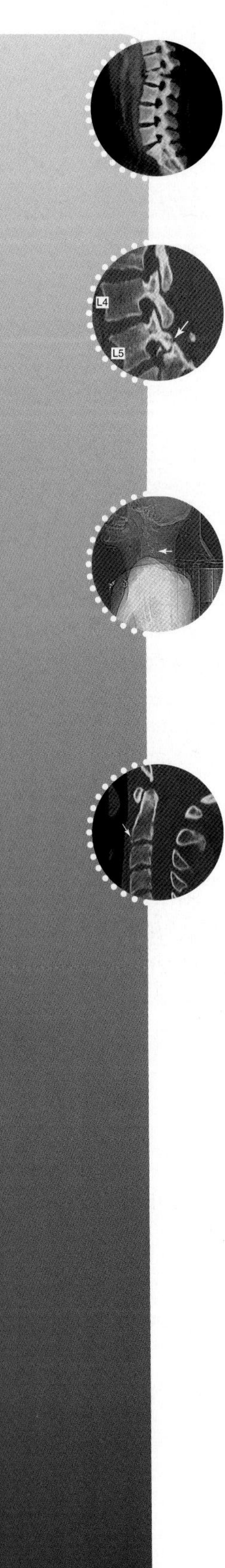

Chapter 6 Chance Fractures

George M. Bridgeforth and Mark Nolden

Chapter 7 Unilateral Facet Dislocations

George M. Bridgeforth and Mark Nolden

Chapter 8 Bilateral Facet Dislocations

George M. Bridgeforth and Mark Nolden

Chapter 9 Teardrop Fracture

George M. Bridgeforth and Mark Nolden

Functional Anatomy

The vertebral column supports the weight of the upper body (i.e., load) and protects the spinal cord. There are 7 cervical vertebrae (C1–C7), 12 thoracic vertebrae (T1–T12), and 5 lumbar vertebrae (L1–L5) (Fig. 1). The sacrum (so-named because it is shaped like a shield) protects the pelvic organs and helps transfer the stress from the load on the pelvic ala (wings) and lower extremities. The sacrum is composed of five bones that are fused together in maturity. The coccyx, the lowermost bone of the spinal column, represents the vestige of the mammalian tail from evolution. It is composed of three to four fused bones.*

The first cervical vertebra is composed of a bony ring without a spinous process. It is commonly referred to as the atlas because it holds up the skull (i.e., globe). The posterior portion of the ring contains two oblong bony plates called the superior facets; these facets help support the occipital condyles at the base of the skull. The second cervical vertebra, which lies beneath the ring of the first cervical vertebra, has a specialized domelike bony process at its center called the dens (odontoid process). The dens (so-named because it is shaped like a tooth) projects through the center of the first cervical ring. The C1–C2 articulation is supported by the surrounding

*A functional spinal unit (FSU) is a term used in biomechanics to study the functional anatomy of the spine. It consists of two adjacent vertebrae, the disc in-between the two vertebral bodies, and the supporting ligaments.

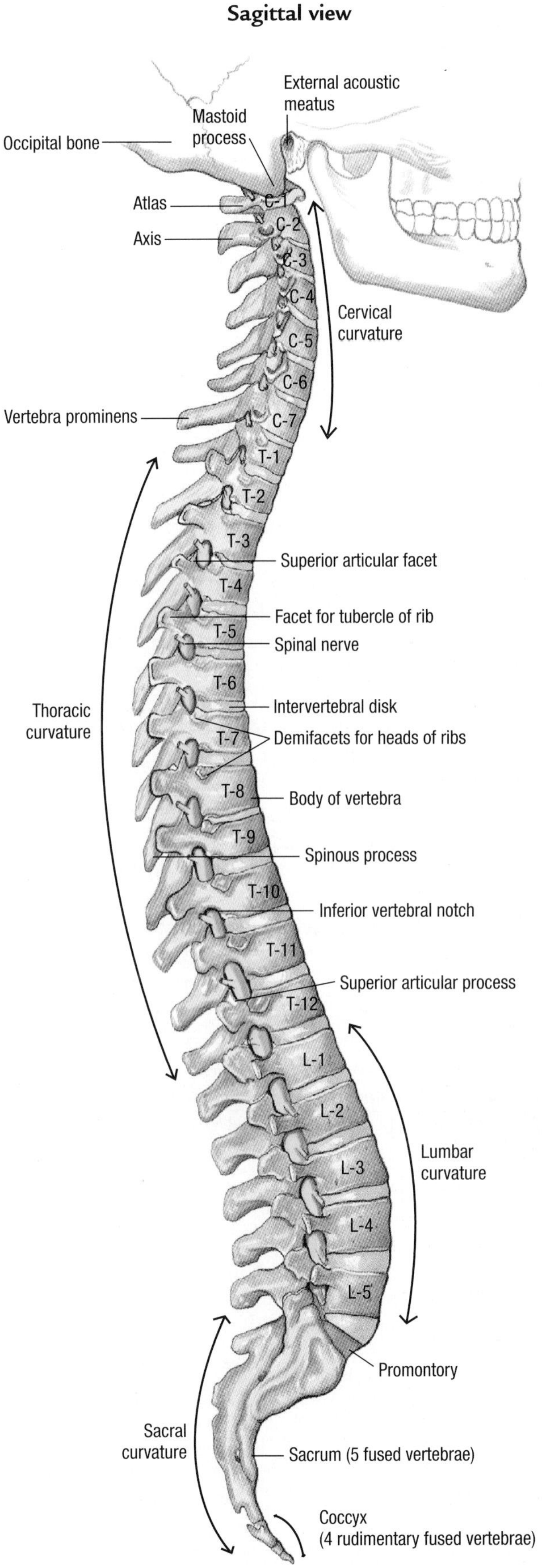

Sagittal view

Figure 1 Vertebral column. Sagittal view. Asset provided by Anatomical Chart Co.

alar ligaments and allows for rotation of the skull, and it assists with flexion, extension, and lateral bending from 0 to 40 degrees. Beginning with the second cervical vertebra and interspaced between each subsequent vertebra from C2 (second cervical vertebra) through L5 (fifth lumbar vertebra) are the vertebral discs.

The vertebral discs have shock-absorbing capabilities. In addition, they help the vertebrae support the upper body. During motion, they provide the cushioning that allows the vertebrae bodies to support the human frame during flexion (bending forward), extension (bending backward), lateral bending (to each side), and rotation. The center of the disc contains a glycoprotein gel–like matrix called the nucleus pulposus. In adults, the nucleus pulposus is approximately 75% water and 25% protein matrix. The glycoprotein matrix is surrounded by a series of fibrocartilaginous rings (approximately 10–20 plates for each disc) called the annulus fibrosis. It should be noted that some of the rings do not extend fully around the total circumference of the nucleus pulposus.

In each plate, the collagen fibers are arranged at an oblique angle (generally between 30 and 60 degrees) to the horizontal plane and are oriented in the same direction. However, some of the overlapping plates contain collagen fibers oriented in opposite direction. This “criss-crossing” orientation of different laminar rings increases the structural support that helps prevent extrusion of the nucleus pulposus during extreme loads (weights) and stresses. Moreover, the herniation of disc material may contribute to inflammation, swelling, and nerve root irritation. Patients with herniated discs may complain of radicular symptoms, including radiating pain, numbness, and weakness.

During spine flexion, anterior compression of the nucleus pulposus occurs, and it extends posteriorly. Under normal circumstances, concentric layers of the annulus fibrosis contain the matrix. A fibrous end plate attaches each disc to the overlying and underling vertebral body. With lateral bending and extension, the load of the body once again compresses the nucleus pulposus and then attempts to expand in the opposite direction.

Each vertebra consists of a vertebral body (excluding the ring-shaped C1) and a posterior arch. Each vertebral body is a load-bearing structure composed of more porous bone in the center surrounded by a thicker structural bone. The cancellous bones allow for vascular channels and nutrients to pass through the central portion of the vertebral body. In addition, the vertebral bodies and the alternating discs protect the anterior portion of the spinal cord. The pedicles connect the vertebral bodies to the posterior arch. The two pedicles and their adjoining lamina, which are composed of cortical bone, form a bony arch that protects the posterior section of the spinal cord.

The transverse processes are two wing-shaped bony projections on either side between the pedicles and the lamina. The posterior neural arch is formed by the pedicles and the lamina. The two transverse processes and a single posterior projection called the spinous processes reinforce each neural arch (with the exception of ring-shaped C1). The transverse process and the spinous process form a bony fortress that helps protect the spinal cord. In addition, they serve as anchoring points for various spinal muscles and ligaments. The facets, transverse processes, and pedicles are jointed on each side by the pars interarticularis.

Each posterior arch from C2 to C5 has two superior and two inferior facets. The facets have oval, slightly concave surfaces that form the joints for each cervical, thoracic, and lumbar vertebra. Each facet has a cartilaginous cushion. The inferior facets of one vertebra articulate with the superior facets of the vertebrae beneath it. In addition, each facet joint is surrounded by a synovial capsule and is lubricated with synovial fluid. Although the spinal column allows for six degrees of freedom, which includes both translational (unidirectional) and rotational movements across three planes, the structural orientation (i.e., degree of angulation) of the facets is different for the cervical, thoracic, and lumbar spine. This difference in each section has a profound effect on the biomechanics of the spine.

Thoracic facets are angulated more in a coronal (i.e., transverse) plane; this orientation allows for greater rotation but limits bending (forward) and extension. In addition, the thoracic vertebrae contain slightly concave plate-shaped cost facets on each side near the junction of the vertebral body and transverse processes. The costal facets allow for the articulation of the ribs with the spinal column. Forward bending is constrained by the rib cage and the posterior ligaments of the spine. Although the cervical and lumbar facets are angulated, they have a greater sagittal orientation (i.e., front to back). This allows for greater flexion. Because of the weight-bearing responsibilities of the lumbar spine, the vertebral bodies, discs, and corresponding facets are larger in the lumbar spine. (The thoracic structures are larger than the cervical structures as well.)

The spinal ligaments provide additional reinforcement; approximately six spinal ligaments support each vertebra. Extending longitudinally from the anterior axis (C2) to the sacrum, the anterior longitudinal ligament anchors the anterior circumferences of the vertebral bodies and the anterior rims of their corresponding discs. It helps prevent anterior displacement of the vertebral bodies and the discs during extension. Extending longitudinally from the posterior axis to the sacrum, the posterior longitudinal ligament runs along the posterior rims of the vertebral bodies and the corresponding disc spaces. Although not as wide as the anterior longitudinal ligament, it helps prevent posterior displacement of the vertebral bodies and ligaments during flexion.

The ligamentum flavum runs between the spinal cord and the lamina. Although it has a higher concentration of elastic fibers than the other spinal ligaments, this contributes to its characteristic yellow color. The ligamentum flavum helps limit displacement of the vertebral arch during flexion. The supraspinous ligament, which runs vertically along the projections of the posterior spinous processes, also limits forward flexion. The supraspinous ligament along with the intertransverse ligaments (which runs between and connects the ipsilateral transverse processes) and the interspinous ligaments (which runs between and connects each spinous process) prevent fanning and displacement of the bony posterior architecture during flexion and rotation.

On either side of two sequential vertebrae is a single foramen. Each foramen allow for the passage of the spinal cord. The spinal cord ends at approximately L1–L2 and continues as a series of fine filaments, which are called the cauda equina (horse's tail).

Approximately 10,000 spinal cord injuries occur in a year. Most primary care physicians, except those in emergency departments and in rural areas, rarely see an acute spinal cord injury. However, more than 250,000 patients live as tetraplegics (quadriplegics) and paraplegics. Thus, it is not uncommon for a primary care physician to care for disabled patients.

In addition, many primary care physicians serve as "gatekeepers" and are the first physicians to see individuals after falls and motor vehicle accidents. Although rare, unstable spinal cord fractures and dislocations may occur without acute neurological impairment. An understanding of the mechanisms of spinal cord injuries and their pathogenesis are essential to providing world-class care. Moreover, primary care physicians with a greater appreciation of the neuropathology of spinal cord injuries are better able to recognize and treat low back pain. Cauda equina injuries from herniated discs, spinal tumors, or metastatic disease constitute medical emergencies that the primary care physician must be able to recognize and refer immediately.

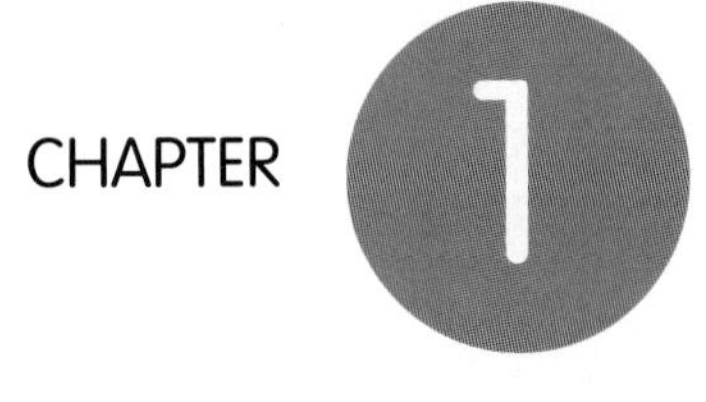

CHAPTER 1 Degenerative Disc Disease

George M. Bridgeforth and Mark Nolden

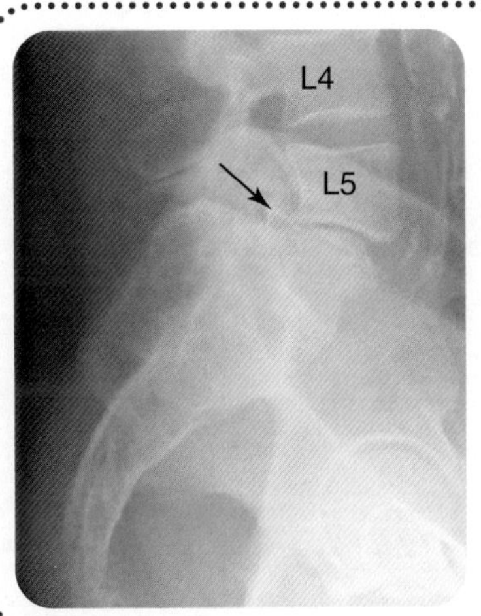

A 66-year-old man presents with chronic back pain and pain in both thighs.

Clinical Presentation

The etiology of low back pain is probably multifactorial. Most people do not engage in regular exercise to strengthen their core abdominal muscles. As a result, excessive loads from obesity, improper lifting techniques, and fatigued muscles from poor core stability place increased strain on the disc and the surrounding neurological structures. Magnetic resonance imaging (MRI) studies in normal individuals without back pain have shown some evidence of degenerative disc disease in about one-third of patients. Therefore, evidence of mild disc protrusions without gross herniations (i.e., pressing on the nerves or the spinal cord) is not sufficient evidence for long-term disability. Routine radiographs for nonradiating low back pain usually are not required during the initial evaluation but should be considered if the patient does not improve by the end of 4 to 6 weeks. The **mechanism of injury** in degenerative disc disease is a non–trauma-related degenerative condition.

Metastatic disease should be suspected in any patient presenting with severe low back pain who is older than 50 years of age (but certainly it has been reported in younger individuals as well—age is not an excluding factor). Constitutional symptoms such as generalized weakness and weight loss, a positive personal history of a preexisting cancer, a family history of cancer, a strong smoking history with pulmonary abnormalities, an undiagnosed breast mass, or new-onset hematuria are indications for an initial radiographic evaluation and further workup (MRI or computed tomography [CT] scan). In addition, the acute onset of radicular findings (numbness, weakness of the lower extremities with a positive straight leg raising [pain that radiates down the leg past the knee with straight leg elevation]) also indicates that additional workup is necessary.

During the history, the examiner should inquire about the severity of the pain, its precipitating and palliative factors, and onset, duration and timing. It is important to inquire whether the pain is radiating or nonradiating. Radicular pain from disc herniations is usually unilateral. Pain that radiates to the groin may be secondary to an L3 radiculopathy or degenerative hip disease. L4 radiculopathies radiate to the skin or the ankle. L5 radiculopathies radiate to the great toe, and S1 radiculopathies radiate to the outside of the foot. In addition, it is

CLINICAL POINTS

- The presence of constitutional symptoms warrants evaluation.
- Metastatic disease should be suspected in any patient with severe low back pain, especially if he or she is older than 50 years of age.
- Middle-aged patients (especially males) who experience the sudden onset of lower extremity motor weakness without low back pain may be experiencing the initial onset of amyotrophic lateral sclerosis.

PATIENT ASSESSMENT

1. Low back pain or stiffness
2. Limited range of motion
3. Possible neurological impairment
4. Radicular findings with a disc herniation (positive straight leg raising, motor weakness, sensory loss, diminished absent reflexes)
5. Cauda equina injury (rare)

important to inquire about motor weakness, especially a foot drop. Ninety percent of radiculopathies affect the L5 or S1 nerve roots (Hoppenfeld, 1976).

Patients with increasingly severe low back pain, radicular pathology, acute foot drop, or incontinence should be evaluated promptly by a specialist. The new onset or a foot drop or a cauda equina syndrome (motor weakness of the lower extremities, sensory impairment of the lower extremities, and bowel or bladder incontinence) constitutes a medical emergency and warrants an immediate referral. Cauda equina injuries are rare.

Radiographic Evaluation

It may not be necessary to order radiographs on initial assessment of nontraumatic cases of low back pain. However, radiographs are recommended for any serious injuries secondary to acute trauma. In addition, radiographs may be

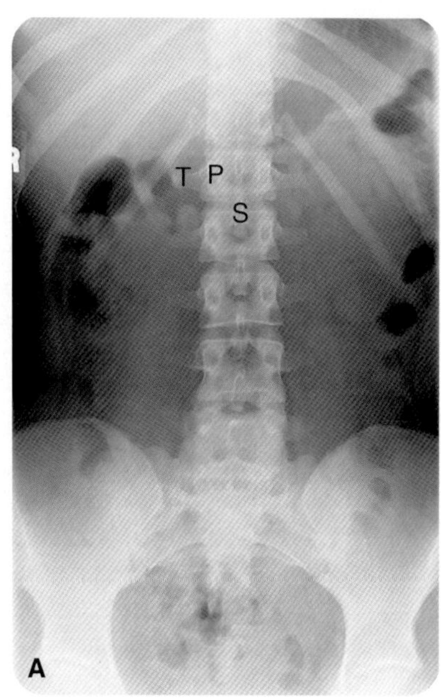

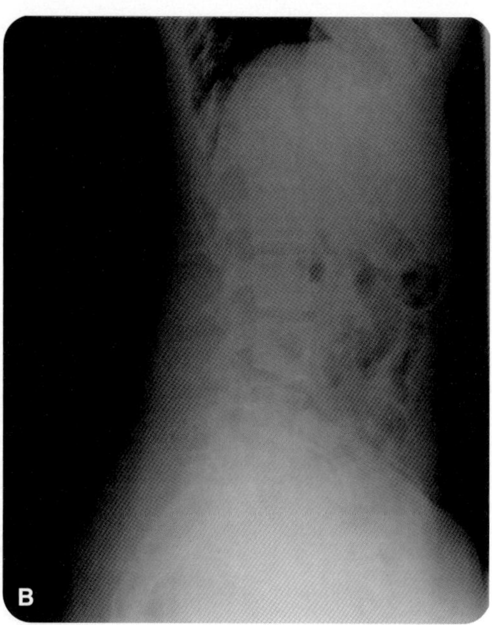

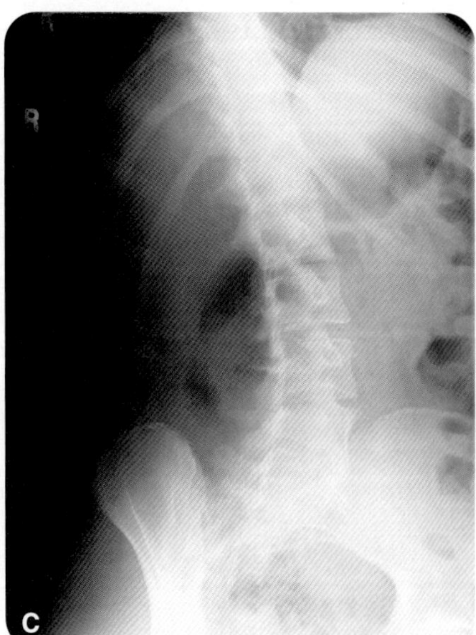

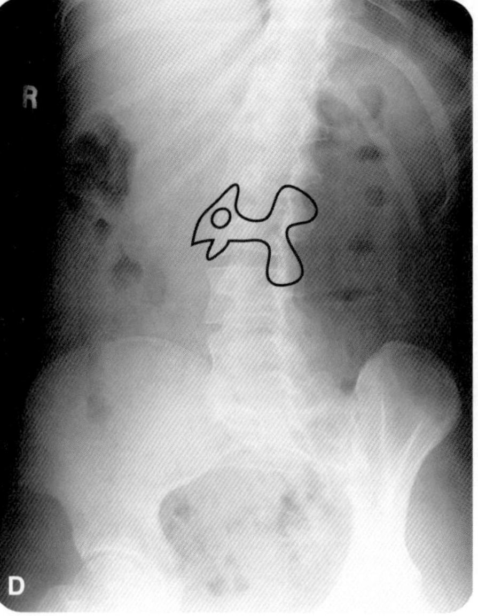

Figure 1.1 A 19-year-old woman without a history of injury presents with back pain of 6-month duration. Normal **(A)** anteroposterior, **(B)** lateral, and **(C** and **D)** bilateral oblique views demonstrate no acute or chronic findings. "Scottie dog" is evident on the oblique projections where the neuroforamina are easily seen. (T = transverse process, P = pedicle and S = spinous process).

NOT TO BE MISSED

- Acute spinal fracture
- Osteoarthritis (usually >50 years)
- Spinal stenosis (usually >50 years)
- Metastatic disease (usually >50 years)
- Pyelonephritis (more common in women)
- Kidney stone
- Abdominal aortic aneurysm
- Bone tumor (rare)
- Osteomyelitis
- Ankylosing spondylitis (more common in men)
- Sacroiliitis
- Cauda equina injury (rare)

considered in patients with severe low back pain who are older than 50 years of age, in patients with metastatic cancer, or in patients whose status deteriorates secondary to low back pain. Tests to order include standard radiographs of the spine—anteroposterior (Fig. 1.1A), lateral (Fig. 1.1B), and oblique views (two; Fig. 1.1C,D). MRI (or CT) may be used in patients with suspected metastatic disease, new-onset radicular symptoms (numbness, weakness, foot drop, diminished or absent reflexes), or focal neurological symptoms.

In figure 1.2, marked multilevel disc space narrowing is apparent. Moreover, multiple discs exhibit a vacuum phenomenon (see figure in introductory case). This finding is a thin hyperlucent line characteristic of severe disc degeneration. In addition, erosion of the inferior end plates, which is secondary to an intravertebral disc herniation (with end plate damage), is visible. These end plate erosions may cause irregularly shaped invaginations into the vertebral body. These invaginations, which may be caudal or cephalic, are called Schmorl nodes. Schmorl nodes are usually located in the center of the superior or inferior end plate (Fig. 1.2). However, they may be seen anteriorly or posteriorly as well. Small osteophytes, which are characteristic of osteoarthritis, may appear along the end plate margins (Fig. 1.3). It should be noted that abdominal aortic aneurysms are uncommon but may be apparent on routine radiographs; clinicians should look for evidence of arterial calcification.

WHEN TO REFER

- Cases of progressive neurological deterioration or cauda equina syndrome (incontinence, loss of bowel tone, loss of libido, perianal [saddle] anesthesia, and weakness of the lower extremities) (immediate referral)
- Metastatic disease without neurological deterioration (prompt referral)
- Mechanical low back pain that does not improve after a 4- to 6-week course of conservative care

SPINAL STENOSIS

There is multilevel spur formation of the vertebral bodies, which is compatible with an osteoarthritis (lateral view). In addition to all of this, one of the most striking findings is the marked narrowing of the foramen secondary to bony overgrowth. Foraminal stenosis may occur at one or multiple levels. Spinal stenosis may be apparent at a single or multiple levels. The narrowed foramen may be appreciated on a lateral or oblique view. Moreover, facet arthropathy (thickened narrowed sclerotic facet joints) should be evident.

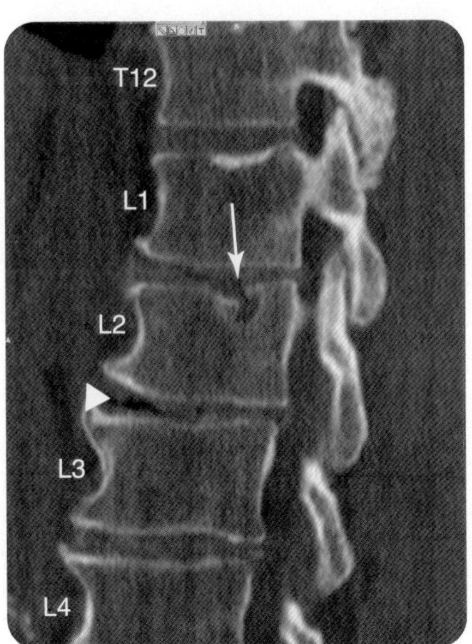

Figure 1.2 A 74-year-old man with low back pain. A selected sagittal reconstructed image from a lumbar spine computed tomography scan demonstrates invagination of the intervertebral disc through the superior end plate of the L2 vertebral body, a Schmorl node. In addition, vacuum phenomenon is observed at the narrowed L2–L3 disc space.

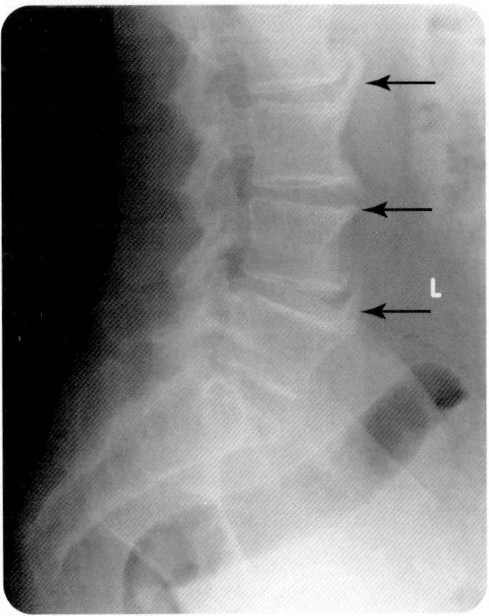

Figure 1.3 A 67-year-old woman without a history of trauma presented with 3-week history of low back pain. A lateral radiograph over the lower lumbar spine demonstrates multiple osteophytes of the lumbar spine.

LIMBUS VERTEBRA

This triangular-shaped bone fragment is generally identified along the anterosuperior vertebral body. Limbus vertebrae are caused by disc herniations. They can be differentiated from acute fractures because the anterosuperior border of the vertebral body is a relatively uncommon place for an acute fracture. Moreover, limbus vertebrae usually have sclerotic margins.

Treatment

Most cases of low back pain respond to conservative care (e.g., pain medication, cold packs, spinal manipulation, or physical therapy). Ninety percent of the cases generally improve within a 4- to 6-week period. Patients with back pain that does not improve with conservative care may benefit from an MRI scan. Surgery should be considered in individuals who show a progressive neurological deficit characterized by increasing pain, numbness, weakness (e.g., foot drop), or bowel and bladder incontinence (cauda equina injury). Severe pain may be caused by central disc herniations in which the disc herniates straight back and may present without focal neurological signs, but these herniations are uncommon.

Suggested Readings

Brant-Zawadzki MN, Deniius SC, Gade GF, Weinstein MP. Low back pain. *Radiology*. 200;217:321–330.

Deyo RA, Weinstein JN. Low back pain. *N Engl J Med*. 2001;344:363–370.

Gillan MG, Gilbert FJ, Andrew JE, et al. Influence of imaging on clinical decision making in the treatment of lower back pain. *Radiology*. 2001;220:393–399.

Hoppenfeld S. *Physical Examination of the Spine and Extremities*. Norwalk, CT: Appleton-Century-Crofts; 1976: 237–264.

Kinkdade S. Evaluation and treatment of low back pain. *Am Fam Physician*. 2007;75:1181–1188.

Maldague B, Noel H, Malghem J. The intravertebral cleft: a sign of ischemic vertebral collapse. *Radiology*. 1978;129:223–229.

Nachemson Al. Newest knowledge of low back pain. A critical look. *Clin Orthop*. 1992;279:8–20.

Pai RR, D'sa B, Raghuveer CV, Kamath A. Neovascularization of the nucleus pulposus: a diagnostic feature of intervertebral disc prolapse. *Spine*. 1999;24:739–741.

Patel AT, Ogle AA. Diagnosis and management of acute low back pain. *Am Fam Physician*. 2000;61:1779–1790.

Saal JA, Saal JS, Herzog RJ. The natural history of lumbar intervertebral disc extrusions treated nonoperatively. *Spine*. 1990;15:683–686.

Seidenwurm D, Litt AW. The natural history of lumbar spine disease. *Radiology*. 1995;195:323–324.

Waddell G, McCulloch JA, Kummel E, Venner RM. Nonorganic physical signs in low back pain. *Spine*. 1980; 5:117–125.

Walling AD. Family Practice International: Radiographs and low back pain. *Am Fam Physician*. 1999;47:194. http://www.aafp.org/afp/990101ap/family.html. Accessed September 12, 2009.

White AA, Panajabi MM. *Clinical biomechanics of the spine*. 2nd ed. Philadelphia, PA: Lippincott Williams & Wilkins; 1990:1–126.

CHAPTER 

Spondylolysis vs. Spondylolisthesis

George M. Bridgeforth and Mark Nolden

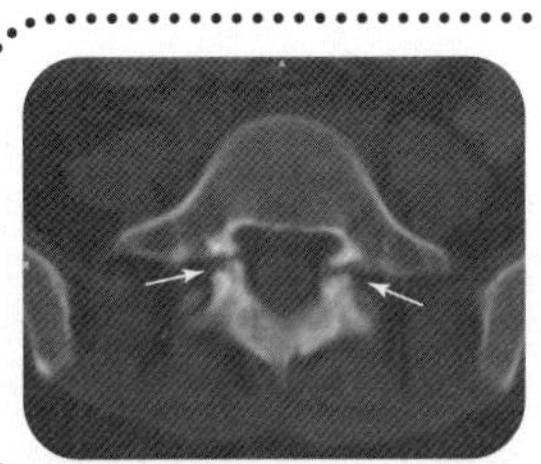

A 40-year-old obese woman presents with hematuria and left flank pain. She denies any numbness, weakness, or bowel or bladder incontinence.

CLINICAL POINTS

- Spondylolysis
  - Most cases are asymptomatic.
  - This stable injury is characterized by a fracture of the pars interarticularis.
  - The condition may be unilateral or bilateral.
- Spondylolisthesis
  - Patients are usually asymptomatic.
  - Symptomatic patients may complain of "something moving in my lower back."
  - Most injuries are stable and are characterized by a bilateral defect in the pars interarticularis.

PATIENT ASSESSMENT

1. Low back pain, aching, and stiffness
2. Nontraumatic spondylolysis: usually asymptomatic radiographic finding
3. Spondylolisthesis: usually does not cause radicular symptoms (numbness and weakness) unless unstable

Clinical Presentation

Most cases of spondylolysis and spondylolisthesis are asymptomatic. They are an incidental finding on detected lumbar sacral radiographs of patients with acute trauma or persistent low back pain. Degenerative spondylolysis or spondylolisthesis usually occurs in patients who are older than 50 years . However, nondegenerative forms may occur in adolescents from contact sports (football) or in gymnasts.

Spondylosis is characterized by a defect in the pars interarticularis (which joins the laminae, the pedicles, and the facets in the posterior vertebral spine) without displacement. Most cases without acute trauma are asymptomatic.

Spondylolisthesis is characterized by anterior displacement of the vertebrae secondary to a defect in the pars interarticularis. Most cases are asymptomatic, but patients with unstable injuries from preexisting trauma or degeneration can develop unstable deficits leading to significant spinal cord damage. Most cases affect the L4–L5 level. Moreover, degenerative spondylolisthesis can be associated with spinal stenosis, neurogenic claudication, radicular pain, or facet arthropathy.

Spinal stenosis may occur as a solo entity without a concomitant spondylolisthesis. Patients with associated neurogenic claudication and spinal stenosis complain of pain, numbness, and weakness affecting both legs. Those with neurogenic claudication are usually older than 50 years. Unlike patients with disc disease, who usually present with unilateral numbness and weakness (affecting one lower extremity), older patients with spinal stenosis present with complaints of bilateral numbness and weakness (affecting both lower extremities). In addition, patients with radicular disc problems have pronounced pain with flexion, which results in increased pressure on the damaged discs. However, patients with spinal stenosis have decreased pain with flexion, which opens the foraminal spaces. Furthermore, unlike patients with disc injuries, patients with spinal stenosis complain of pain with extension. This may be due to narrowing of the foramen or associated facet arthropathies. Another key clinical clue is that radicular pain from disc injuries is generally aggravated by straight leg raising. With spinal stenosis, the findings are variable and depend on whether there is underling disc pathology. A negative straight leg raising test in an older patient with bilateral radicular symptoms points toward spinal stenosis.

An abdominal examination should be performed initially on all patients with low back pain (e.g., aneurysm, cholecystitis, pancreatitis) Also, the presence

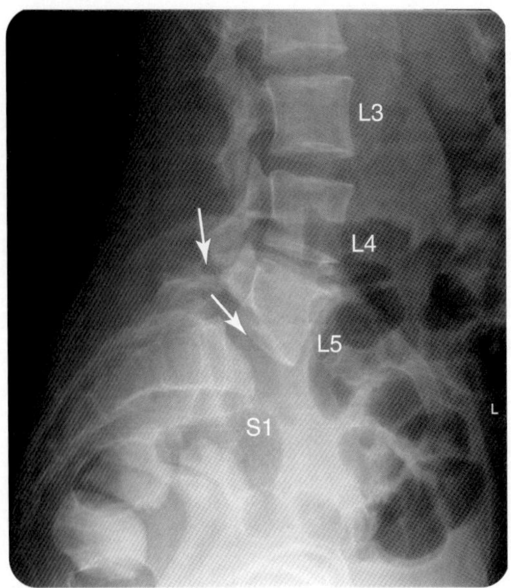

Figure 2.1 Lateral radiograph focused over the L5-S1 disc level in the patient described in the case presentation demonstrates the pars interarticularis defect with minimal anterior displacement of L5 over S1.

of good pulses would point away from vascular claudicating, which is usually seen in heavy smokers. Finally, it is important to note that spinal stenosis may also occur in the cervical spine.

Radiographic Evaluation

Anteroposterior, lateral, and oblique (two views) radiographs should be ordered. For severe spinal trauma, a computed tomography scan is necessary. With chronic spondylolisthesis, flexion and extension views should also be obtained.

A spondylolysis is characterized by a separation of the pars interarticularis without displacement. The pars interarticularis is the bony isthmus that connects the superior and inferior facets of each individual vertebra. However, if there is displacement of the vertebral body (best identified on the lateral radiographs), the condition is called a *spondylolisthesis* (Fig. 2.1).

A chronic defect (fracture) in the pars interarticularis (spondylolysis) is best appreciated on the oblique view (Fig. 2.2). On this view, the superior facet forms the ear of the "Scottie dog." The pedicle forms the eye, and the inferior facet forms the front leg. The nose is formed by the ipsilateral transverse process. The back leg is formed by the opposite inferior facet. If there is a break in the neck of the "Scottie dog" or a collar (characterized by a thin sclerotic line without vertebral displacement) around the "Scottie dog," the patient has a spondylolysis. Acute injuries are characterized by thin oblique line without sclerotic margins. However, chronic injuries have sclerotic margins that are characterized by surrounding thick white regions. Sometimes, this injury may be suspected by a poorly defined sclerotic pedicle on one or both sides or at one level on the anteroposterior radiograph.

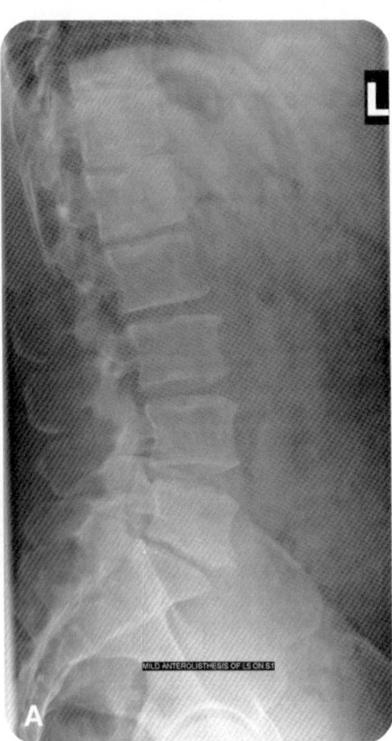

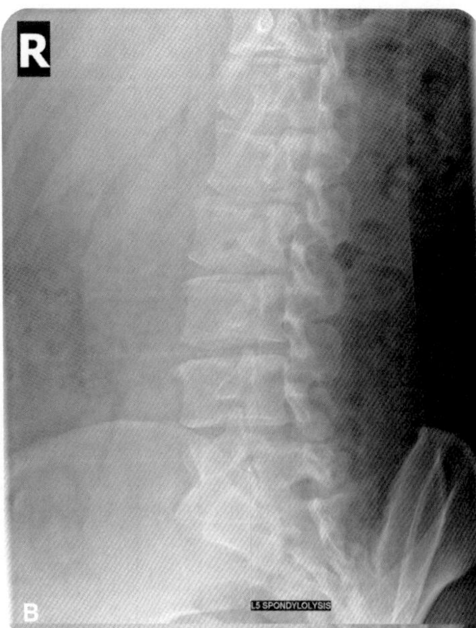

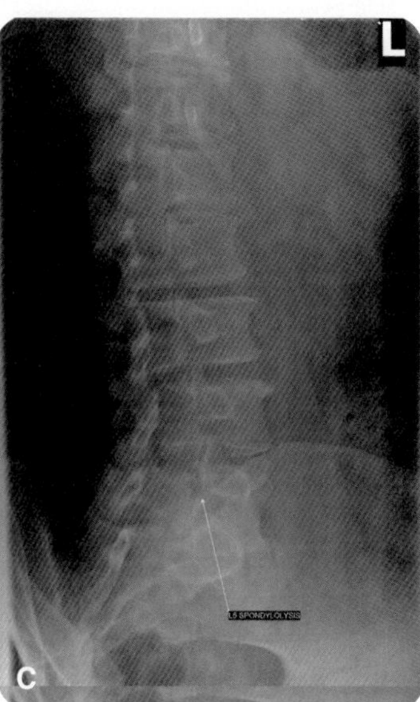

Figure 2.2 Bilateral L5 spondylolysis seen on the oblique views of the lumbar spine radiograph. Notice that the neck of the "Scottie dog" has irregular lucency representing the fracture line. These are most likely chronic as sclerosis is present. Mild anterolisthesis of L5 of S1 is seen on the lateral view of this patient. (Courtesy of Richard Kim, MD).

NOT TO BE MISSED

- Acute spinal fracture
- Degenerative disc disease
- Osteoarthritis (usually >50 years)
- Spinal stenosis (usually >50 years)
- Metastatic disease (usually >50 years)
- Facet arthropathy (facet narrowing with sclerotic facets)
- Pyelonephritis (more common in women)
- Kidney stone
- Abdominal aortic aneurysm
- Bone tumor
- Osteomyelitis
- Ankylosing spondylitis (more common in men)
- Sacroiliitis
- Cauda equina injuries (rare)

Table 2.1 Grading System in Spondylolisthesis

GRADE	DEGREE OF DISPLACEMENT
1	Up to 25%
2	25%–50%
3	50%–75%
4	>75%

If there is evidence of lumbar vertebral displacement (without a vertebral fracture) secondary to a defect in the pars interarticularis, then a spondylolisthesis should be suspected. The examiner should looks on the oblique views for a break in the neck of the "Scottie dog." A spondylolisthesis is a bilateral injury. Generally, it affects the lower lumbar vertebrae. There are four grades for a spondylolisthesis. The grading system is based on the degree of lateral displacement of the lumbar vertebral bodies as identified on the lateral view (Table 2.1).

Treatment

Initial treatment for spondylolysis is conservative, unless there is an acute fracture. The patient should not engage in sports and other activities until the pain subsides. Nonsteroidal anti-inflammatory drugs may reduce pain and inflammation. A regimen of exercise and/or physical therapy helps increase pain-free movement and improve flexibility and muscle strength. Primary care physicians do see spondylosis, spondylolisthesis, and spinal stenosis. Most of these cases are nonsurgical and are managed by these physicians.

Most cases of spondylolisthesis without neurological loss are stable and respond to conservative care (e.g., pain medication, cold packs, physical therapy). However, for a chronic spondylolisthesis, flexion and extension views should be checked for instability (characterized by increased vertebral body displacement on flexion and extension radiographs). Unstable cases of spondylolisthesis with progressive neurological dysfunction are candidates for a posterior decompressive laminectomy with or without a single-level fusion. Patients with instability should be referred to a spine specialist. Acute injuries are uncommon. However, with severe acute spinal cord injuries, the patient should be placed on a spine board (and in a hard collar if there is a cervical injury) and referred immediately to a high-level emergency treatment facility.

Spina bifida occulta, which is a congenital abnormality, is characterized by an incomplete fusion of the spinous process at L5. Generally, it is seen as an incidental finding noted on the radiographs. Spina bifida occulta is usually the result of incomplete development of the spinous process at the L5 level (Fig. 2.3). Generally, it is best appreciated on the anteroposterior radiograph (Fig. 2.4). The condition is thought to be related to low folate levels (secondary to increased needs) in pregnant women. It does not require treatment.

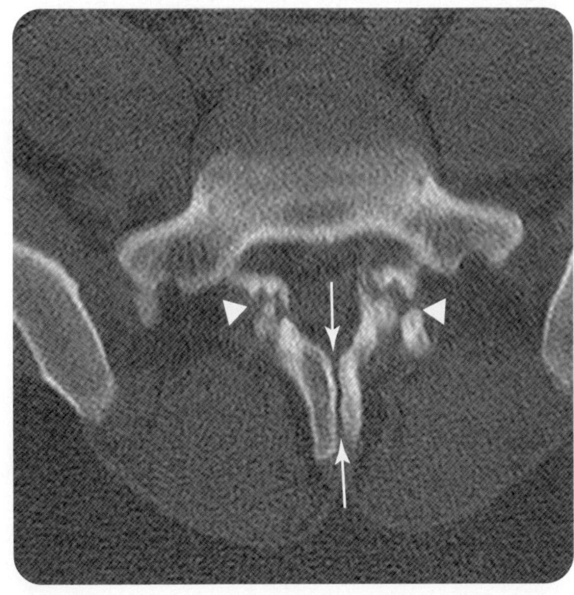

Figure 2.3 Selected axial computed tomography image through L5 on bone windowing in a 38-year-old woman with left-sided back pain demonstrates chronic bilateral pars interarticularis defects and nonunion of the spinous process at this level, spina bifida occulta.

WHEN TO REFER

- Any acute traumatic spine fracture (immediate referral)
- Evidence of spinal instability with increased separation on flexion versus extension (lateral) views
- Increased separation with flexion
- Any cervical separation, whether acute or chronic (immediate referral)

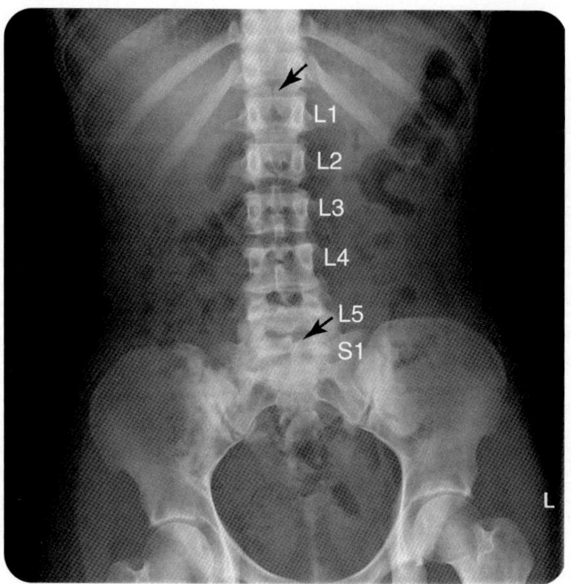

Figure 2.4 The anteroposterior view of the lumbar spine in a 20-year-old woman complaining of back pain after being assaulted illustrates spina bifida occulta at L1 and L5.

Suggested Readings

Brant WE, Helms CA. *Fundamentals of Diagnostic Radiology*. 3rd ed. Philadelphia, PA: Lippincott Williams & Wilkins; 2007:326–329.

Fredrickson BE, Baker D, Holick WJ, Yuan HA, Lubicky JP. The natural history of spondylolysis and spondylolisthesis. *J Bone Joint Surg Am*. 1984;66(5):699–707.

Greenspan A. *Orthopedic Imaging*. Philadelphia, PA: Lippincott Williams & Wilkins; 2004:394–401, 464–466.

Harris JH, Harris WH, Noveline RA. *The Radiology of Emergency Medicine*. 3rd ed. Baltimore, MD: Lippincott Williams & Wilkins; 1993:273–276.

Hu SS, Tribus CB, Diab M, Ghanayem AJ. Spondylolisthesis and spondylolysis. *J Bone Joint Surg*. 2008;90:656–671.

Watter WC, Bomo CM, Gilbert TJ, Keiner DS. An evidence-based clinical guideline for the diagnosis and treatment of degenerative lumbar spondylolisthesis. *Spine J*. 2009;9(7):605–606.

Weinstein JN, Lurie JD, Tosteson T, et al. Surgical versus nonsurgical treatment for lumbar degenerative spondylolisthesis. *New Engl J Med*. 2007;356:2257–2270.

Weinstein JN, Lurie JD, Tosteson TD, Zhao W. Surgical compared with nonoperative treatment for degenerative spondylolisthesis: four-year results in the Spine Patient Outcomes Research Trial (SPORT) randomized and observational cohorts. *J Bone Joint Surg Am*. 2009;91(6):1295–1304.

CHAPTER 3

Comminuted Vertebral Body Fractures

George M. Bridgeforth and Mark Nolden

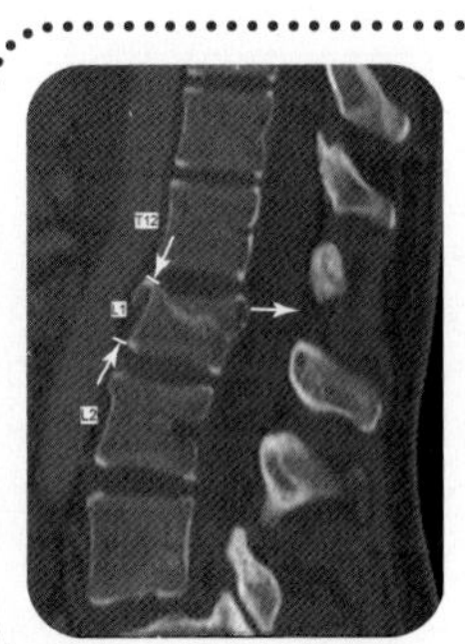

A 23-year-old woman, who drank a six-pack of beer before swinging over a brook on a rope, slipped and fell into the water below, landing on her feet without losing consciousness. She complains of back pain.

Clinical Presentation

All patients with high-impact spinal cord injuries from trauma, motor vehicle accidents, sports, and recreational or competitive diving have unstable spinal injuries until proven otherwise. In addition, there is a strong correlation of traumatic brain injuries associated with these cases. All patients with an acute spinal cord injury who are mentally obtunded or have an impaired mental status from drug or alcohol intoxication have a traumatic brain injury until proven otherwise. For most trauma cases, a noncontrast computed tomography (CT) scan is sufficient to rule out an acute subdural hematoma. Box 3.1 lists the indications for a head CT.

Various clinical clues may help differentiate between an acute spinal cord injury and a traumatic brain injury. Although it is uncommon, patients with an acute spinal cord injury may present without neurological impairment. Primary care physicians need to know how to distinguish between stable and unstable injuries.

In most cases of acute spinal cord injury, a neighboring fracture or dislocation is usually evident.

Acute spinal cord injuries usually present with bilateral neurological impairments. Although diffuse brain damage following closed head injuries may present with bilateral upper motor signs, the impairment caused by a spinal cord injury is usually below a specific neurological level. Upper motor neuron signs are characterized by motor weakness, spasticity, hyperreflexia, and upgoing plantar (Babinski) responses, and they are usually associated with a sensory impairment. In contrast, head injuries are usually associated with an impaired mental status, bilateral upper motor neuron signs with diffuse damage, or unilateral upper motor neuron signs on the opposite side with focal damage. In addition, acute cranial nerve impairments affecting the speech, vision, or hearing are common.

Patients with acute spinal cord injuries above the midthoracic level exhibit acute spinal shock. Acutely, spinal shock is characterized by hypotension (blood pressures less than 100/70 mm Hg), motor weakness, poor or absent reflexes, loss of voluntary bowel tone (the patient does not exhibit a forceful strain during a rectal examination), and sensory impairment. These findings are below the level of the spinal cord injury. Several days later, when the

CLINICAL POINTS

- Patients with narrow cervical spinal canals may have a central spinal stenosis.
- A head CT may be indicated after high-impact spinal injuries.
- A spinal CT may be indicated if there is evidence of the following:
  - Extreme pain
  - Focal tenderness
  - Focal neurological signs of spinal trauma (acute weakness, numbness, loss of reflexes, loss of bowel tone)
  - Evidence of spinal ecchymosis, hematomas, or crepitus
- Not all patients with acute spinal cord injuries exhibit neurologic impairment.

Box 3.1 Indications for Computed Tomography of the Head

Severe headache with focal neurological signs or acutely impaired cranial nerve signs (sudden onset of visual, speech, or hearing disturbances)

Head injury with recurrent nausea and vomiting

Obtunded mental status including drug or alcohol intoxication or short-term cognitive-memory impairments

Poor result on Glasgow Coma Scale

Skull fracture

Major traumatic injuries above the clavicle

Age more than 60 years

Coagulation disorder (or taking anticoagulants)

Acute onset of seizure

patient recovers from spinal shock, they then exhibit upper motor neuron signs below the level of the spinal cord injury. Patients with spinal cord injuries below the midthoracic region develop acute paraplegia of the lower extremities. The bowel and bladder problems affecting paraplegics are different than those affecting tetraplegics (quadriplegics).

Traditionally, the Frankel classification, a functional classification, was used to group acute spinal cord injuries into four major classes (Box 3.2). The American Spinal Injury Association (ASIA) classification ,which is presented in greater detail in Chapter 4, has replaced the Frankel classification. The ASIA classification system adds a Class E, in which both motor and sensory functions are normal.

It is important to remember that it is possible to have serious fracture or dislocation of the spine despite normal neurological function. An individual with an unstable spinal cord injury to the vertebral column may have normal or near-normal neurological function. Therefore, all patients who are subject to acute spinal cord trauma have unstable injuries to the spine until proven otherwise by a history, a thorough neurological assessment, initial radiographs, and a CT scan.

If a spinal fracture is suspected, the patient should be immobilized on a spine board. Moreover, if there is accompanying head, cervical, or upper chest wall trauma, the neck should be placed in a hard cervical collar as well. The patient should be referred immediately to a high-level emergency trauma center, and a CT scan should be obtained.

PATIENT ASSESSMENT

1. Look for moderate to marked focal tenderness at the fracture site. Bruising may or may not be present.
2. With acute injuries, examine carefully for weakness, sensory loss, loss of bowel tone, and loss of reflexes.
3. Always assume an unstable spinal cord fracture until proven otherwise.

Box 3.2 Functional Classification of Acute Spinal Cord Injuries

Class A: complete motor and sensory loss below the level of the spinal cord injury

Class B: preserved sensory function but not motor function below the level of the spinal cord injury

Class C: preservation of motor function below the level of the spinal cord injury, although it is nonfunctional

Class D: preservation of functional motor strength below the level of the spinal cord injury

NOT TO BE MISSED

- Back contusion
- Spinal fracture
- Degenerative disc disease
- Foraminal stenosis
- Metastatic disease (especially in patients >50 years; usually in lumbar spine, pelvis, ribs, and hips)
- Aortic aneurysms (thoracic and lumbar injuries)
- Ankylosing spondylitis (more common in men)
- Osteomyelitis (rare)
- Bone tumor

Radiographic Evaluation

Some experts note that cervical spine radiographs may not be indicated for patients who are not involved in high-impact collisions. Such radiographs are not necessary in the following instances:

- The patient is fully alert and oriented.
- There are no accompanying head injuries or impaired level of consciousness.
- There is no evidence of drug or alcohol impairment.
- There is no cervical pain.
- The neurological examination is normal.
- There are no accompanying distracting injuries (i.e., a different injury that could possibly distract the patient from "complaining" about an acute spinal cord injury).

If any of these criteria are not met, radiographs are clearly indicated. Until there is malpractice legislation that protects physicians from following these guidelines, all physicians should use their own discretion. Tests to order include the following radiographs: anteroposterior (minor trauma only), lateral (minor trauma only), and oblique views (minor trauma only). Initial radiographs may not rule out a fracture or dislocation. If the examiner suspects a spinal cord injury, a CT is indicated. Following a high-impact collision with signs of even mild cervical discomfort, the physician should strongly consider obtaining radiographs followed by a CT scan. Inexperienced examiners who are unfamiliar with acute spinal cord injuries should not obtain flexion/extension views. They should see that the patient is stabilized on a spine board and cervical collar and transferred to a regional trauma facility.

The following points are important:

- For cervical injuries, the examiner must be able to see all the way down to the C7–T1 interspace. If this is not visible, a swimmer's view should be obtained.
- Odontoid (open mouth) views should be included in any cervical spine trauma series. This view should be examined carefully for an odontoid fracture.
- Finally, flexion and extension views should be obtained only by experienced practitioners with solid background in assessing acute spinal cord injury trauma. The flexion and extension radiographs are taken laterally and are examined carefully for signs of increased displacement.

Increased displacement between the corresponding vertebrae or interspinous distance (between two adjoining spinous processes) is evidence of instability until proven otherwise. On a normal cervical radiograph (lateral view), the angle between two adjacent spinous processes should not exceed 11 degrees. Moreover, the relationship between the anterior longitudinal ligament line, the posterior longitudinal ligament line, the spinolaminar line, and the spinous process line should remain intact even in flexion and extension views (Fig. 3.1). Evidence of increased fanning (i.e., the spinous processes spread wide open like a fan) on the lateral or the flexion view strongly suggests a disruption of the posterior ligament complex. Disruptions of the posterior ligament complex are usually associated with unstable spinal cord injuries, and failure to stabilize the patient (hard collar and a spine board) may result in permanent quadriplegia or death.

Vertebral body fractures may present in various ways. A comminuted vertebral body fracture is a fracture that is characterized by three or more fragments. A burst fracture is a type of comminuted fracture in which the bony fragments are dispersed in all directions. This type of fracture is discussed in greater detail in Chapter 4. A comminuted fracture is not a burst fracture if there is a comminuted fracture of the vertebral body but the vertebral height is preserved and fractured fragments are not dispersed in all directions.

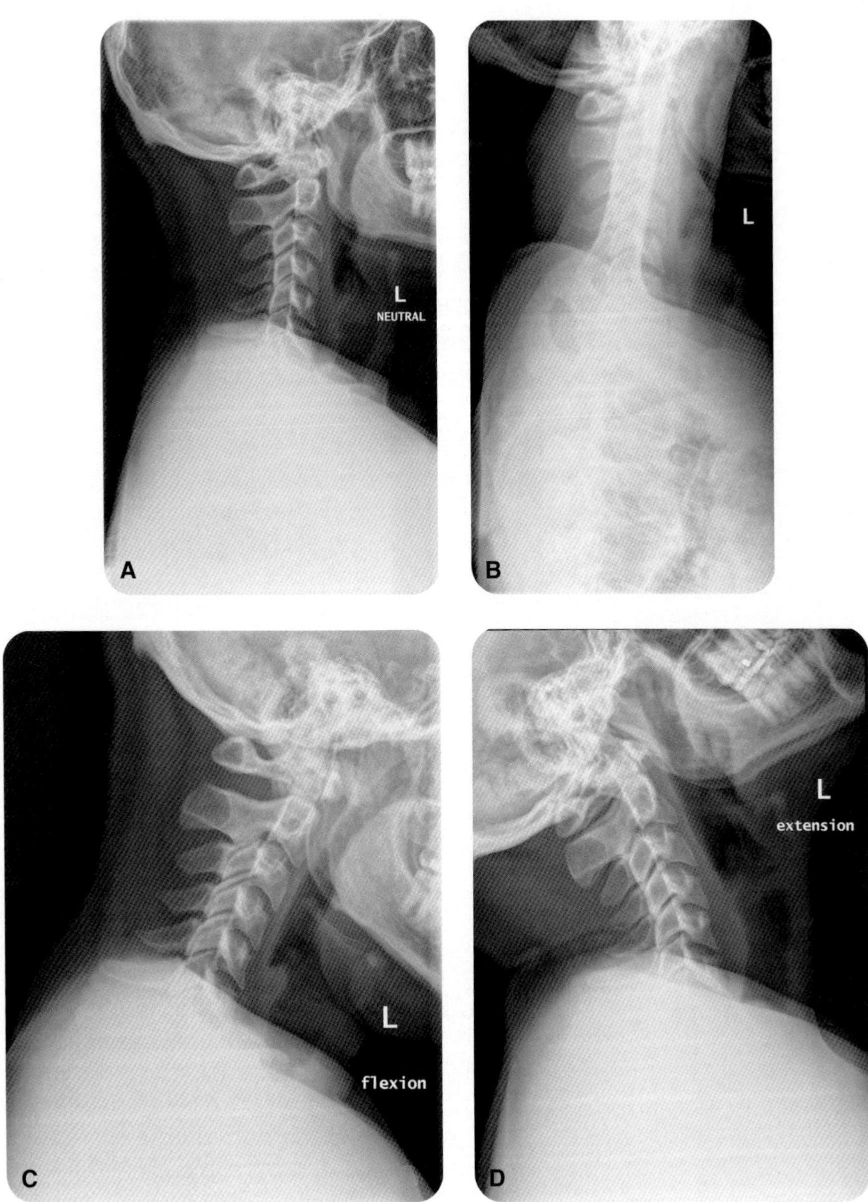

Figure 3.1 A 23-year-old man with neck pain after a motor vehicle collision. **(A)** Lateral, **(B)** swimmer's, **(C)** flexion, and **(D)** extension views do not demonstrate a fracture or subluxation. A magnetic resonance imaging scan of the cervical spine does not demonstrate an acute injury.

Stability not only is determined by the type of fracture and its associated findings—dislocations or disruptions of the supporting ligamentous structures—but also is based on the three-column model of Denis. The first column is made up of the anterior longitudinal ligament and the first two-thirds of the vertebral bodies (and its adjacent discs). The second column is made up of the posterior one-third of the vertebral bodies (and the adjacent discs) and extends to the posterior longitudinal ligament. The third column is made up of the bony and supporting ligamentous structures posterior to the posterior longitudinal ligament. This includes pedicels, laminae, facets, transverse processes, spinous processes, and their surrounding ligaments.

Fractures or dislocations involving one column are generally considered to be stable injuries. Fractures involving all three columns are unstable. Fractures involving two columns should be considered to be unstable until proven otherwise (Fig. 3.2). When a column is fractured or has disrupted ligaments, the

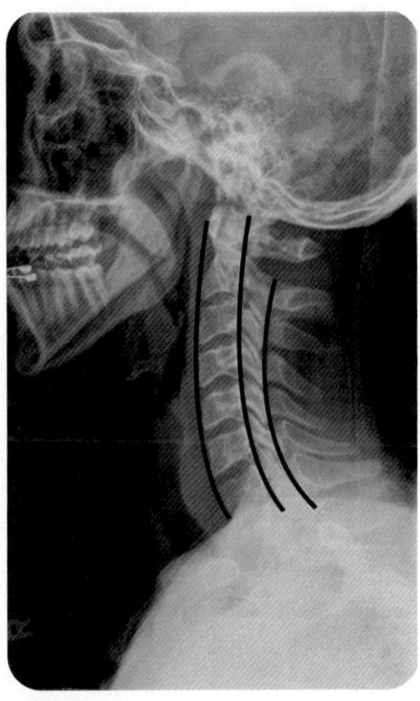

Figure 3.2 A 20-year-old man presents after a motor vehicle collision. Initial plain radiograph examination of the cervical spine questions prevertebral soft tissue prominence, which is proven normal by computed tomography. Notice the preservation of the three columns. (Courtesy of Mitesh Trivedi, MD.)

columns move as independent entities, and significant spinal cord impairment or death may result. With high-impact injuries, radiographs alone may not be sufficient to rule out a vertebral fracture. In an emergency setting, the patient should be stabilized, and a "stat" CT scan should be obtained.

If there is a fracture or displacement involving two or three columns of Denis, one can assume that there is instability. Even a fracture involving one column of Denis may still be unstable; a "stat" CT scan must be obtained. Vertebral body fractures involving the first column of Denis may appear stable. However, there may be torn spinal ligaments in the posterior complex, which is an unstable injury. When it is present, it is necessary to look for fanning of the spinous processes on the lateral radiograph. The fanning may increase with flexion views.

It is important to note that up to 15% of vertebral fractures may not appear on routine radiographs. Therefore, it is strongly recommended that all individuals with severe spine (cervical, thoracic, or lumbar) trauma should be immobilized. This is especially true if they have bruises over the spine, marked focal tenderness, associated head injuries, drug or alcohol intoxication, or associated acute neurological deficits.

Treatment

Patients with stable spinal factures are generally treated with a halo vest (for cervical injuries) or a thoracic lumbar orthosis (for lower thoracolumbar injuries). Patients who are paraplegics and in a thoracic lumbar orthosis brace generally require about 3 months of rehabilitation, and those who are tetraplegics (quadriplegics) and in a halo vest are hospitalized in a spinal cord injury unit for approximately 6 months. Paraplegic individuals without severe traumatic brain injuries usually become fully independent. They are able to drive using adaptive driving equipment and are fully independent with wheelchair transfers (transfer to and from a wheel chair) and the basic activities of daily living. On the other hand, tetraplegic individuals need motorized wheelchairs and require assistance with wheelchair transfer and activities of daily living. The absence of severe neurological impairment may allow individuals who had acute spinal cord injuries to engage in activities fully, but they may still have problems with spasticity of the lower extremities as well bowel and bladder dysfunction.

WHEN TO REFER 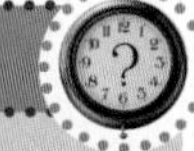

- Serious acute spinal trauma requiring stabilization warrants immediate referral.

Unstable spinal fractures generally require an open reduction and internal fixation. The duration of hospitalization for severe spinal cord injuries varies with the degrees of neurological impairment. Patients with severe spinal cord injuries (especially cervical injuries) should always be assessed for associated traumatic brain injuries as well.

Suggested Readings

Blackmore CC, Emerson SS, Mann FA, Koepsell TD. Cervical spine imaging in patients with trauma: determination of fracture risk to optimize use. *Radiology*. 1999;211:759–765.

Blacksin MF, Lee HJ. Frequency and significance of fractures of the upper cervical spine detected by CT in patients with severe neck trauma. *AJR Am J Roentgenol*. 1995;165:1201–1204.

Denis F. The three column spine and its significance in the classification of acute thoracolumbar spinal injuries. *Spine*. 1983;8:817–831.

Haydel MJ, Preston CA, Mills TJ, et al. Indications for computed tomography in patients with minor head injury. *New Engl J Med*. 2000;343:100–105.

Holdsworth F. Review article fractures, dislocations, and fracture-dislocations of the spine. *J Bone Joint Surg Am*. 1970;52:1534–1551.

Keene JS, Goletz TH, Lilleas F, Alter AJ, Sackett JF. Diagnosis of vertebral fractures: a comparison of conventional radiography, conventional tomography, and computed axial tomography. *J Bone Joint Surg Am*. 1982;64:586–594.

Marar BC. The pattern of neurological damage as an aid to the diagnosis of the mechanism in cervical spine injuries. *J Bone Joint Surg Am*. 1974;56:1648–1654.

Norton WL. Fractures and dislocations of the cervical spine. *J Bone Joint Surg Am*. 1962;44:115–139.

Novelline RA, Rhea JT, Rao PM, Stuk JL. Helical CT in emergency radiology. *Radiology*. 1999;213:321–339.
Saboori M, Ahmadi J, Farajzadegan Z. Indications for brain CT in patients with minor head injury. *Clin Neurol Neurosurg*. 2007;109:399–405.
Sliker CW, Mirvis SE, Shanmuganathan K. Assessing cervical spine stability in obtunded blunt trauma patients: review of medical literature. *Radiology*. 2005;234:733–739.
Vaccaro AR, Kim DH, Brodke DS, et. al. Diagnosis and management of thoracolumbar spine fractures. *J Bone Joint Surg Am*. 2003;85:2456–2470.
White AA, Panjabi MM. *Clinical Biomechanics of the Spine*. 2nd ed. Philadelphia, PA: Lippincott Williams & Wilkins; 1990:169–345.
Wintermark M, Mouhsine E, Theumann N, et al. Thoracolumbar spine fractures in patients who have sustained severe trauma: depiction with multi-detector row CT. *Radiology*. 2003;227:681–689.
Woodring JH, Lee C. Limitation of cervical radiography in the evaluation of acute cervical trauma. *J Trauma*. 1994;36(3):458–459.

CHAPTER 4

Wedge Fractures

George M. Bridgeforth and Mark Nolden

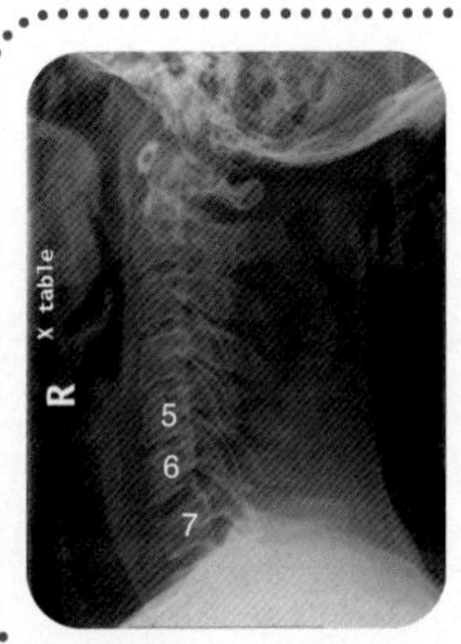

A 53-year-old restrained male driver is involved in a motor vehicle collision. He presents with posterior neck pain.

CLINICAL POINTS

- Wedge compression fractures are caused by spinal flexion.
- Neurological signs of spinal shock (numbness, weakness, absent reflexes, loss of bowel tone) may occur.

PATIENT ASSESSMENT

1. Check for associated head, thoracic, and abdominal injuries. Patients with acute spinal cord trauma may have traumatic brain injuries or damage to other major organs as well.
2. Always check patient's neurovascular status.
3. With acute trauma, always assume spinal instability until proven otherwise.

Clinical Presentation

Patients with clinically significant spinal cord injuries may present acutely without or without discernable neurological impairment. They may have low blood pressure associated with acute tetraplegia (quadriplegia) as well as loss of reflexes and bowel tone, which are classic indicators of spinal shock. Spinal shock is usually seen with severe spinal cord injuries above the midthoracic area.

The neurological examination is based on the last intact neurological level, and a functional classification is determined on the basis of the Frankel classification (see Chapter 3) and the American Spinal Injury Association (ASIA) classification. The ASIA classification system includes five levels (Box 4.1).

Wedge fractures are usually stable injuries caused by excessive flexion. They occur more commonly in the cervical region. The most common levels or cervical spinal cord injury are C5 and C6. If a tetraplegic patient exhibits loss of motor function with intact sensation extending to the S4–S5 region (i.e., the perianal region), he or she is a class B tetraplegic. If the patient has accompanying nonfunctional motor weakness (less than grade 3) below the level of the spinal cord injury, he or she is a class C tetraplegic. If the patient has at least half of the muscles with functional movement (grade 3 or greater) below the level of the spinal cord injury, he or she is a C5 class D tetraplegic. A C5 class A tetraplegic has intact biceps function (C5 muscle) but motor and sensory impairment below that level. A C6 class A tetraplegic has intact biceps function (C5) and wrist extension (C6) but motor and sensory impairment below that level. Higher-level tetraplegic patients are usually ventilator dependent.

Radiographic Evaluation

Wedge fractures are compression fractures that are characterized by a triangular-shaped compression deformity of the anterior vertebral body. The compression of the vertebral body generally involves the first column of Denis. The compression deformity is appreciated best on the lateral view. As noted earlier, the first column extends from the anterior longitudinal ligament to two-thirds of the vertebral body. Usually, wedge compression fractures are considered to be stable injuries. However, if an examiner identifies a wedge (pie-shaped) fracture of the anterior vertebral body on a radiograph (best appreciated on a lateral

Box 4.1 American Spinal Injury Association (ASIA) Modified Classification System of Spinal Damage

Class A: complete motor and sensory loss

Class B (incomplete injury): intact sensation (but not motor function) below the level of the injury and includes the sacral region S4–S5

Class C (incomplete injury): nonfunctional motor strength preserved below the neurological level of injury and more than half of the key muscles below the neurological level with a grade less than 3 (i.e., a grade 3 muscle can exhibit full range of motion against gravity but not resistance applied by the examiner)

Class D (incomplete injury): functional motor strength preserved below the neurological level of injury—at least half of the key muscles with a grade greater than or equal to 3 or better.

Class E: normal sensation and intact motor function

view), the examiner must not automatically assume stability. Flexion/extension radiographs should not be obtained by practitioners who are not familiar with treating acute spinal cord injuries (see Fig. 4.1).

Wedge fractures are generally stable fractures. Stable fractures do not show evidence of vertebral body displacement with flexion/extension views. If there is marked compression of the anterior two-thirds of the vertebral body (>40%) or if the fracture pattern extends across the entire vertebrae into the second column of Denis, the examiner should suspect a burst fracture.

Flexion rotation injuries (with compression) may result in a compression fracture of the anterior vertebral body, which is associated with a disruption of the posterior ligaments. With this type of injury, flexion radiographs show an increase in the interspinous space (between two adjacent spinous processes). If there is a disruption of the posterior longitudinal ligament (second column) and the posterior ligaments (third column), the injury is unstable. The third

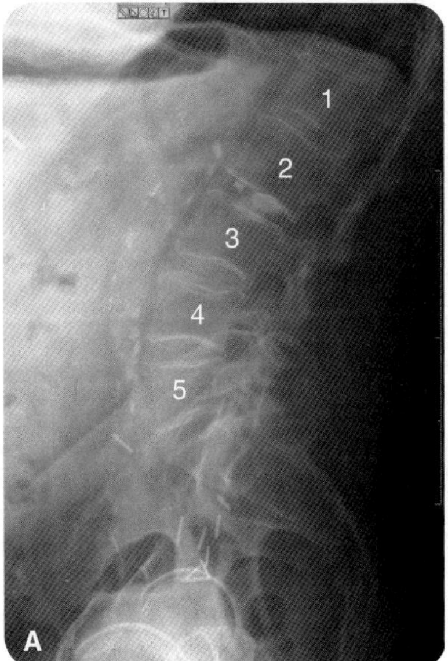

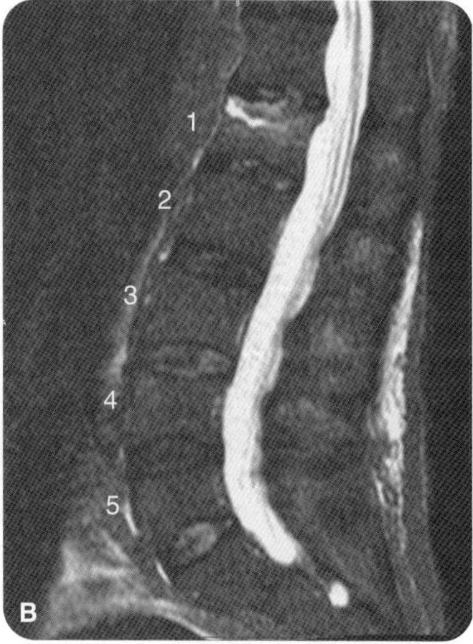

Figure 4.1 A 69-year-old man presents with low back pain for 2 days without a history of trauma. **(A)** Lateral radiograph of the lumbar spine demonstrates generalized bone demineralization and loss of the vertebral body height at L1. **(B)** A selected sagittal STIR image of the lumbar spine in the same patient demonstrates abnormal fluid signal in the L1 vertebral body, which is consistent with an acute wedge fracture.

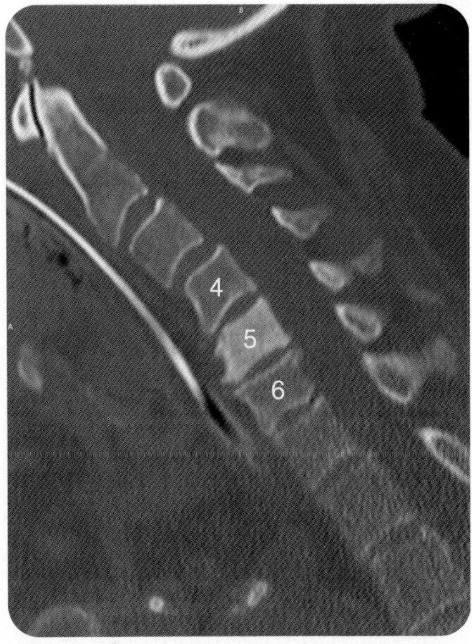

Figure 4.2 A 60-year-old woman with metastatic lung cancer presents with neck pain. A selected sagittal computed tomography image of the cervical spine demonstrates anterior wedging of the C5 vertebral body, which is diffusely sclerotic from bony metastasis.

NOT TO BE MISSED

- Fracture involving two (or three) columns of Denis
- Evidence of vertebral displacement with an acute fracture
- Involvement of 40% or more of the vertebral body
- Vertebral body fracture associated with separation or fanning of the spinous processes on the lateral radiograph

column comprises all structures that are posterior to the posterior longitudinal ligament. In any event, patients with acute spinal cord injuries should be stabilized. Their injuries should be evaluated with a computed tomography scan (Fig. 4.2). Radiographs alone may miss underlying spinal fractures.

WHEN TO REFER

- All acute spinal cord injuries require immediate referral.

Treatment

Generally, most cervical wedge compression fractures are treated with a halo vest. Most lumbar compression fractures are treated using a thoracolumbar orthosis brace. However, if there is evidence of instability of the posterior ligamentous structures, then the risk of a kyphotic deformity (curvature of the spine in the shape of a reverse C) increases over time. Surgical stabilization may be indicated.

Suggested Readings

Acheson MB, Livingston RR, Richardson ML, Stimac GK. High-resolution CT scanning in the evaluation of cervical spine fractures: comparisons with plain film examinations. *AJR Am J Roentgenol*. 1987;148:1179–1185.

Berlin L. CT versus radiology for initial evaluation of cervical spine trauma: what is the standard of care? *AJR Am J Roentgenol*. 2003;180:911–915.

Blackmore CC. Clinical predictions rules in trauma imaging: who, how, and why? *Radiology*. 2005;235:371–374.

Flanders AE, Schaefer DM, Doan HT, Mishkind MM, Gonzalez CF, Northrup BE. Acute spine trauma: correlation of MR imaging finds with degree of neurologic deficit. *Radiology*. 1990;177:25–33.

Holdsworth F. Review article fractures, dislocations and fracture-dislocations of the spine. *J Bone Joint Surg Am*. 1970;52:1534–1551.

Novelline RA, Rhea JT, Rap PM, Stuk JL. Helical CT in emergency radiology. *Radiology*.1999;213:321–339.

Rao SK, Wasyliw C, Nunez DB Jr. Spectrum of imaging findings in hyperextension injuries of the neck. *Radiographics*. 2005;25:1239–1254.

Thompson WL, Stiell IG, Clement CM, Brison RJ. Association of injury mechanisms with the risk of cervical spine fractures. *CJEM*. 2009;11:14–22.

White AA, Panjabi MM. *Clinical Biomechanics of the Spine*. Philadelphia, PA: Lippincott Williams & Wilkins; 1990:170–351.

Yuh WT, Zacher CK, Barloon TJ, Sato Y, Sickels WJ, Hawes DR. Vertebral compression fractures: distinction between benign and malignant causes with MR imaging. *Radiology*. 1989;172:215–218.

CHAPTER 5

Burst Fractures

George M. Bridgeforth and Mark Nolden

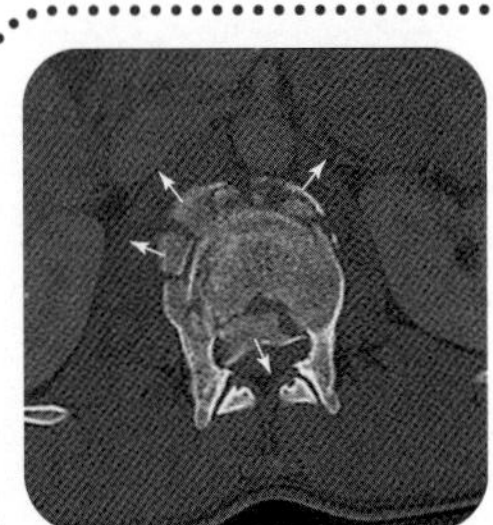

A 21-year-old man falls 30 ft down an elevator shaft without losing consciousness. He reports some problems with sensation and motor function below the waist.

Clinical Presentation

Burst fractures are traumatic spinal injuries that involve vertebral breakage. They may occur as a result of cervical injuries from diving accidents or from rollover accidents in which the driver was not wearing a seat belt. The **mechanism of injury** involves an axial load impact against a rock or a shallow river or against the roof of a vehicle as it rolls over. Cervical burst fractures may also be seen in contact sports injuries—in football, from an illegal technique called "spearing," in which the top of the helmet is used as a weapon during a flying block or a tackle.

As expected, impact injuries to the cervical spine may be associated with traumatic brain injuries. Therefore, the neurological examination should document any associated head trauma. Computed tomography (CT) scans of the cervical region and the head are indicated. Patients with severe neurological damage from cervical may present obtunded and in spinal shock. Severe cervical injuries may result in permanent tetraplegia (quadriplegia) once the patient recovers from spinal shock within 48 to 72 hours. A Jefferson fracture is a burst fracture of the first cervical ring (vertebrae). These fractures are usually fatal.

Burst fractures caused from falls in which the heels or buttocks strike the ground first may cause damage to the lower thoracic to upper lumbar vertebrae. Usually these occur between T10 and L2, but burst fractures as low as L5 have been reported. Patients with cervical or thoracolumbar burst fractures may fall into any one of the five American Spinal Injury Association (ASIA) spinal injury groups (see Chapter 4). Signs of an unstable burst fracture include acute neurological impairment, kyphosis (forward angulation of the spinal column greater than 20 degrees), acute subluxation (dislocation of the spinal column), and a 50% or greater encroachment of the spinal canal. A complete neurological examination, initial radiographs, and a CT scan are used to assess stability. The comprehensive neurological assessment should be conducted while the patient has been immobilized on a spine board with a hard cervical collar. It is important to examine the patient for other traumatic injuries to the major organs as well.

Severe thoracolumbar injuries may present acutely with loss of motor and sensory function below the umbilicus (T10 level). Severe thoracolumbar injuries may result in permanent paraplegia. Falls during which the patient lands feet first are associated with unilateral or bilateral heel fractures (10% of heel fractures are bilateral). Complete paraplegics with acute spinal cord injuries lose lower extremity sensation, so the presence of any bruising or

CLINICAL POINTS

- Burst fractures are caused by axial loads (downward forces).
- Neurological impairment may occur as a result of burst fractures.
- Cervical axial load injuries may be associated with traumatic brain injuries.
- Thoracolumbar injuries may be associated with abdominal trauma.
- Numbness and weakness occurs at and below the level of the spinal cord injury.
- Bladder, bowel, and sexual impairment may result.

PATIENT ASSESSMENT

1. Check for neurological impairment.
2. Always check for bilateral calcaneal injuries from falls.
3. Always assume spinal instability until proven otherwise. Patients with severe trauma should be immobilized in a hard cervical collar and on a spine board.
4. Always check neurovascular status carefully.

swelling of the heels warrants radiographic analysis of the affected foot or feet. However, patients with normal neurological function manifest heel pain unless they are obtunded from a traumatic brain injury, drug, or alcohol intoxication. Ten percent of calcaneal fractures from falls are bilateral.

Radiographic Evaluation

Tests to order, depending on the type and severity of the trauma, include the following:

- **Acute cervical trauma (minor):** anteroposterior (AP), lateral (must be able to see the C7-T-1 interspace vertebrae), and oblique radiographs. A swimmer view is used to visualize the C7 vertebrae if it is not identified on the lateral projection. An odontoid view (open mouth view), used to evaluate fractures of the odontoid process, is also necessary. Flexion/extension views should be read only by experienced spinal care providers. Flexion and extension radiographs are never taken until the initial radiographs have been evaluated first (Fig. 5.1).
- **Acute thoracolumbar trauma (minor):** AP, lateral, and oblique radiographs (two oblique views). Flexion and extension radiographs should be taken only if necessary.
- **Acute cervical** and **thoracolumbar trauma (severe):** CT scan "stat"

Burst fractures are comminuted dispersion fractures of the vertebral body; they are caused by an axial load. Unlike wedge compression fractures, which are limited to the anterior column of Denis, burst fractures are characterized by a comminuted fracture involving the anterior and the middle columns of Denis. The comminuted fractures may be identified on an AP view as compressed vertebrae. In addition to the decreased vertebral height, there is an outward dispersion of the vertebral fragments. This dispersion is characterized by an increase in the interpedicular space (a horizontal measurement taken from pedicle to pedicle in a single vertebra).

On the lateral view, the examiner can identify a comminuted fracture of the entire vertebral body. Unlike wedge compression fractures, which affect mainly the anterior column of Denis, the examiner should look for flattening and dispersion of the entire vertebral body with retropulsion posteriorly of the middle

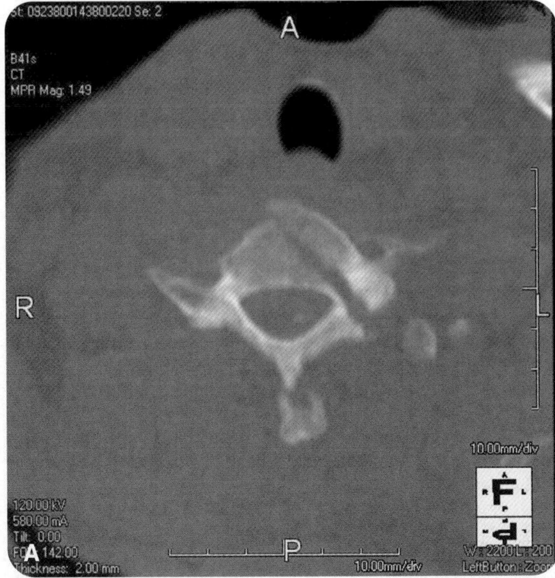

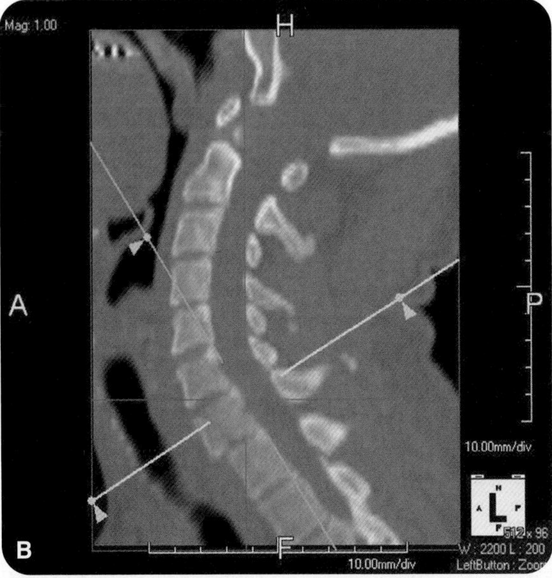

Figure 5.1 While tubing in the Atlantic Ocean, a 48-year-old man is swept into the sand by a wave. **(A)** Sagittal reformatted image of the cervical spine. **(B)** Maximum intensity projection image through the C7 vertebral body, demonstrating an acute burst fracture.

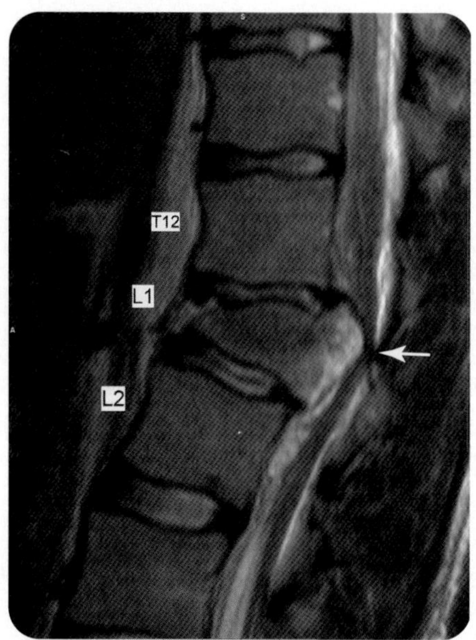

Figure 5.2 Selected T2-weighted sagittal image in the patient in the introductory case demonstrating 12-mm retropulsion of the posterior fracture fragment, resulting in compression and edema of the conus.

column (Fig. 5.2). This retropulsion is one of the hallmarks of a burst fracture. In contrast, a wedge compression fracture involves the anterior half to two-thirds of the vertebral body, and there is no evidence of retropulsion of the bony fragments seen on the lateral view. However, if there is anterior and middle column involvement characterized by a dispersed comminuted fracture, one must suspect a burst fracture. The lateral projection shows a comminuted fracture of the entire vertebral body. Associated findings include a decreased vertebral height associated with an increased distance from the anterior to the posterior vertebral body.

Unlike wedge compression fractures, burst fractures generally do not involve the posterior column. Wedge compression fractures may or may not have torn posterior ligaments. When the posterior ligaments are torn, they result in an increased space (fanning) between the spinous processes on a flexion view. Wedge fractures that involve the anterior column (flexion injuries) are usually stable. However, wedge fractures with posterior ligament disruption (flexion rotation injuries) are unstable. As previously stated, unstable burst fractures are characterized by kyphosis, acute subluxation, or a 50% or greater encroachment of the spinal canal.

The posterior (third column of Denis) is usually spared unless there is a strong rotational component associated with the axial load causing damage to the posterior complex (i.e., torn spinal ligaments). A good example would be a flexion rotation injury of the spine following a direct impact to the skull.

Treatment

Stable injuries of the thoracolumbar spine may be treated with a thoracolumbar orthosis brace for 8 to 10 weeks (a turtle shell), which is worn for 2 months. The patient then undergoes several months of physical therapy. Some spinal dislocation may be apparent after removal of the brace, but if no further major dislocation of subluxation occurs, no addition external stabilization may be necessary.

Unstable fractures require surgical stabilization. Length of recovery depends on type of injury and associated neurological deficits. The type of approach (anterior vs. posterior) is made on a case-by-case basis but usually involves bone grafts (strut) with a titanium plate fixation. Patients who develop a progressive kyphotic deformity following a posterior approach may have to have a second stabilization performed via an anterior approach.

Quadriplegics may be in a spinal rehabilitation facility for 5 to 6 months. Paraplegics may be in rehabilitation for 2 to 3 months.

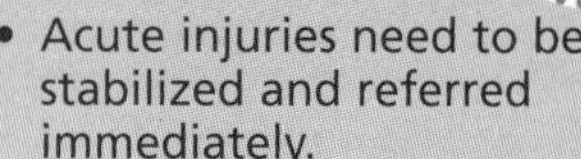

WHEN TO REFER

- Acute injuries need to be stabilized and referred immediately.

NOT TO BE MISSED

- Associated traumatic head injuries (especially with cervical trauma)
- Heel fractures associated with thoracolumbar burot fractures (from falls)
- Bowel and bladder impairment may still exist after neurological recovery

Suggested Readings

Akbarnia BA, Crandal DG, Burkus K, Matthews T. Use of long rods and a short arthrodesis for burst fractures of the thoracolumbar spine: a long-term follow-up study. *J Bone Joint Surg Am.* 1994;76(11):1629–1635.

Andreychik DA, Alander DH, Senica KM, Stauffer ES. Burst fractures of the second through fifth lumbar vertebrae: clinical and radiographic results. *J Bone Joint Surg Am.* 1996;78(8):1156–1166.

Atlas SW, Regenbogern V, Rogers LF, Kim KS. The radiographic characterization of burst fractures of the spine. *AJR Am J Roentgenol.* 1986;147:575–582.

Bono CM, Vaccaro AR, Hurlbert RJ, et al. Validating a newly proposed classification system for thoracolumbar spine trauma: looking to the future of the thoracolumbar injury classification and severity score. *J Orthop Trauma.* 2006;20(8):567–572.

Denis F. The three column spine and its significance in the classification of acute thoracolumbar spinal injuries. *Spine.* 1983;8:817–831.

Finn CA, Stauffer ES. Burst fracture of the fifth lumbar vertebra. *J Bone Joint Surg Am.* 1992;74(3):398–403.

Greenspan A. *Orthopedic Imaging.* 4th ed. Philadelphia, PA: Lippincott Williams & Wilkins; 2004:385–397.

Harris JH, Harris WH, Novelline RA. *The Radiology of Emergency Medicine.* 3rd ed. Baltimore, MD: Lippincott Williams & Wilkins; 1993:266–271.

Holdworth F. Review article fractures, dislocations and fracture-dislocations of the spine. *J Bone Joint Surg Am*. 1970;52:1534–1551.
Hsu JM, Joseph T, Ellis AM. Thoracolumbar fracture in blunt trauma patients: guidelines for diagnosis and imaging. *Injury*. 2003;34(6):426–433.
Kilcoyne RF, Mack LA, King HA, Ratcliff SS, Loop JW. Thoracolumbar spine injuries associated with vertical plunges: reappraisal with computed tomography. *Radiology*. 1983;146(1):137–140.
Kösling S, Dietrich K, Steinecke R, Klöppel R, Schulz HG. Diagnostic value of 3D CT surface reconstruction spinal fractures. *Eur Radiol*. 1997;7:61–64.
Leone A, Guglielmi G, Cassar-Pullicino VN, Bonomo L. Lumbar intervertebral instability: a review. *Radiology*. 2007;245:62–77.
Maynard FM, Bracken MB, Creasey G, et al. International Standards for Neurological and Functional Classification of Spinal Cord Injury: American Spinal Injury Association. *Spinal Cord*. 1997;35:266–274.
Novelline RA, Rhea JT, Rao PM, Stuk JL. Helical CT in emergency radiology. *Radiology*. 1999;213:321–339.
Vaccaro AR, Kim DH, Brodke DS, et. al. Diagnosis and management of thoracolumbar spine fractures. *J Bone Joint Surg Am*. 2003;85:2456–2470.
White AA, Panjabi MM. *Clinical Biomechanics of the Spine*. Philadelphia, PA: Lippincott Williams & Wilkins; 1990:244–258.
Wilcox RK, Boerger TO, Allen DJ, Barton DC. A dynamic study of thoracolumbar burst fractures. *J Bone Joint Surg Am*. 2003;85:2184–2189.
Wintermark M, Mouhsine E, Theumann N, et. al. Thoracolumbar spine fractures in patients who have sustained severe trauma: depiction with multi-detector row CT. *Radiology*. 2003;227:681–699.
Wood K, Butterman G, Mehbod A, Garvey T. Operative compared with nonoperative treatment of a thoracolumbar burst fracture without neurological deficit. *J Bone Joint Surg Am*. 2003;85:773–781.
Yuh WT, Zachar CK, Barloon TJ, et al. Vertebral compression fractures: distinction between benign and malignant causes with MR imaging. *Radiology*. 1989;172:217–218.

CHAPTER 6

Chance Fractures

George M. Bridgeforth and Mark Nolden

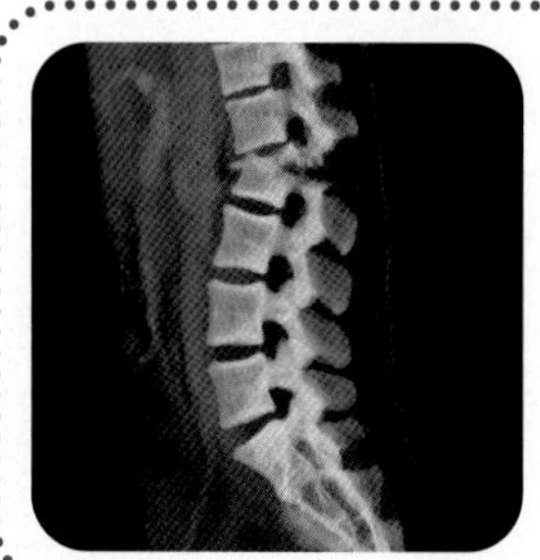

A 42-year-old restrained female passenger presents with back and chest pain after a motor vehicle collision, which took the life of her 4-year-old child.

SECTION 1 Spine

Clinical Presentation

Chance fractures are uncommon injuries, and they have become even less likely since the introduction of combination shoulder strap-lap seat belts. In older vehicles, where the seat belt does not include a shoulder strap, and in an accident, the patient can be thrown forward against the seat belt, which functions like a restraining fulcrum. As the patient is thrown forward and upward, there is a disruption of the spinal column through all three columns of Denis. The **mechanism of injury** is flexion distraction. The majority of injuries affect the lower thoracic to upper lumbar vertebrae. Ligamentous injuries may be seen, especially if there is an associated rotational component to the injury. Surprisingly, neurological injuries are uncommon and occur in approximately 15% of cases. Usually, these injuries are characterized by a paraplegia below T10 level (the umbilicus) or a cauda equina injury.

Individuals with complete T10 paraplegia (American Spinal Injury Association [ASIA] class A) present with a total loss of neurological function below the umbilicus (navel). This includes a complete loss of motor function, total sensory loss, and loss of sexual, bowel, and bladder function.

Individuals with an incomplete spinal cord injury (T10 paraplegia [ASIA class B]) have a loss of motor function but intact sensory function, which includes the sacral segments. This would be a very unusual level but sensation of the legs and perianal sensation would be intact. Impaired sexual function and bowel and bladder incontinence are still present.

Individuals with an incomplete spinal cord injury (T10 paraplegia [ASIA class C]) have motor weakness of the lower extremities (with less than 50% of the key muscles having a grade less than 3/5). Once again, there is accompanying impaired sexual, bowel, and bladder function.

Individuals with an incomplete spinal cord injury (T10 [ASIA class D]) would exhibit functional motor strength in the lower extremities (at least 50% of the muscles or more would exhibit grade 3/5 or stronger motor function). However, these injuries may still be accompanied by impaired sexual, bowel, and bladder function.*

CLINICAL POINTS

- This compression injury is caused by violent forward flexion.
- Once known as the "seat belt injury," this fracture is now less common.
- Survivors usually have paraplegia, with lower motor neuron damage to the bowel and bladder.
- Other serious injuries to the abdominal organs (ruptured liver, spleen, aorta, kidneys) may occur.

*Patients with cervical spinal cord injuries develop upper motor neuron damage to the bowel and bladder once they recover from spinal shock. Patients with thoracolumbar injuries have lower motor neuron damage to the bowel and bladder. The two conditions are managed differently. A complete discourse on this subject is beyond the focus of this text.

PATIENT ASSESSMENT

1. Assess carefully for neurovascular compromise (loss of pulses, cold cyanotic limbs).
2. Assess for other abdominal organ injuries (aortic tears, as well as liver, kidney, and spleen damage).
3. Look for bruising of the abdomen and the chest wall.

Individuals with acute cauda equina injuries present with mixed picture of upper motor neuron (injury to the central nervous system) and lower motor neuron (injury to nerve roots and peripheral nerves). There may be acute traumatic low back pain with an asymmetrical motor and sensory impairment of the lower extremities. There is an acute loss of voluntary bowel tone on a rectal examination (i.e., patients cannot generate a forceful tone when they bear down). In addition, there is perianal saddle anesthesia, which is characterized by a loss of sensation to pinprick in the gluteal region surrounding the anus. In addition, there is a loss of the anal wink reflex (i.e., a contraction of the anal sphincter that occurs when the anal rim is stroked with a cotton swab). Acute spinal core injuries to the lower thoracic and lumbar regions (or acute cervical injuries with spinal shock) are initially characterized by similar findings (saddle anesthesia, loss of voluntary bowel tone, loss of the anal wink reflexes); however, an asymmetrical motor sensory impairment of the lower extremities leads the examiner more toward a cauda equina injury.

As expected, the rate of associated abdominal injuries is high—reported to be 50% or more. There may be associated damage to the aorta, liver, spleen, uterus, thoracic ribs, diaphragm, or kidneys. Therefore, a surgical consultation and a computed tomography (CT) of the abdomen (or possibly the head) are indicated.

Radiographic Evaluation

It is necessary to obtain the following tests:

- Lateral and anteroposterior radiographs of the spine
- CT scans for acute thoracolumbar trauma (severe)
  - Abdominal CT
  - Head CT (if the patient is acutely intoxicated, has an associated injury above the clavicle, or has an impaired mental status)
  - Spinal CT with sagittal reconstructions (Fig. 6.1).

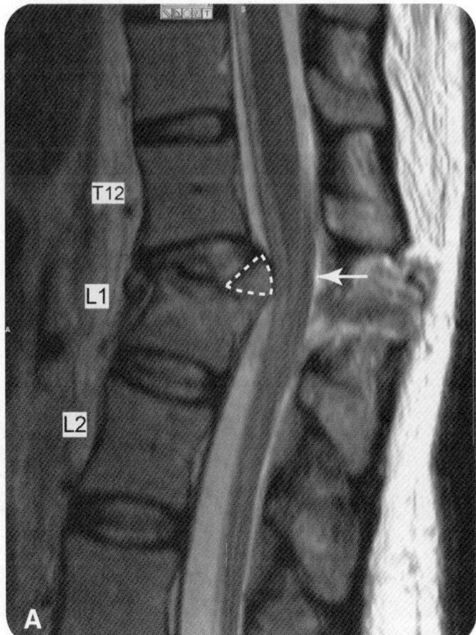

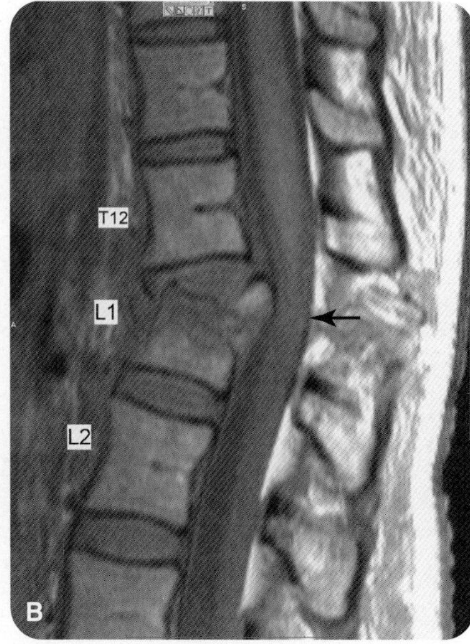

Figure 6.1 **(A)** Sagittal T1-weighted and **(B)** T2-weighted magnetic resonance images of a 51-year-old man involved in a serious motor vehicle accident, demonstrating the Chance fracture at L1 and the superior retropulsion causing posterior displacement of the cauda equina.

NOT TO BE MISSED

- Associated heat injuries
- Associated organ damage
- Burst fractures with acute paraplegia

WHEN TO REFER

- Possibly unstable injuries should be stabilized and referred immediately.

Chance fractures are unstable injuries that result in the disruption of all three columns of Denis. It is necessary to look for disruption (with or without displacement) affecting all three columns of Denis on the lateral radiograph. These injuries are characterized by a flexion distraction that occurs against a fixed fulcrum. On a lateral radiograph, the horizontal fracture line extends through the spinous process, lamina, pedicle, and the vertebral body. In addition, from a biomechanical standpoint, the thoracic vertebrae receive additional support from the ribs, which act like a buttressing strut, preventing the anterior displacement of the thoracic vertebrae. T11 and T12 (the 11th and 12th thoracic ribs) articulate with the floating ribs, which do not provide a bracing function. In addition to all of this, the thoracic facets are oriented in an anteroposterior (coronal) configuration. This configuration not only allows for lateral bending but also provides additional support against an anterior subluxation of the vertebral columns. Facet orientation begins to change as the vertebrae transition from T12 to L1. In the lumbar vertebrae, the facets are angulated in a front to back (sagittal) direction to allow for forward bending and extension. The orientation of the lumbar facets does not provide effective buttressing at the (seat belt) level of injury (see Fig. 6.2).

Treatment

Patients who do not opt for surgical fixation may be treated with a fiberglass or plaster cast. Those who do not respond to more conservative treatment are candidates for surgical stabilization.

Severe injuries causing disruption of all three columns are unstable injuries. Generally, they are treated by surgical fixation. With pedicle screw fixation, the rod is anchored one level above and below the fractured vertebrae. Rod-hook fixations may involve placing the rods two levels above and below the injured vertebrae. In addition, there is a hybrid device consisting of hooks above the injured vertebrae with pedicle screws below (Goodrich). Patients need to be monitored for a progressive kyphotic deformity (forward angulation of the spine).

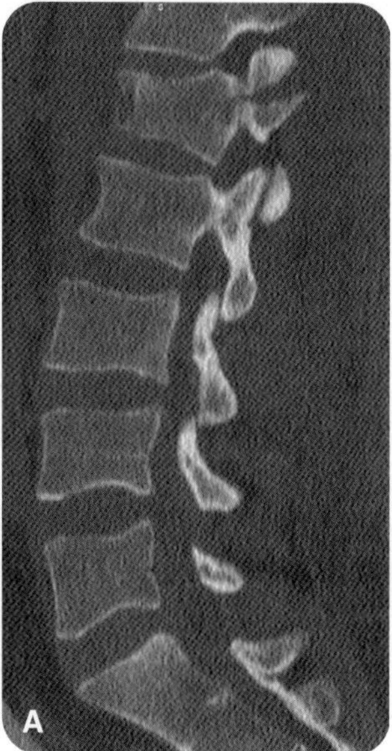

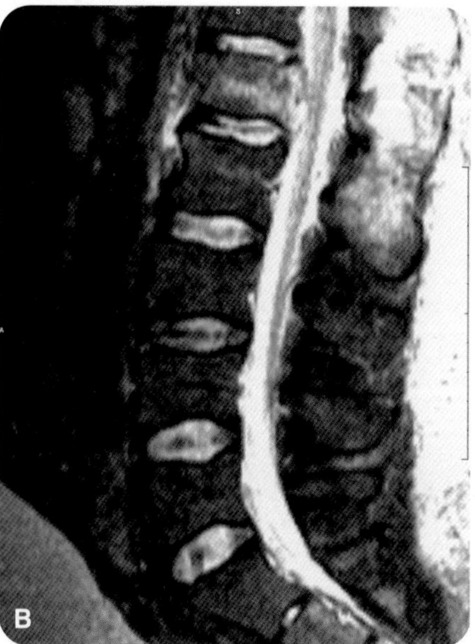

Figure 6.2 A 34-year-old intoxicated man presents with mild back pain after his motor vehicle rolls over. **(A)** Sagittal reconstructed computed tomography image of the lumbar spine demonstrates an acute Chance fracture through L1. **(B)** Sagittal STIR image of the lumbar spine in the same patient demonstrates extensive edema along the fracture site.

Suggested Readings

Bernstein MP, Mirvis SE, Shanmuganathan K. Chance-type fractures of the thoracolumbar spine: imaging analysis in 53 patients. *AJR Am J Roentgenol*. 2006;187:859–868.

Brant WE, Helms CA. *Fundamentals of Diagnostic Radiology*. 3rd ed. Philadelphia, PA: Lippincott Williams & Wilkins; 2007:1108.

Chance GQ. Notes on a flexion fracture of the spine. *Br J Radiol*. 1948;21:452–453.

Goodrich JA. Chance fracture: treatment. http://www.emedicine.medscape.com/article/1263663-treatment. Accessed September 11, 2009.

Greenspan A. *Orthopedic Imaging*. 4th ed. Philadelphia, PA: Lippincott Williams & Wilkins; 2004:392–393.

Harris JH, Harris WH, Novelline RA. *The Radiology of Emergency Medicine*. 3rd ed. Baltimore, MD: Lippincott Williams & Wilkins; 1993:254, 260–262.

Leone A, Guglielmi G, Cassar-Pullicino VN, Bonomo L. Lumbar intervertebral instability: a review. *Radiology*. 2007;245:62–77.

McKinnis LN. *Fundamentals of Orthopedic Radiology*. Philadelphia, PA: FA Davis; 1997:149–154.

CHAPTER 7 Unilateral Facet Dislocations

George M. Bridgeforth and Mark Nolden

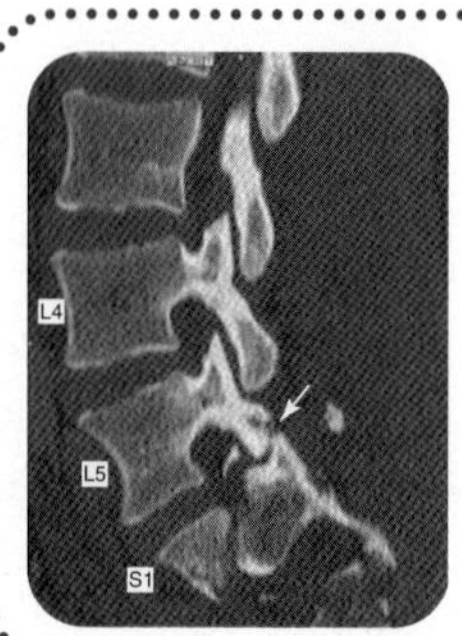

A 19-year-old man was an unrestrained backseat passenger in an automobile involved in a collision with another motor vehicle. He now presents with left sacral and left groin pain.

Clinical Presentation

The most common cause of unilateral facet injuries are motor vehicle accidents, followed by contact sports injuries. The **mechanism of injury** involved in this spinal injury is flexion/rotation. Unlike bilateral facet injuries, most unilateral facet injuries are stable and occur in the midcervical region. Facet injuries to the lumbar spine are less common and are more likely to be associated with spinal fractures. However, the unilateral cervical facet injuries may also be associated with facet fractures. Therefore, all patients should be stabilized on a spine board with a hard collar. Instability should always be assumed until proven otherwise.

The most common clinical presentation with a unilateral facet dislocation is radicular cervical pain. The flexion rotation injury causes the superior facet to slide over the inferior facet. The inferior facet is forced caudally and cause nerve root impingement of the neuroforamen beneath the inferior facet. This bony impingement where the nerve root exists from the vertebral column produces radicular symptoms. In selected cases, there may an accompanying disc protrusion as well.

Patients with C5 (fifth cervical nerve root irritation) have pain and numbness that radiates to the deltoid region (outside of the shoulder). Differential diagnosis includes C5 radiculopathies from disc herniations without facet dislocations as well as such shoulder injuries as acute humeral head, upper shaft fractures, humeral dislocations, and acute rotator cuff tears. A facet dislocation may be misdiagnosed as an acute shoulder injury or a herniated cervical disc. A thorough musculoskeletal examination followed by radiological studies can be very helpful.

Patients with C5 radiculopathies from unilateral facet dislocations of herniated discs usually demonstrate decreased sensation along the lateral deltoid (outside of the shoulder at the head of the humerus) to pinprick. In the acute setting following a cervical injury, it is not advised to assess cervical range of motion until an unstable spinal injury has been ruled out. Patients with acute radiculopathies from herniated discs often have impaired cervical range of motion as well. Later findings with severe radiculopathies from unilateral facet dislocations or herniated discs include biceps weakness (weak elbow flexion with the handheld palm facing upward) on the affected side and a diminished or absent biceps (C5) reflex.

CLINICAL POINTS

- Common causes of unilateral facet dislocations are motor vehicle accidents and contact sports injuries.
- Radiculopathy occurs on the side of the unilateral facet dislocation.
- Some patients with radiculopathies present with diminished sensation of the fingers.
- These types of dislocations may be associated with a traumatic brain injury.

C6 radiculopathies from unilateral facet dislocations or cervical herniations lead to pain and/or numbness that radiates to the thumb and index finger (Hoppenfeld six shooter). Later stages may manifest weakness with wrist extension (C6–C7 muscle function) and a diminished or absent brachioradial reflex (C6) at the wrist is very helpful. C7 radiculopathies have numbness that radiates to the middle finger. Marked nerve root involvement may present with weakness of grip strength and triceps function (weak elbow extension). Additional findings may include diminished or absent triceps reflex on the affected side. Early radiculopathies have deceased sensation of the middle finger. Marked nerve root involvement present with weakness of wrist flexion as well. C8 injuries radiate to the little finger. Early radiculopathies present with diminished sensation of the little finger.

Patients with cervical (or lumbar) stenosis usually present with bilateral radiculopathies affecting both upper extremities. In addition, there may involvement affecting more than one spinal level. Radiographs show narrowed foramen (exit canals for the spinal nerves) on the lateral radiographs and on the oblique radiographs.

With all acute cervical injuries, it is imperative that the examiner evaluates the lower extremities for upper motor neuron signs. Most nerve root injuries are lower motor neuron injuries. Lower motor neuron injuries are characterized by sensory loss, motor weakness, hyporeflexia, or areflexia (diminished or absent) reflexes. On the other hand, upper motor neuron injuries involve damage to the central nervous system (brain or spinal cord).

Unlike lower motor neuron injuries, upper motor neuron injuries are characterized by weakness, hyperactive reflexes, upgoing plantar responses (positive Babinski reflexes in the feet), clonus (recurrent jerking reflexes), and clasp-knife spasticity (increased muscle tone that eventually yields to marked resistance applied by an examiner across a joint). Patients with cervical injuries who have bilateral upper motor neuron signs affecting the lower extremities have either accompanying acute cervical spinal cord injuries or severe bilateral head injuries. With acute cervical injuries, this should prompt further evaluation with computed tomography (CT) of the head and the cervical spine.

Radiographic Evaluation

The following tests should be ordered depending on the type and severity of injury:

- **Acute cervical trauma (minor):** anteroposterior (AP), lateral (must be able to see to the C7–T1 interspace vertebrae), and oblique radiographs. A swimmer view is used to visualize C7 if it is not identified on the lateral projection. An odontoid view (open mouth view), used to evaluate fractures of the odontoid process, is also necessary. Flexion and extension radiographs should never be taken until the initial radiographs have been evaluated first.
- **Acute thoracolumbar trauma (minor):** AP, lateral, and oblique radiographs (two oblique views). Again, flexion and extension radiographs should be taken only if necessary and after the initial radiographs have been evaluated first.
- **Acute cervical** and **thoracolumbar trauma (severe):** CT scan "stat." In the acute setting, cervical spine radiographs followed by a CT scan help demonstrate a unilateral facet dislocation and document the degree of cervical protrusion versus an injury from a pure cervical herniation (Figs. 7.1 and 7.2). Also, patients with acute cervical injuries that radiate to the shoulder and those who have evidence of shoulder impairment (acute pain, swelling, bruising, tenderness, decreased range of motion) should have accompanying shoulder radiographs as well to rule out an associated shoulder fracture, acromioclavicular joint injury, or shoulder dislocation. The presence of pain, limited shoulder range of motion, and a positive drop arm test is indicative

PATIENT ASSESSMENT

1. Look for nerve root impingement with radicular symptoms secondary to a locked dislocated facet.
2. Most unilateral facet dislocations are stable. However, always assume instability until proven otherwise.
3. Rule out associated head, shoulder, and thoracic trauma, especially with cervical injuries.
4. Check for nerve root irritation (i.e., pinched nerve) at the site of the injury.
5. Always check neurovascular status carefully.

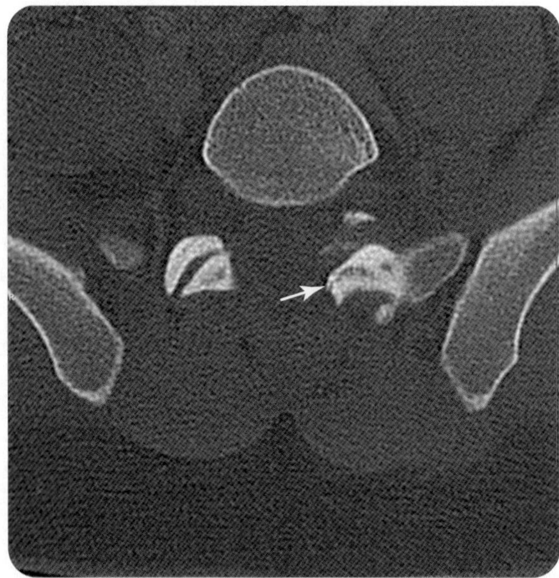

Figure 7.1 Axial computed tomography image demonstrating an abnormal appearance of the left L5–S1 facet and normal articulation on the right.

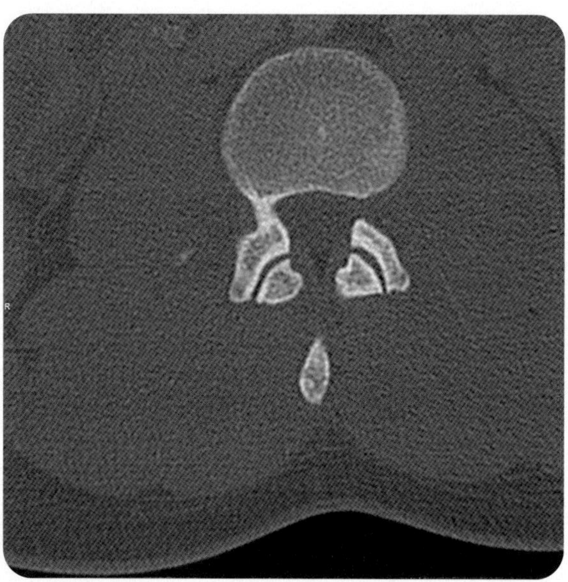

Figure 7.2 Axial computed tomography image at L2–L3 demonstrating normal bilateral articulating facets.

of a rotator cuff tear. In such cases, magnetic resonance imaging studies of the shoulder are indicated. If there is an associated head injury, it is necessary to obtain a CT scan of the head as well (rule out a fracture vs. a subdural hematoma).

Unilateral facet dislocations are generally stable injuries. In many cases, the anteroposterior view shows a rotated spinous process that points to the side of the dislocation. On the lateral view, there is a step off deformity which may represent up to a 25% (anterior) displacement of the anterior vertebral body. If the degree of vertebral displacement exceeds 25%, the examiner should suspect an unstable injury with associated fractures and significant damage to the posterior column (the spinal structures that are distal to the posterior longitudinal ligament). Most facet injuries affect the cervical region. Although lumbar facet injuries are uncommon, they may be associated with facet and transverse process fractures as well. The examiner should suspect an unstable fracture:

- If there is more than 25% displacement of the anterior vertebral body relative to the neighboring superior and inferior vertebral bodies.
- If there are extensive fractures involving at least two spinal columns of Denis.
- If there is fanning of the posterior spinous process identified on the lateral view. The latter finding would indicate extensive tears in the posterior ligament complex in the neighboring vertebrae (see Fig. 7.3).

NOT TO BE MISSED

- Cervical strain
- Cervical contusion
- Acute cervical fracture
- Degenerative arthritis
- Cervical radiculopathy
- Cervical stenosis
- Cervical osteomyelitis (intravenous drug abusers)

Treatment

Most unilateral facet injures can be "unlocked" by traction or by manipulation. Unilateral facet injuries that cannot be unlocked by conservative means are treated surgically.

Initially, a closed reduction is attempted with halo traction. If this is unsuccessful, a reduction may be attempted by a spinal surgeon while the patient is under general anesthesia. Patients with extensive cervical injuries my be placed in a halo vest for up to 3 months. However, if a closed reduction is

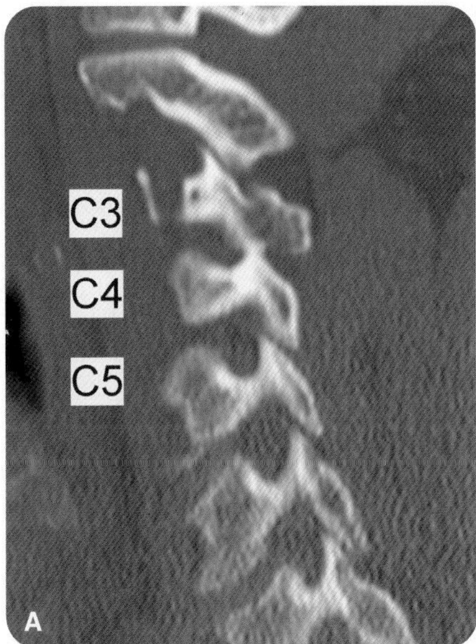

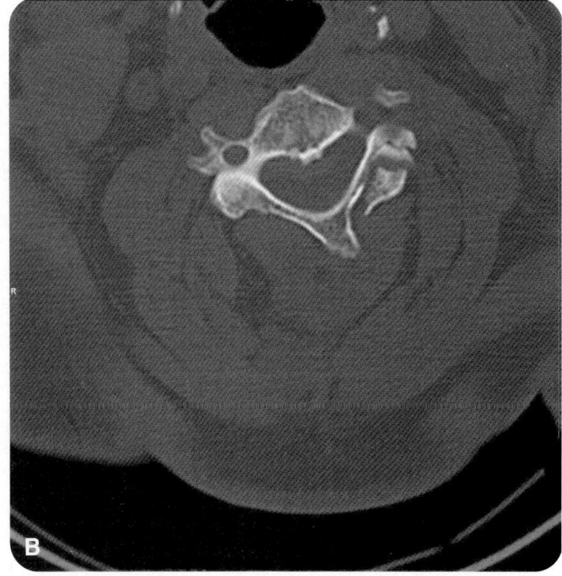

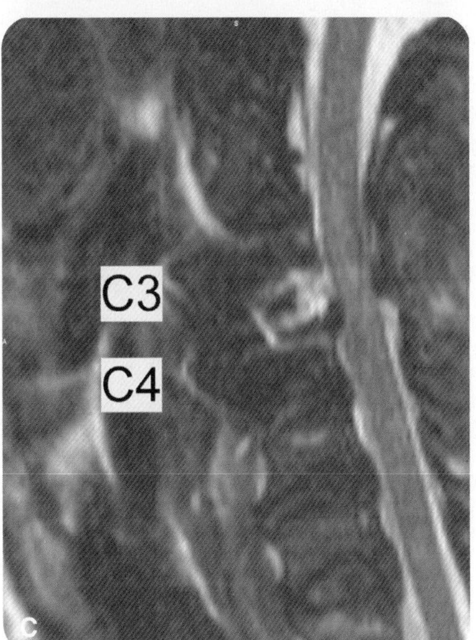

Figure 7.3 A 56-year-old unrestrained male driver experiences neck pain, paralysis and numbness below the chest after a motor vehicle collision. **(A)** Sagittal and **(B)** axial computed tomography images demonstrate a unilateral locked facet at C3–C4 on the left. **(C)** A sagittal STIR image from magnetic resonance imaging demonstrates cord compression and cord edema at C3 in the same patient.

unsuccessful, the patient may undergo an open reduction which consists of posterior wiring and bone graft placement. Following surgery, patients are placed in a halo vest for a 3 month period. Another indication for surgical stabilization are patients who were initially treated conservatively, but are developing a progressive kyphotic deformity (anterior angulation). These patients are stabilized with a cervical fusion that is performed an anterior or posterior approach.

WHEN TO REFER

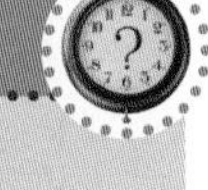

- All cases should be referred immediately.

Suggested Readings

Blacksin MF, Lee HJ. Frequency and significant of fractures of the upper cervical spine detected by CT in patients with severe neck trauma. *AJR Am J Roentgenol.* 1995;165:1201–1204.

Brant-Zawadzki M, Miller EM, Federle MP. CT in the evaluation of spine trauma. *AJR Am J Roentgenol.* 1981; 136:369–375.

Clark CT, Igram CM, El-Khoury GY, Ehara S. Radiographic evaluation of cervical spine injuries. *Spine.* 1988; 13:742–747.

Gellad FE, Levine AM, Joslyn JN, Edwards CC, Bosse M. Pure thoracolumbar facet dislocation: clinical features and CT appearance. *Radiology.* 1986;161:505–508.

Halliday AL, Hendernson BR, Hart BL, Benzel EC. The management of unilateral mass/facet fractures of the subaxial cervical spine: the use of magnetic resonance imaging to predict instability. *Spine*. 1997;22: 2614–2621.

Rao SK, Wasyliw C, Nunez D. Spectrum of imaging findings in hyperextension injuries of the neck. *Radiographics*. 2005;25:1239–1254.

Sekhon LHS, Fehlings MG. Epidemiology, demographics and pathophysiology of spinal cord injury. *Spine*. 2001;26:S2.

Thompson WL, Stiell IG, Clement CM, Brison RJ. Association of injury mechanisms with the risk of cervical spine fractures. *CJEM*. 2009;11:14–22.

White AA, Panjabi MM. *Clinical Biomechanics of the Spine*. 2nd ed. Philadelphia, PA: Lippincott Williams & Wilkins; 1990:170–242.

CHAPTER

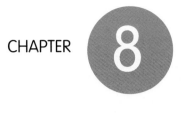

8 Bilateral Facet Dislocations

George M. Bridgeforth and Mark Nolden

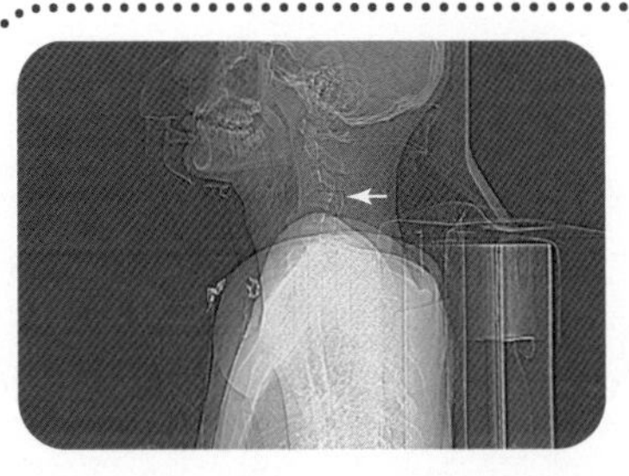

An 18-year-old man is involved in a motor vehicle collision in which he is rear-ended. He is disoriented and complains of severe cervical pain as well as weakness and numbness of the arms and legs.

CLINICAL POINTS

- This condition is considered unstable.
- Associated neurological deficits are usually present; cervical injuries may cause quadriplegia.
- Disk herniation may occur.

Clinical Presentation

Bilateral facet dislocations are unstable injuries characterized by disruption of the posterior ligament complex and damage to the anterior and posterior longitudinal ligaments. The cervical canal is no longer intact. The **mechanism of injury** is hyperflexion. Most of the injuries affect the midcervical region. Thoracic and lumbar injuries are rare but have been reported. As a result of the soft tissue damage, neurological injury is common.

Within 48 to 72 hours, the acute spinal shock is followed by upper motor neuron signs of motor (deltoid) weakness, hyperreflexia, clonus (oscillating reflexes), spasticity, and upgoing plantar responses (upgoing big toe when the soles of the feet are stroked with a reflex hammer). High-level spinal cord injuries (C2–C4) are characterized by damage to the phrenic nerve and severe permanent respiratory impairments. Patients with high-level injuries are ventilator-dependent tetraplegics (quadriplegics). Unlike paraplegics, tetraplegics cannot live independently. Even after extensive training, they require assistance with daily living.

PATIENT ASSESSMENT

1. With acute injuries, possible weakness, sensory loss, loss of sphincter tone, and loss of reflexes
2. Associated head injuries and organ damage
3. Progressive paralysis

Radiographic Evaluation

Tests to order, for both acute cervical trauma and acute thoracolumbar trauma include anteroposterior, lateral, and oblique views (two). In cases of cervical injury, it is necessary to see to C7. Optional radiographs include the following:

- Swimmer view, which is used to visualize the disc space between C-7 and T-1 (C7) if it is not identified on the lateral projection
- Flexion/extension views, which should be obtained only by experienced spinal care providers. Flexion and extension radiographs are *never* taken until the initial radiographs have been evaluated first for instability.

On the lateral view, vertebral body displacements of more than 50% are indicative of bilateral facet dislocations (Fig. 8.1). Moreover, the dislocated superior facets are "perched" on top of the inferior facets (like birds wings sitting on a fence). In these cases, the superior facets may actually appear anterior to the inferior facets. Unlike unilateral facet injuries, bilateral dislocated facet injuries are unstable. As previously stated, they are associated with torn

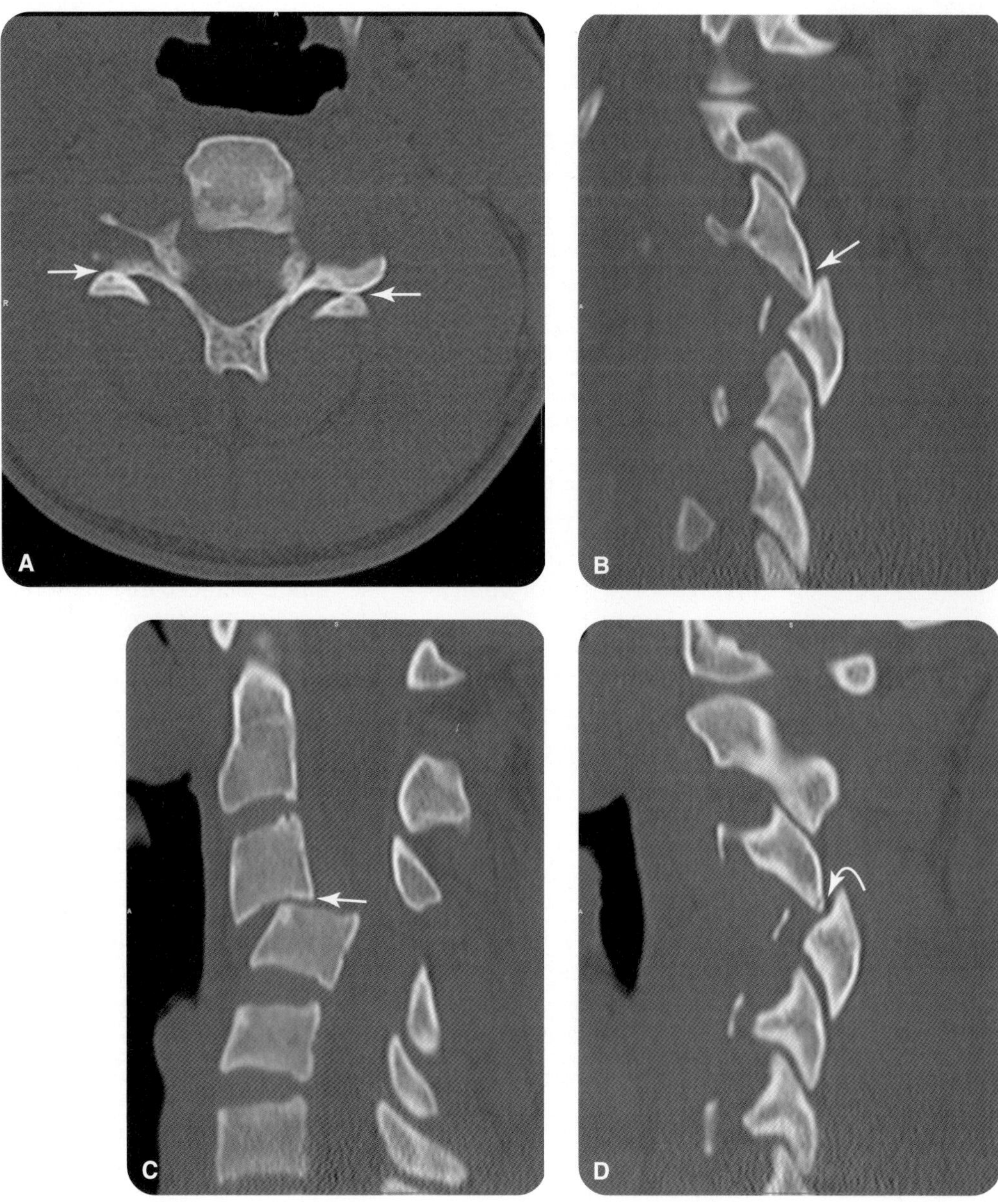

Figure 8.1 (A) An axial computed tomography image in the patient in the introductory case, demonstrating the "reverse hamburger" sign of bilateral locked facets. More apparent on soft tissue windows (not shown) is a 6-mm epidural hematoma at this level. **(B–D)** Selected sagittal CT images through the cervical spine demonstrate similar findings.

NOT TO BE MISSED

- Cervical strain
- Cervical contusion
- Acute cervical fracture
- Degenerative arthritis
- Cervical radiculopathy
- Cervical stenosis
- Cervical osteomyelitis (intravenous drug abusers)

posterior complex ligaments (i.e., the surrounding and supporting ligaments posterior to the posterior longitudinal ligament) as well as damaged anterior and posterior longitudinal ligaments (Fig. 8.2). There is significant damage to all three columns of Denis.

In addition, there may be an accompanying disc herniation, which can be evaluated by a "stat" computed tomography (CT) scan. Patients with accompanying disorientation, obtundation, and acute drugs or alcohol intoxication should also have a head CT obtained to check for associated traumatic brain injury.

Treatment

Bilateral facet dislocations are unstable injures with a high rate of redislocation in addition, there is a high risk for developing a kyphotic deformity (i.e., a

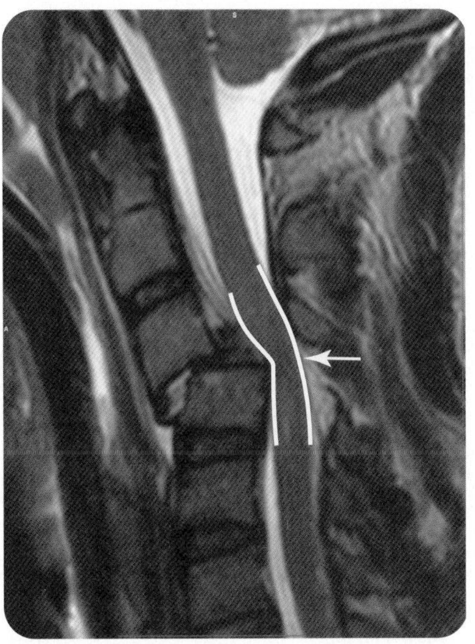

Figure 8.2 A T2-weighted magnetic resonance image through the bilateral jumped facets at C3 on C4 in the patient in the introductory case demonstrates ligamentous injury and prevertebral edema. There is severe cord compression at this level.

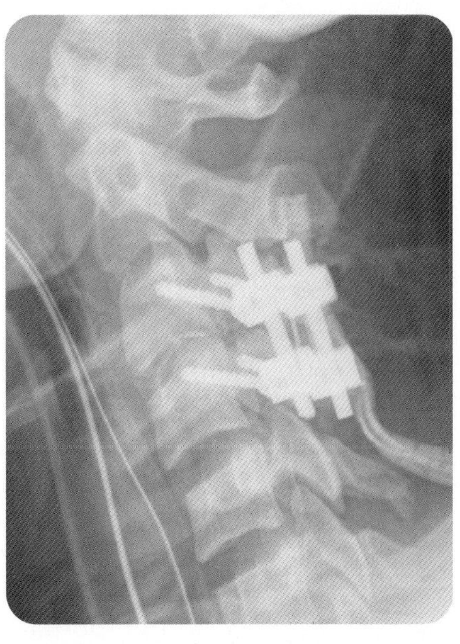

Figure 8.3 A lateral radiograph of the cervical spine after posterior spinal fusion at C3–C4.

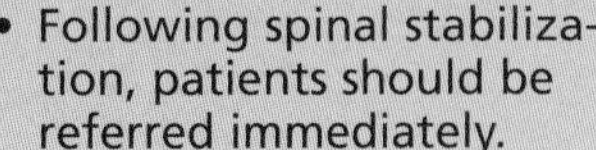

WHEN TO REFER

- Following spinal stabilization, patients should be referred immediately.

progressive anterior angulation of the spine). An anterior or a posterior fusion may be required for stabilization (Fig. 8.3). Patients who are not surgical candidates may be placed in a halo vest for 3 months. The patient's neurologic condition may improve after realignment.

Suggested Readings

Blacksin MF, Lee HJ. Frequency and significant of fractures of the upper cervical spine detected by CT in patients with severe neck trauma. *AJR Am J Roentgenol.* 1995;165:1201–1204.

Brant-Zawadzki M, Miller EM, Federle MP. CT in the evaluation of spine trauma. *AJR Am J Roentgenol.* 1981;136:369–375.

Clark CT, Igram CM, El-Khoury GY, Ehara S. Radiographic evaluation of cervical spine injuries. *Spine.* 1988;13:742–747.

Gellad FE, Levine AM, Joslyn JN, Edwards CC, Bosse M. Pure thoracolumbar facet dislocation: clinical features and CT appearance. *Radiology.* 1986;161:505–508.

Halliday AL, Hendernson BR, Hart BL, Benzel EC. The management of unilateral mass/facet fractures of the subaxial cervical spine: the use of magnetic resonance imaging to predict instability. *Spine.* 1997;22:2614–2621.

Holdsworth F. Review article fractures, dislocations, and fracture-dislocations of the spine. *J Bone Joint Surg.* 1970;52:1534–1551.

Mara BC. The pattern of neurological damage as an aid to the diagnosis of the mechanism in cervical-spine injuries. *J Bone Joint Surg.* 1974;56:1648–1654.

Norton WL. Fractures and dislocations of the cervical spine. *J Bone Joint Surg.* 1962;44:115–139.

Ohashi K, El-Khoury GY. Musculoskeletal CT: recent advances and current clinical applications. *Radiol Clin North Am.* 2009;47(3):387–409.

Rao SK, Wasyliw C, Nunez D. Spectrum of imaging findings in hyperextension injuries of the neck. *Radiographics.* 2005;25:1239–1254.

Sekhon LHS, Fehlings MG. Epidemiology, demographics and pathophysiology of spinal cord injury. *Spine.* 2001;26:S2.

Thompson WL, Stiell IG, Clement CM, Brison RJ. Association of injury mechanisms with the risk of cervical spine fractures. *CJEM.* 2009;11:14–22.

White AA, Panjabi MM. *Clinical Biomechanics of the Spine.* 2nd ed. Philadelphia, PA: Lippincott Williams & Wilkins; 1990:170–242.

CHAPTER 9

Teardrop Fracture

George M. Bridgeforth and Mark Nolden

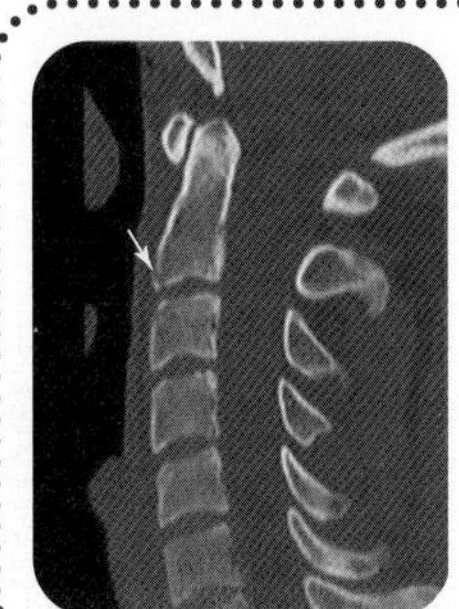

A 21-year-old unrestrained male driver is transported to the emergency department after a rollover motor vehicle collision.

Clinical Presentation

Teardrop fractures are fractures of the strike cervical spine that affect the anterior inferior end plate. The **mechanism of injury** may be flexion (unstable) or extension (stable). A flexion teardrop fracture is the most severe fracture of the cervical spine. Often, such injuries occur after dives into shallow pools of water. These injuries are characterized by damage to all three columns of Denis. In addition, there is a very strong association with an acute anterior cord syndrome secondary to the acute infarction of the anterior spinal artery. Patients with an anterior cord syndrome have damage to the anterior two-thirds of the spine with posterior column sparing. Therefore, they present with acute tetraplegia (quadriplegia). Spinal shock may occur. Clinically, the patients with spinal shock have low blood pressure. In addition, they manifest bilateral motor weakness below the level of the spinal cord injury, as well as loss of pinprick, sexual function, and bowel tone. However, with an anterior spinal cord injury, position sense and vibration sense are preserved because the posterior columns (fasciculus cuneatus and gracilis, which receive their blood supply from the posterior spinal artery) are spared.

In addition, secondary injuries such as associated thoracic and abdominal trauma may result. Severe sequelae such as tetraplegia may also occur. C2 through C4 tetraplegics (quadriplegics) are known as high-level tetraplegics. They have impaired respiratory function as a result of phrenic nerve damage and impaired thoracic expansion from their spinal cord injuries. If these patients survive, they remain ventilator dependent.

On the other hand, extension teardrop injuries are generally stable. There is no disruption of the posterior ligament complex. Because the posterior ligament complex is intact, there is no protrusion of the vertebral body into the spinal canal.

CLINICAL POINTS

- Instability should always be assumed until proven otherwise.
- Kyphosis occurs at the level of injury in patients with flexion teardrop fractures.
- Unstable injuries may be associated with anterior cord syndrome.

Radiographic Evaluation

Tests to order, for both acute cervical trauma and acute thoracolumbar trauma, include anteroposterior, lateral, and oblique views (two). In cases of cervical injury, it is necessary to see to C7. Optional radiographs include the following:

- Swimmer view, which is used to visualize the disc space between the seventh cervical vertebrae (C7) and first thoracic vertebrae (T1) if it is not identified on the lateral projection

PATIENT ASSESSMENT

1. Acute tetraplegia (quadriplegia) in severe cases, with spinal shock
2. Possible weakness, sensory loss, loss of sphincter tone, and loss of reflexes
3. Posterior column sparing (light touch, vibration, and position sense remain intact despite profound weakness and loss of pinprick) in anterior spinal cord injuries
4. Associated head and thoracic trauma in cervical injuries

NOT TO BE MISSED

- Cervical strain
- Cervical contusion
- Acute cervical fracture
- Degenerative arthritis
- Cervical radiculopathy
- Cervical stenosis
- Cervical osteomyelitis (intravenous drug abusers)

- Flexion/extension views, which should be obtained only by experienced spinal care providers. Flexion and extension radiographs are *never* taken until the initial radiographs have been evaluated for instability first.
- Odontoid view (open mouth view), which is used to evaluate odontoid fractures

Teardrop fractures are triangular fractures that involve the anterior inferior vertebral body (Figs. 9.1A,B). If there is a triangular-shaped fragment that involves the anterior superior vertebral body, then limbus vertebrae should be suspected and ruled out. Teardrop fractures from flexion injuries (Fig. 9.2) are generally unstable and involve the anterior inferior vertebral body; this is best appreciated on the lateral view. The involvement of all three columns of Denis is characterized by a disruption of the posterior ligament complex (the posterior longitudinal ligament, ligamentum flava, transverse spinal ligaments, interspinous ligaments, and supraspinous ligament). The ligamentous disruption is most easily seen on the lateral radiograph. Moreover, the torn posterior ligament complex is characterized by an increased space between the spinous processes at the level of injury. This increased separation may be more readily apparent on flexion/extension views.

There may be posterior displacement of the vertebral body (second column of Denis) associated with a teardrop fracture at the anterior inferior border (first column). The posterior displaced vertebral body may cause an impaction injury to the spinal cord. This impaction may result in an anterior cord syndrome. The impaction injury causes damage to the anterior spinal artery. Patients with this condition may present with acute tetraplegia (quadriplegia) and spinal shock, with sparing of the posterior columns.

In extension teardrop fractures, lateral radiographs show a teardrop fracture of the anterior inferior vertebral body without evidence of vertebral displacement. In addition, there is no displacement between the spinous processes. Because this is a stable injury, the middle and posterior columns of Denis are intact.

In cases of acute, severe cervical or thoracolumbar trauma, a computed tomography (CT) scan should be obtained "stat." It may also be necessary to obtain a CT scan of the head if there is an associated traumatic brain injury.

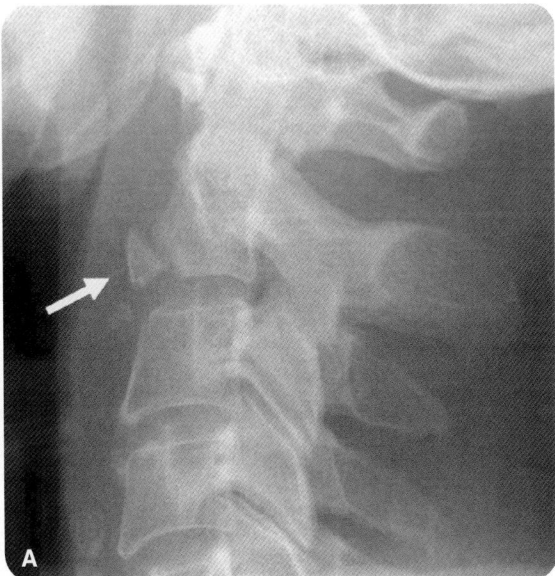

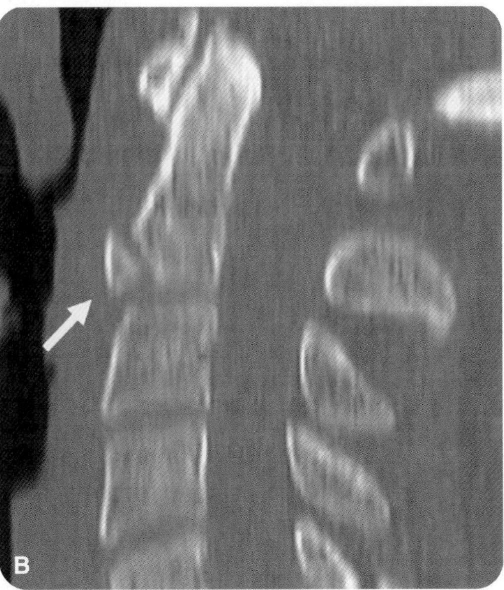

Figure 9.1 Hyperextension teardrop fracture of C2. **(A)** Lateral cervical radiograph and **(B)** sagittal multiplanar CT reformation show a triangular fragment arising from the anterior inferior margin of C2 (*white arrows*). (From Schwartz ED, Flanders AE, eds. *Spinal Trauma: Imaging, Diagnosis, and Management.* Philadelphia, PA: Lippincott Williams & Wilkins, 2007.)

WHEN TO REFER

- Following spinal stabilization, patients should be referred immediately for a "stat" CT scan.
- Referral is not necessary for those with limbus vertebra, which is associated with disc deterioration.

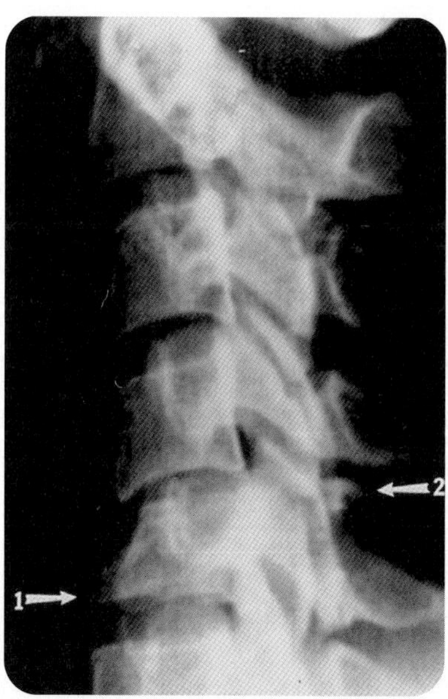

Figure 9.2 This patient sustained a whiplash injury with resultant flexion injury. A typical flexion teardrop fracture is demonstrated at (*1*). An increased interspinous distance and an associated avulsion fracture of the posterior elements of C5 is demonstrated at (*2*). (From Swischuk L. *Emergency Radiology of the Acutely Ill or Injured Child*. 2nd ed. Baltimore, MD: Lippincott Williams & Wilkins; 1986:674, reprinted with permission.)

Treatment

Patients should be immobilized in a hard collar by using a spine board. Those with stable injuries of the cervical spine may be placed in a halo vest. Use of a neck collar for comfort and mild activity restriction for a few weeks may be necessary. Those with unstable injuries may require an open reduction and internal fixation to stabilize the injury and prevent kyphosis, pain, and further neurologic deterioration.

Suggested Readings

Acheson MB, Livingston RR, Richardons ML, Stimac GK. High-resolution CT scanning in the evaluation of cervical spine fractures: comparison with plain film examinations. *AJR Am J Roentgenol*. 1987;148: 1179–1185.

Bovill EG, Eberle CF, Day L, Aufranc OE. Dislocation of the cervical spine without spinal cord injury. *JAMA*. 1971;218:1288–1290.

Clark CR, Igram CM, El-Khoury GY, Ehara S. Radiographic evaluation of cervical spine injuries. *Spine*. 1988;13: 742–747.

Davis SJ, Teresi L, Bradley WG, Ziemba MA, Bloze AE. Cervical spine hyperextension injuries: MR findings. *Radiology*. 1991;180:245–251.

Graeber M, Kathol M. Cervical spine radiographs in the trauma patient. *Am Fam Physician*. 1999;59(2):331–342.

Holdsworth F. Review article fractures, dislocations, and fracture-dislocations of the spine. *J Bone Joint Surg Am*. 1970;52:1534–1551.

Lee JS, Harris JH, Mueller CF. The significance of prevertebral soft tissue swelling in extension teardrop fracture of the cervical spine. *Emerg Radiol*. 1997;4(3):132–139.

Marar BC. Hyperextension injuries of the cervical spine: the pathogenesis of damage to the spinal cord. *J Bone Joint Surg Am*. 1974;56:1655–1662.

Nepper-Rasmussen J. CT of dens axis fractures. *Neuroradiology*. 1989;31:104–106.

Novelline RA, Rhea JT, Rao PM, Stuk JL. Helical CT in emergency radiology. *Radiology*. 1999;213:321–339.

Schneider RC, Kahn EA. Chronic neurological sequelae of acute trauma to the spine and spinal cord, I: the significance of the acute-flexion or tear-drop fracture-dislocation of the cervical spine. *J Bone Joint Surg Am*. 1956;38:985–997.

Sliker CW, Mirvin SE, Shanmuganathan K. Assessing cervical spine stability in obtunded blunt trauma patients: review of the medical literature. *Radiology*. 2005;234:733–739.

Stabler A, Eck J, Penning R, et al. Cervical spine: postmortem assessment of accident injuries—comparison of radiographic, MR imaging, anatomic and pathologic findings. *Radiology*. 2001;221:340–346.

Thompson WL, Stiell IG, Clement CM, Brison RJ. Association of injury mechanism with the risk of cervical spine fractures. *CJEM*. 2009;11:14–22.

Woodring JH, Lee C. Limitations of cervical radiography in the evaluation of acute cervical trauma. *J Trauma*. 1994;34:32–39.

SECTION 2

Hip

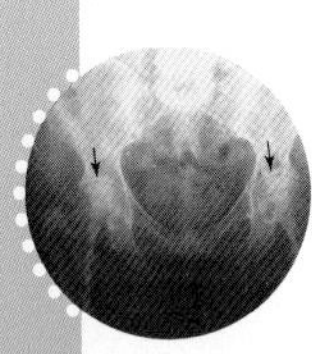

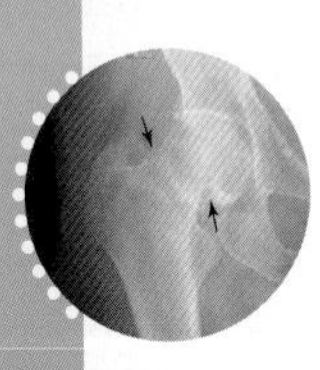

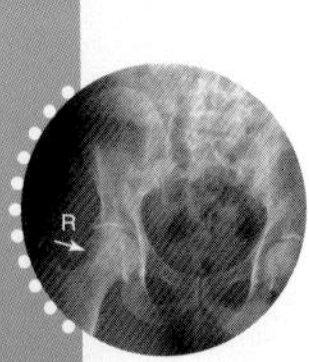

Functional Anatomy

The hip is a multiplanar ball-and-socket joint. The rounded head of the femur articulates with the acetabular fossa. At the center of the femoral head, there is a small, rounded depression called the fovea; the ligamentum teres connects the humerus with the acetabulum (Fig. 1). The acetabulum is a concave socket formed by the fusion of the ischium, the pubis, and the ilium. The surface area of this articulation is enhanced by a horseshoe-shaped cartilaginous rim called the labrum. This cartilaginous collar not only allows for a deeper pocket but also for smoother range of motion. Moreover, this protective cushion helps prevent wear and tear of the joint over time. The range of motion of the hip allows for movement with four degrees of freedom (across three planes). The range

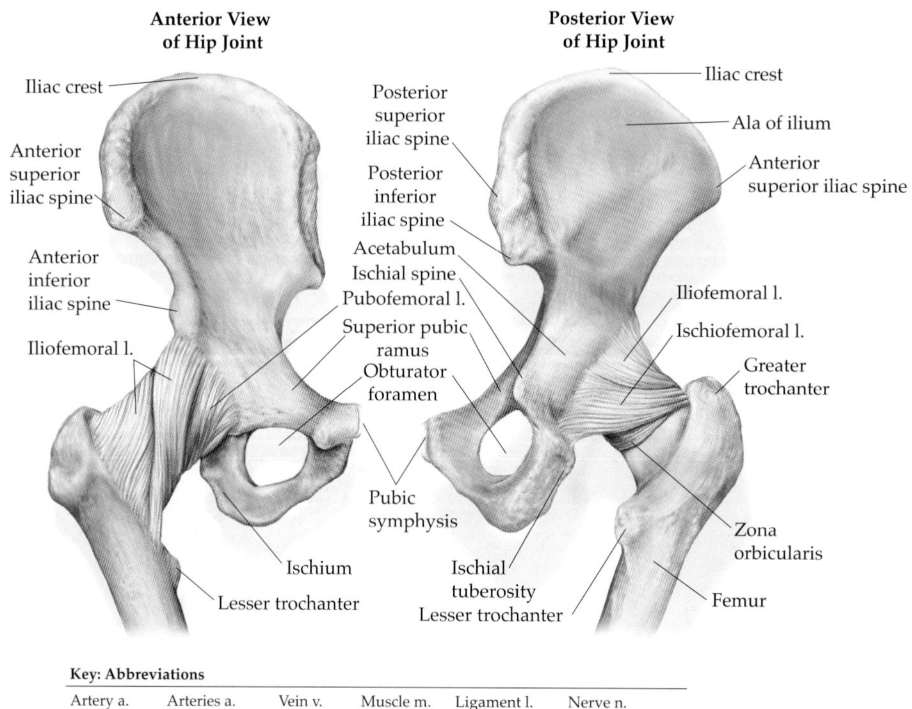

Figure 1 Anterior and posterior views of hip joint. Asset provided by Anatomical Chart Co.

of motion includes flexion (elevation of the thigh toward the head), extension (movement of the thigh in the opposite direction [toward the buttocks]), adduction (movement of the thigh medially), abduction (movement of the thigh laterally), circumduction (movement of the thigh in a clockwise or counterclockwise motion), and internal and external rotation. The base of the acetabulum is formed by the transverse acetabular ligament, which makes up its floor. This ligament helps prevent inferior subluxation of the femoral head.

The hip joint is surrounded by a dense fibrous capsule, which covers the nonarticulating head of the humerus and two-thirds of the neck. Moreover, the hip joint is supported by three extracapsular (i.e., lying outside of the joint capsule) ligaments: the iliofemoral, the ischiofemoral, and the pubofemoral ligaments. The strong Y-shaped iliofemoral ligament helps maintain upright posture while standing.

The heads of both femurs are load-bearing surfaces. In other words, they help support the weight (i.e., load) of the upper body. During standing and ambulation, the load from the upper body is transferred to the femoral head, through each bony neck and the down the load-bearing shafts of each femur and each tibia. The femoral neck is the weakest part of the hip and is subject to fracture because it has a poor nutrient arterial supply and is a major stress point during traumatic injuries. In addition, the femoral neck is composed of trabecular bone, which is less suited than laminar bone for transmitting loads (i.e., body weight).

The upper surface of the femoral shaft has two oblong-shaped bony prominences—the greater and lesser trochanters. The lesser trochanter lies inferiorly and medially to the greater trochanters. The trochanters serve as the bony attachments that anchor many of the major supporting muscles of the hip.

The angle of inclination is an angle formed by the intersection of the longitudinal axis of the femoral shaft and the femoral neck. Patients with angles of inclination approaching 90 degrees (i.e., coxa vara) have knock-knees. The femoral shafts are internally rotated and anatomically adducted. On the other hand, patients with an angle of inclination approaching 150 to 160 degrees have coxa valga and are bow legged. This condition may be associated with externally rotated femurs as well.

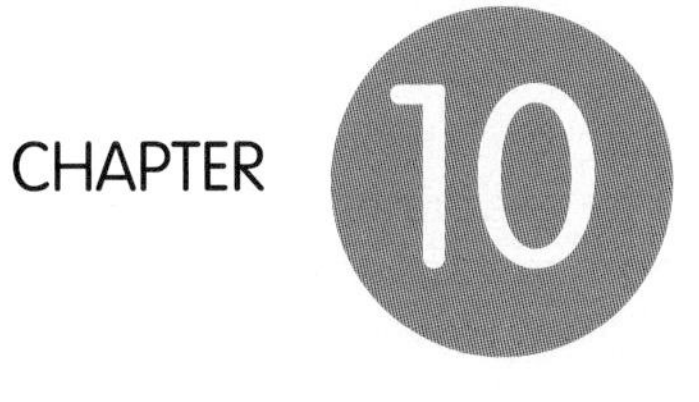

Degenerative Hip Disease (Osteoarthritis)

George M. Bridgeforth, Kevin Bozic, and Jay Patel

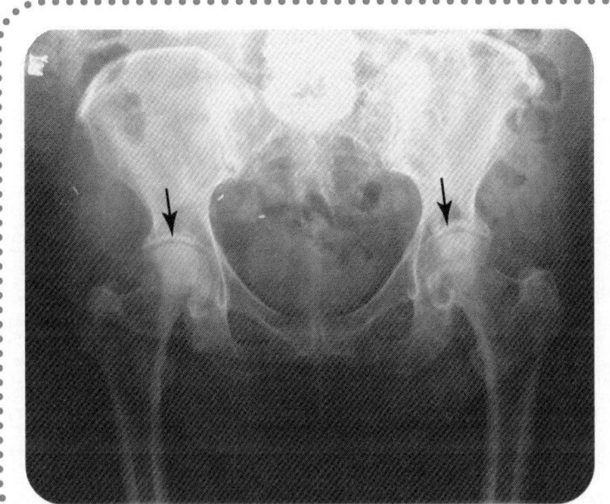

A 79-year-old obese woman presents with left hip pain after a fall. She has difficulty walking.

Clinical Presentation

Degenerative disease of the hip, a large weight-bearing joint, may affect elderly patients or patients who have been taking steroids for long periods. Complaints of long-term hip or groin pain are not uncommon. Reports of morning stiffness are very common, usually with osteoarthritis. The **mechanism of injury** is a degenerative process. Usually degenerative joint disease is bilateral; however, one hip may be affected more severely than the other. It is helpful if other signs of osteoarthritis are present. Common findings include hypertrophy of the knees and the presence of Heberden nodes (joint hypertrophy) of the distal interphalangeal joints affecting some of the fingers. Patients with degenerative hip disease have impaired range of motion of the affected hip. Patients exhibit limited flexion as well as internal and external rotation. Moreover, they have an antalgic gait. In mild cases, the limp may be slight. In severe cases, the pain can be severe, and complaints of falling are common. Hip fractures from falls frequently occur in elderly patients, and these are associated with significant morbidity and mortality.

CLINICAL POINTS

- Patients often complain of chronic hip pain.
- A history of morning stiffness is frequent.
- Both hips are usually affected.

Two helpful clinical tests are the Stinchfield test and the Faber test. A Stinchfield test is performed with the patient in supine position. The patient is asked to elevate his or her leg (with the knee straight) to 20 or 30 degrees. A positive test (which indicates intracapsular pathology) is characterized by hip pain or groin pain. If the patient does not complain of pain, the examiner may apply a steady downward force at the ankle in the direction of the examining table. In that case, pain that is reproduced at the ipsilateral hip or groin represents a positive test. The Stinchfield test is different than the Lasègue test, a straight leg-raising test used for back pain. With a positive Lasègue test, the patient complains of radicular low back pain that radiates from the back down the leg, generally at an elevation of 30 to 60 degrees. The Stinchfield test is also different from the Lhermitte test. In a positive Lhermitte test, low back pain radiates down the opposite (i.e., nonelevated) leg. It indicates radicular pathology on that side.

When screening for osteoarthritis, some examiners may prefer to use a Faber (Patrick test). **Faber** stands for (hip) **f**lexion, **ab**duction, and **e**xternal **r**otation. In this maneuver, the leg is placed into a frog leg position. In other words,

PATIENT ASSESSMENT

1. Positive Stinchfield test (pain with active straight leg raise)
2. Pain-limited passive range of motion
3. Antalgic gait (limp)

the hip is placed into abduction by placing the foot across the opposite knee. After stabilizing the opposite pelvis with one hand, the examiner applies pressure against the bent knee in a downward direction toward the examining table. Pain in the groin or the hip indicates hip pathology. However, pain along the sacroiliac joint indicates sacroiliac pathology. Patients with intra-articular pathology from an avascular necrosis may present with similar clinical findings; further radiologic evaluation is warranted.

Patients with hip fractures exhibit moderate to marked pain and tenderness to palpation. Clinical findings such as acute swelling and ecchymosis (i.e., bruising) may represent a recent fracture. There is impaired range of motion with an antalgic gait as well. Patients with contusions presents with similar findings but there is no evidence of a fracture.

Patients with metastatic disease may present with similar findings of severe hip pain, with impaired range of motion. Unexplained weight loss, a history of cancer, or a family history of cancer may be an important clue. The majority of metastatic diseases are caused by breast, lung, and prostate cancers. They metastasize to the hip, spine, and pelvis. Metastatic diseases may not be apparent on the initial radiographs. However, if the patient has other clinical findings such as a palpable breast mass, lung mass, hematuria (kidney cancer), or a prostrate nodule, then computed tomography (CT) with 2-mm sections might be warranted. Some clinicians prefer bone scans, but a positive bone scan is usually followed by a CT scan anyway. If there is an associated degenerative arthritis, a bone scan may not distinguish between the two conditions.

A trochanteric bursitis is characterized by focal pain and soreness over the greater trochanter. Essentially, it is a diagnosis of exclusion (radiographs do not reveal any fractures). It is treated with cold pain and analgesic medication. Severe cases may require a steroid injection into the trochanteric bursa. Rheumatoid arthritis may be identified by rheumatoid changes affecting other joints such as knees, wrists, metacarpals, pip joints, and ulnar deviation of hands.

Osteomyelitis of the hip is rare. The examiner should look for a portal of infection (e.g., open hip fractures, intravenous drug abuse). The patients manifest marked constitutional signs: elevated fevers, chills, and diaphoresis (sweating) with severe pain.

It is important to examine elderly patients for other signs of bruising or fractures, because elder abuse should be suspected if multiple areas of unexplained bruising are encountered. The elderly are more prone to develop osteoporosis; therefore, even minor falls may cause a serious hip fracture. For this reason, polypharmacy should always be monitored, especially in the elderly.

NOT TO BE MISSED

- Hip contusion/fracture
- Dislocation
- Trochanteric bursitis
- Avascular necrosis
- Metastatic disease
- Rheumatoid arthritis
- Osteomyelitis
- Bone tumors

Radiographic Evaluation

Plain radiographs of the hip(s) (anteroposterior [AP] and lateral [frog leg]) views should be ordered. There are four radiological hallmark findings for degenerative joint disease (osteoarthritis), which are listed as follows:

- Narrowing of the joint space
- Subchondral sclerosis
- Osteophyte (bone spur) formation
- Subchondral cyst formation (see Fig. 10.1)

All four findings need not be present. For example, in early degenerative joint disease, there may be narrowing of the joint space associated with early subchondral sclerosis and osteophyte formation. The subchondral sclerosis is a reactive process to the articular thinning. Essentially, the bone is trying to repair itself. Moreover, subchondral cysts may be difficult to identify. The joint space narrowing and the early osteophyte formation manifest themselves as mild joint hypertrophy. These findings are best appreciated on the AP view.

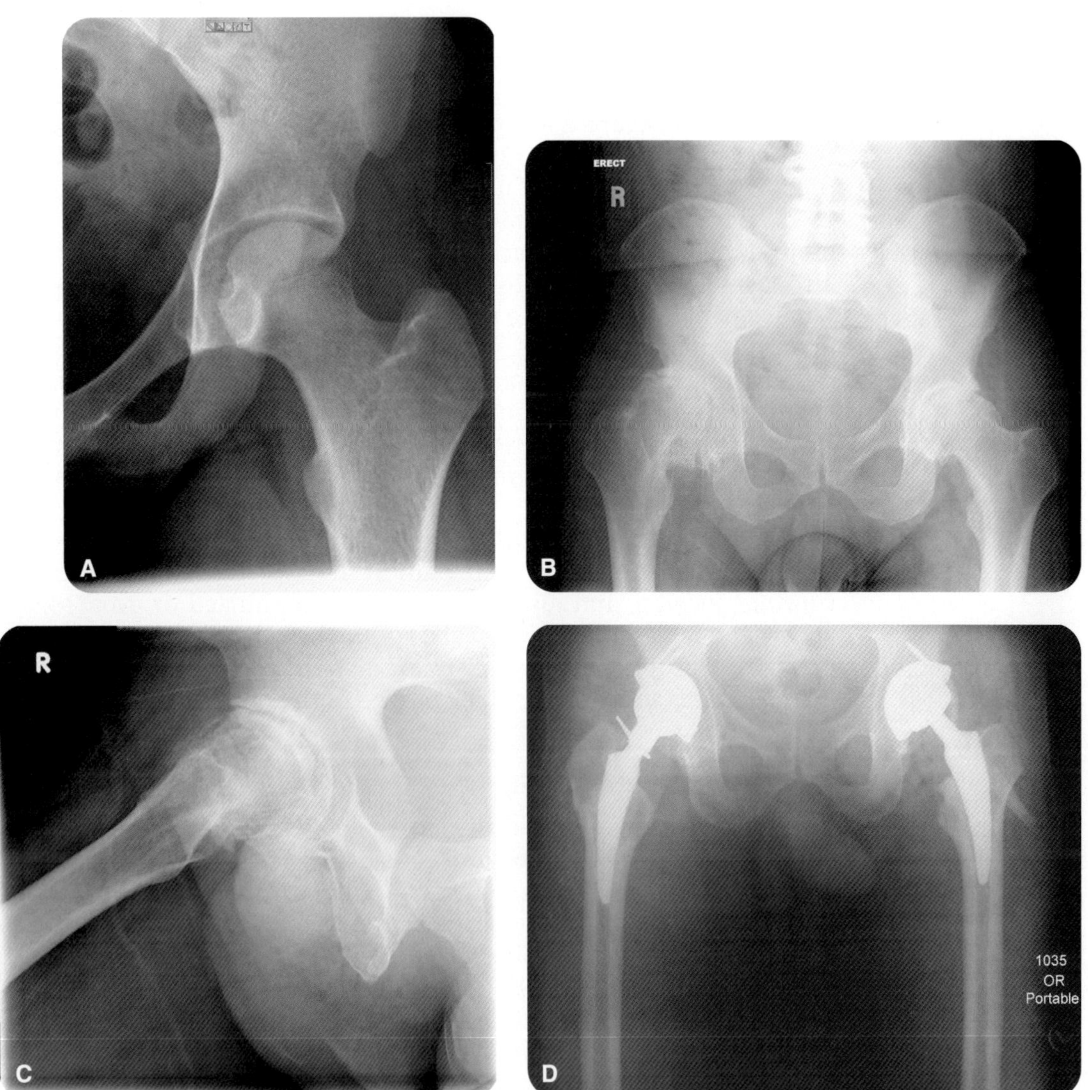

Figure 10.1 **(A)** A 19-year-old woman with sickle cell disease presents with hip pain, which magnetic resonance imaging proves negative for avascular necrosis. Note the smooth contour of the femoral head and acetabulum in the normal left hip. The joint space is preserved, and there are no bony osteophytes. Compare with a 53-year-old man with severe bilateral hip pain **(B)**, which is an anteroposterior radiograph of the pelvis demonstrating bilateral osteoarthritis, which is more severe on the right. **(C)** A frog-leg view of the right hip joint demonstrates near-total narrowing of the joint space, subchondral sclerosis, osteophytes, and subchondral lucencies, probably representing subchondral cysts. **(D)** An anteroposterior radiograph of the bilateral hip joints nearly two years after the initial examination demonstrates bilateral total hip prostheses.

In addition, it is necessary to look for evidence of degenerative joint disease elsewhere. Usually, knees, hips, and the distal phalanges of the hands and feet are commonly affected. (In general, osteoarthritis is a bilateral condition.) Heberden nodes are hypertrophic osteophytic changes of the distal interphalangeal joints of the hands and are usually present on the clinical examination as well. Moreover, it is important to check the pelvis and the spine for metastatic conditions, especially in older patients (older than 50 years).

Treatment

NONSURGICAL APPROACHES

The treatment course for hip osteoarthritis begins with conservative management. Initially, treatment includes weight loss, physical therapy, anti-inflammatory medications, and activity modification.

Reducing weight reduces the load through the hip joint, which can reduce pain and the rate at which the hip joint degenerates. For patients who weigh more than 300 lb, weight loss is recommended prior to hip replacement because even if this measure does not achieve pain relief, many surgeons believe that the risks of surgery, including infection, implant failure, and dislocation of the prosthesis, are too high in morbidly obese patients.

Strengthening of the musculature not only around the hip joint but also around the trunk, lower back, knees, and ankles improves gait mechanics. It is also useful for patients to experience physical therapy before a total hip replacement (THR) because they will be undergoing an aggressive therapy regimen postoperatively.

Common agents used for pain control include nonsteroidal anti-inflammatory agents (NSAIDs) (ibuprofen, naproxen, meloxicam, nabumetone, diclofenac, etodolac, indomethacin). Patients who cannot tolerate NSAIDS may be treated with acetaminophen or tramadol. The long-term use of narcotics should be discouraged.

Patients with arthritis of the hip can often modify their daily activities and exercise regimen to reduce the pain in the hip. High-impact activities such as running, jogging, and jumping should be minimized or avoided. Low-impact activities such as swimming, walking, and bicycling are recommended alternatives. In addition, some patients are able to reduce the pain in the hip and increase their activities by using a cane in the opposite hand.

SURGICAL APPROACHES

If conservative treatment has failed, the patient should be referred to an orthopedic surgeon for evaluation and consideration for operative management. The mainstay of surgical treatment for arthritis of the hip is THR. Hip replacement involves removal of the arthritic femoral head and acetabular cartilage and implantation of a femoral and acetabular prosthesis (an artificial prosthetic replacement).

The femoral component is a stemmed prosthesis that fits into the femoral canal after the surgeon removes the femoral neck. A femoral head prosthesis is then attached to the top of the femoral prosthesis to mimic the "ball" part of the hip joint. The acetabular component is a cup that is placed into the location of the existing acetabular socket after it is prepared by reaming the existing damaged cartilage and underlying bone. A plastic polyethylene, ceramic, or metal liner is then inserted into the cup to enable smooth motion between the ball and socket.

The 1994 National Institutes of Health consensus statement on THR reported, "THR is an option for nearly all patients with diseases of the hip that cause chronic discomfort and significant functional impairment." Historically, this has included patients 60 to 75 years of age who have hip pain that limits their ability to walk or rise from a chair or prevents them from sleeping and performing their activities of daily living. However, with advances in technology and surgical technique, younger patients with disabling hip disease are now also considered candidates for hip replacement. Often, these are patients with a history of a hip fracture, avascular necrosis, rheumatoid arthritis, or congenital abnormalities of the hip. Although improvements in surgical techniques and implant materials have allowed for increased longevity of hip replacements, younger patients who undergo hip replacement frequently still require revision surgery at some point in their lives. For younger patients, as with older patients, hip replacement is usually considered only after more conservative measures such as pain medication, physical therapy, and less-invasive surgeries have been attempted first. Very elderly patient (older than 75 years) can also undergo THR, although a detailed health examination is required to ensure that the patient is an appropriate surgical candidate.

Other surgical options include pelvic osteotomy, hip resurfacing, and hip arthroscopy. Osteotomies, which involve cutting and reorienting the bones around the hip joint, are used occasionally in young patients who may benefit from a total hip arthroplasty but have more than 30 years of life expectancy. Osteotomies are ways to surgically cut and realign the bones around the hip joint to redistribute the joint forces in a way that makes it easier for the patient to move the hip and to slow the degeneration of the hip. There are many different types of osteotomies, each tailored to specific hip mechanical problems. The outcomes for osteotomies are mixed. For some patients, an osteotomy may buy the patient additional time before eventually undergoing a THR. Osteotomies are becoming rarer as improvements in prosthetic design and surgical technique have increased the durability of a primary THR.

Hip resurfacing is a technique that can be used to treat hip arthritis and avascular necrosis of the femoral head in younger patients with good bone quality. It involves "capping" the femoral head with a metal prosthesis and allowing this capped femoral head to articulate with the patient's own acetabulum or an acetabular prosthesis. In previous decades, hip resurfacing had fallen out of favor due to poor outcomes because of the materials used in the past. Recent modifications with metal components and improvements in surgical techniques have brought resurfacing back to the attention of surgeons and patients. Patients who have collapse of the femoral head, poor bone quality, or large bone cysts are considered poor candidates for hip resurfacing. In addition, resurfacing is typically reserved for patients younger than 65 years, with a body mass index less than 35 and a good bone quality.

The main advantage of hip resurfacing compared with THR is the preservation of bone stock in the femur. Because the femur is capped, very little of the femur bone is removed. If revision surgery is every required, there is more of the patient's own femoral bone remaining, which can make revision surgery easier in hip resurfacing patients than in patients who have previously undergone THR. For this reason, hip resurfacing has a theoretical benefit for younger patients who may need revision surgery in the future, because conversion to a THR is still possible. However, once someone has a THR, hip resurfacing is no longer an option. Another advantage of hip resurfacing is that a larger-diameter femoral head prosthesis is used, which could theoretically reduce the rate of postoperative dislocation rates.

One of the major drawbacks of hip resurfacing is the risk of femoral neck fracture, which requires conversion to THR. The rate of fracture has been reported to be 0% to 4%. Other disadvantages include the uncertainty of long-term outcomes, potential for loosening of the prosthesis, and the fact that the few surgeons have extensive experience with performing this surgery. Results from the Australian hip registry suggest that the survival rate of hip resurfacing implants is lower than the survival rate for hip replacement implants during the first 5 years following surgery. Hip resurfacing is not appropriate for many patients who require hip surgery, and patients who are interested in hip resurfacing should seek consultation with an orthopedic surgeon.

Hip arthroscopy involves using an arthroscopic camera and instruments to inspect and repair the hip joint. The procedure involves first creating small portals into the hip joint through which the camera and instruments can be introduced. Results of hip arthroscopy are heavily dependent on the specific condition being treated. Although in certain cases hip arthroscopy to remove loose bodies or to reshape the femoral neck (for a condition called femoroacetabular impingement) may slow the progression of osteoarthritis, in general, it is *not* recommended for patients who have diffuse arthritic changes in their hip. Complications with hip arthroscopy can occur in 1% to 6% of cases and include damage to nerves (from stretching or direct trauma) and direct trauma to the joint when using arthroscopic instruments. Nerve injury caused by stretching during positioning is usually temporary.

WHEN TO REFER

- Patients with severe hip osteoarthritis who have difficulty ambulating and climbing stairs and have failed a trial of conservative therapy
- Elderly patients with a history of sudden or recurrent falls, who may have motor weakness secondary to a stroke. A comprehensive neurologic examination that checks for upper motor neuron signs (motor weakness, hyperreflexia, upgoing plantar responses) coupled with a pattern of sensory weakness should be performed. Other metabolic conditions such as uncontrolled diabetes may contribute to the unsteadiness and should be excluded as well.

Suggested Readings

Archibeck M, White R. What's new in adult reconstructive knee surgery. *J Bone Joint Surg Am.* 2002;84: 1719–1726.

Buergi ML, Walter WL. Hip resurfacing arthroplasty: the Australian experience. *J Arthroplasty.* 2007;22(7) (suppl 3):61–65.

D'Ambrosia RD. Epidemiology of osteoarthritis. *Orthopedics.* 2005;28(2)(suppl)s201–s205.

Fanc C, Teh J. Imaging of the hip. *Imaging.* 2003;15:205–216.

Felson DT. An update on the pathogenesis and epidemiology of osteoarthritis. *Radiol Clin North Am.* 2004; 42(1):1–9.

Greenspan A. *Orthopedic Imaging: A Practical Approach.* 4th ed. Philadelphia, PA: Lippincott William & Wilkins; 2004:446–451.

Hamel MB, Toth M, Legedza A, Rosen MP. Joint replacement surgery in elderly patients with severe osteoarthritis of the hip or knee: decision making, postoperative recovery, and clinical outcomes. *Arch Intern Med.* 2008;168(13):1430–1440.

Harris JH, Harris WH, Novelline RA. *The Radiology of Emergency Medicine.* 3rd ed. Baltimore, MD: Lippincott Williams & Wilkins; 1993:790–804.

Manaster BJ. Adult chronic hip pain: radiographic evaluation. *Radiographics.* 2000;20:s3–s25.

McKinnis LN. *Fundamentals of Orthopedic Radiology.* Philadelphia, PA: FA Davis; 1997:230–231.

Rosen P, Doris PE, Barkin RM, Barkin SZ, Markovchick VJ. *Diagnostic Radiology in Emergency Medicine.* St Louis, MO: Mosby; 1992:188–189.

Saint Clair SF, Higuera C, Krahs V, et al. Hip and knee arthroplasty in the geriatric population. *Clin Geriatr Med.* 2006:22(3):515–533.

CHAPTER 11

Hip Fractures

George M. Bridgeforth, Kevin Bozic, and Jay Patel

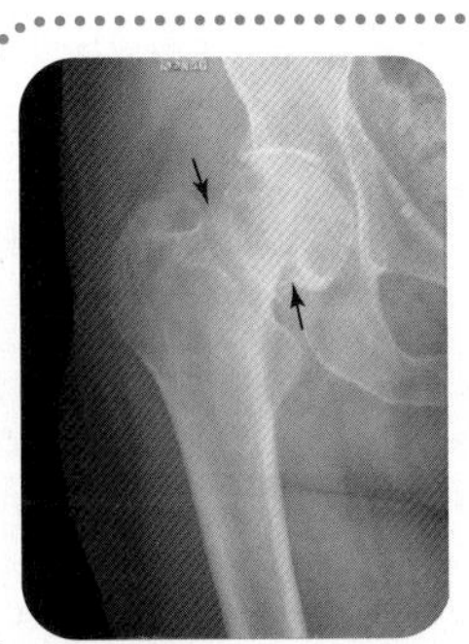

A 97-year-old woman presents with left hip pain after falling.

Clinical Presentation

Hips are one of the more common fractured joints; according to Medicare epidemiological studies, hip fractures account for up to 45% of all fractures. The overall cause of hip fractures, as well as hip dislocations, is impact. In individuals younger than 60 years, hip fractures are commonly caused by motor vehicle accidents. In individuals older than 60 years, hip fractures are usually caused by falls. According to the Centers for Disease Control and Prevention, 90% of the hip fractures in adults 65 years of age and older result from falls. There is a higher risk of hip fractions and dislocations in the elderly, especially in Caucasian women with osteoporosis. The mortality rate in the elderly is substantial; 15% to 20% of such patients with hip fractures die within 1 year.

There are two types of hip fractures: intracapsular and extracapsular. Intracapsular hip fractures occur above the intertrochanteric line (a line drawn from the greater to the lesser trochanter on the anteroposterior [AP] view), and extracapsular fractures occur below this point. Intertrochanteric and subtrochanteric fractures occur at or below the intertrochanteric line. Intertrochanteric and subtrochanteric fractures are described according to the number of fractured segments (two to four). The **mechanisms of injury** involved in hip fractures are

- Subcapital fractures (intracapsular): impaction
- Transcervical fractures (intracapsular): clockwise rotation of the femoral head against a counterclockwise rotation of the femoral neck
- Intertrochanteric fracture (extracapsular): generally from a fall in which there was a direct blow to the hip
- Subtrochanteric fractures (extracapsular): impaction

Approximately 85% to 90% of hip dislocations are posterior, and the remaining are anterior.

The clinical hallmark of a hip fracture is the presence of marked pain, swelling, and tenderness, with an inability to bear weight on the affected side. The clinical examination usually reveals pain-limited range of motion, with marked guarding and apprehension by the patient. It is critical to conduct and document a thorough neurovascular examination that assesses motor weakness, sensory loss, areflexia, and loss of voluntary rectal tone (lower motor neuron injury is generally associated with displaced pelvic fractures). Other causes

CLINICAL POINTS

- The elderly are at higher risk for falls. Routinely reviewing medications and arranging for home health visits for geriatric patients are important preventive steps.
- Most (85%) of hip dislocations are posterior (best appreciated on lateral view).
- Hip fractures are divided into intracapsular and extracapsular types.
- A thorough neurovascular examination should always be conducted.

of the clinical manifestations include hip contusions, avascular necrosis (AVN), degenerative osteoarthritis, and trochanter bursitis.

AVN may be difficult to detect during the initial examination. Radiographic findings may not be apparent for several weeks. In this case, magnetic resonance imaging may help detect an occult fracture or an early AVN. The diagnosis of AVN or an occult fracture should be suspected in any patient who presents with severe hip or groin pain that is not improving. The situation may be complicated by the fact many elderly patients have limited ambulation secondary to degenerative osteoarthritis. The incidence of AVN is greater with intracapsular and displaced hip fractures.

One of the major problems is that severe contusions, hip fractures, dislocations, or AVN may be complicated by bleeding into injured hip. It is important to monitor vital signs carefully for evidence of hemodynamic instability. It is essential to critically review the medications for polypharmacy and limit medications that may cause unwarranted sedation, lightheadedness, and dizziness.

Many elderly patients may be taking multiple medications (especially for high blood pressure); therefore, hypotension with tachycardia is common during the initial presentation. A "stat" complete blood cell count that examines the hemoglobin level and the hematocrit level is an important part of the workup.

Radiographic Evaluation

Radiographs should include AP and lateral (frog leg) views. Hip dislocations are appreciated best on the lateral (frog leg) view. With posterior dislocations, the possibility of a fracture of the posterior acetabular lip caused by the impact from the dislocated femoral head should be checked for very carefully. On the AP view, anterior displacement (10%–15% of the dislocations) may be characterized by a slight medial displacement of the femoral head. It is necessary to look for a subtle effacement of the acetabular space (the cartilaginous cushion that separates the acetabulum from the femoral head).

Hip fractures are divided into intracapsular and extracapsular fractures:

- Intracapsular
  - Capital (uncommon)
  - Subcapital (common)
  - Transcervical (uncommon)
- Extracapsular
  - Intertrochanteric
  - Subtrochanteric
  - Trochanteric

The anatomical classification of intracapsular hip fractures and extracapsular hip fractures is based on the intertrochanteric line. The intertrochanteric line is drawn from the greater trochanter to the lesser trochanter. Fractures above the intertrochanteric line are intracapsular. Fractures at or below the intertrochanteric line are extracapsular. Intracapsular fractures have a higher risk of femoral AVN (up to one-third of cases). In addition, the risk of femoral AVN is higher with displaced fractures (Harris).

SUBCAPITAL FRACTURES (INTRACAPSULAR)

On an AP view, subcapital fractures may be characterized by a foreshortened femoral neck. The short femoral neck has a sclerotic rim, which is characterized by an increased density due to impacted bone. Normally, the femoral head sits directly on top of the femoral neck like a scoop of ice cream on a cone. Any displacement of the femoral head may indicate a subcapital fracture (Fig. 11.1).

PATIENT ASSESSMENT

1. It is necessary to look for marked pain, swelling, and tenderness. Bruising may or may not be present.
2. Pain with limited range of motion may be evident.
3. Patients may have pain with limited weight-bearing with an impaired gait.
4. Neurovascular status, including rectal tone, should be checked carefully. Associated lower motor neuron injuries to the pelvis may cause loss of bowel and bladder function with impaired voluntary rectal tone, acute motor weakness, sensory impairment, and diminished (or absent reflexes) of the affected extremity.

NOT TO BE MISSED

- Hip strain/contusion
- Hip fractures
- Metastatic disease
- Trochanteric bursitis
- AVN
- Paget disease
- Hematoma
- Abscess
- Osteomyelitis
- Bone tumors (uncommon)

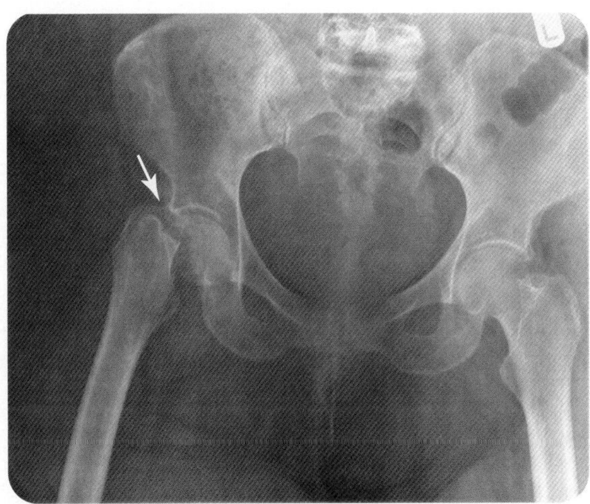

Figure 11.1 Anteroposterior radiograph of the hip, demonstrating an impacted and superiorly displaced subcapital fracture of the right femur in a 58-year-old woman with osteoarthritis and an inability to bear weight on her right side.

TRANSCERVICAL FRACTURES (INTRACAPSULAR)

An AP view may demonstrate an increased varus (inward displacement) deformity of the femoral neck.

INTERTROCHANTERIC FRACTURE (EXTRACAPSULAR)

An intertrochanteric fracture is characterized by a line that extends from the greater trochanter to the lesser trochanter. A nondisplaced fracture may be very subtle and should be screened for carefully.

SUBTROCHANTERIC FRACTURES (EXTRACAPSULAR)

A subtrochanteric fracture is a fracture that is distal to the intertrochanteric line (see earlier text). It is important to note that intertrochanteric and subtrochanteric fractures may be divided by the number and the type of fragments.

- Two-part fracture: a solitary fracture with a separate fragment
- Three-part fracture: a proximal femoral fracture associated with a secondary fragmentation of either the greater or lesser trochanter
- Four-part fracture: a proximal femoral fracture associated with fragmentation of both the greater and lesser trochanter

Treatment

The patient should be referred to orthopedics immediately for treatment. Closed reduction with pinning versus hip replacement depends on many factors, including the type of injury and the age of the patient. Surgical intervention can include closed reduction with percutaneous pinning, open reduction internal fixation, hemiarthroplasty, and total hip arthroplasty (Fig. 11.2). In a young patient and/or active patient, femoral neck fractures are often associated with high-energy trauma (e.g., motor vehicle collision, fall from height) and are considered an emergency because of the risk of AVN due to transient disruption of the blood supply. These fractures are often treated by closed or open reduction with internal fixation.

Hemiarthroplasty or total hip arthroplasty is used less commonly in young patients with femoral neck fractures because of the high rate of failure due to

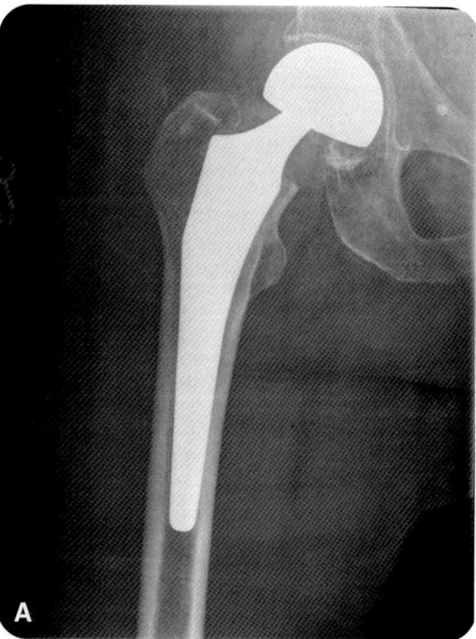

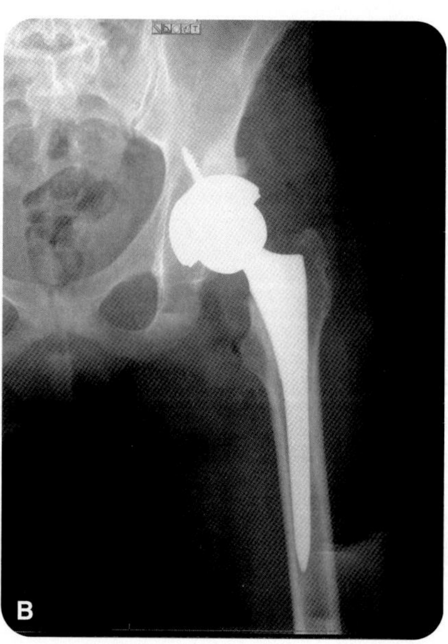

Figure 11.2 **(A)** Anteroposterior postoperative radiograph from the patient in the introductory case, demonstrating a right hip hemiarthroplasty. **(B)** Anteroposterior postoperative radiograph from a different patient, demonstrating a total left hip arthroplasty.

wear and mechanical loosening, the risk of dislocation, and the worse functional outcome. In older patients, hemiarthroplasty and total hip arthroplasty are preferred because the patient is able to weight-bear immediately, reducing the associated morbidities from hospitalization. Surgical intervention should be undertaken as soon as the patient is medically stabilized and cleared for surgery. Total hip arthroplasty is considered in patients who were active at baseline or when a patient has evidence of hip osteoarthritis prior to the femoral neck fracture. Postoperatively, all patients should be treated with chemical and/or mechanical venous thromboembolism prophylaxis.

Although the healing potential of intertrochanteric and subtrochanteric fractures is high, internal fixation to prevent the development of varus or external rotation malunions is required. Fixation techniques include intramedullary or plate fixation. Similarly, postoperative chemical and/or mechanical venous thromboembolism prophylaxis is appropriate, and early ambulation is encouraged.

WHEN TO REFER

An orthopedic surgeon should evaluate the following:

- Femoral neck fractures
- Extracapsular fractures such as intertrochanteric or subtrochanteric fractures

Other conditions for referral are as follows:

- Open fractures (immediate referral)
- All cases of AVN
- Any cases of neurovascular compromise ("stat" referral)

Suggested Readings

Anglen JO, Weinstein JN. Nail or plate fixation of intertrochanteric hip fractures: changing pattern of practice. *J Bone Joint Surg*. 2008;90:700–707.

Brunner LC, Eshilian-Oates L. Hip fractures in adults. *Am Fam Physician*. 2003;67:537–542.

Centers for Disease Control and Prevention. Hip fractures among older adults. http://www.cdc.gov. Accessed September, 2009.

Cummings SR, Nevitt MC, Browner WS, et al. Risk factors for hip fracture in white women. *New Engl J Med*. 1995;332:767–774.

Dominguez S, Liu P, Mandell RC, Richman PB. Prevalence of traumatic hip and pelvic fractures in patients with suspected hip fractures and negative initial standard radiographs—a study of emergency department patients. *Acad Emerg Med*. 2005;12(4):366–369.

Framer ME, White LR, Brody JA, Bailey KR. Race and sex differences in hip fracture incidence. *Am J Public Health*. 1984;74(12):1374–1380.

Grisso JA, Kelsey JL, Strom BL, O'Brien LA. Risk factors for hip fracture in black women. *New Engl J Med*. 1994;330(22):1555–1559.

Harris JH, Harris WH, Novelline RA. *The Radiology of Emergency Medicine*. 3rd ed. Baltimore, MD: Lippincott Williams & Wilkins; 1993:790-804, 808–810.

Hayes WC, Myers ER, Robonovitch SN, et al. Etiology and prevention of age-related hip fractures. *Bone*. 1996;18(1)(suppl):77s–86s.

Koval KJ, Zuckerman JD. Hip fractures, I: overview and evaluation and treatment of femoral neck fractures. *J Am Acad Othop Surg*. 1994;2:141–149.

Koval KJ, Zucerkman JD. Hip fractures, II: evaluation and treatment of intertrochanteric fractures. *J Am Acad Orthop Surg*. 1994;2:150–156.

Perron AD, Miller MD, Brady WJ. Orthopedic pitfalls in the ed: radiographically occult hip fractures. *Am J Emerg Med*. 2002;20(3):234–237.

Rao SS, Cherukuri M. Management of hip fractures: the family physician's role. *Am Fam Physician*. 2006;73: 2195–2202.

Roche JJW, Wenn RT, Sahota O, Moran CG. Effect of comorbidities and postoperative complications on mortality after hip fracture in elderly people: prospective observational cohort study. *BMJ*. 2005;331: 1374–1378.

Schwartz AV, Nevitt MC, Brown BW, Kelsey JL. Increased falling as a risk factor for fractures among older women: the study of osteoporotic fractures. *Am J Epidemiol*. 2005;161(2):180–185.

Stevens JA, Olson S. Reducing falls and resulting hip fractures among older women. *MMWR Recomm Rep*. 2000;49(RR-2):3–12.

Tornetta P, Mostafavi HR. Hip dislocations: current treatment regimens. *Orthop Surg*. 1997;5:27–36.

Zuckerman JD. Hip fracture. *New Engl J Med*. 1996;334:1519–1525.

CHAPTER 12

Avascular Necrosis

George M. Bridgeforth, Kevin Bozic, and Jay Patel

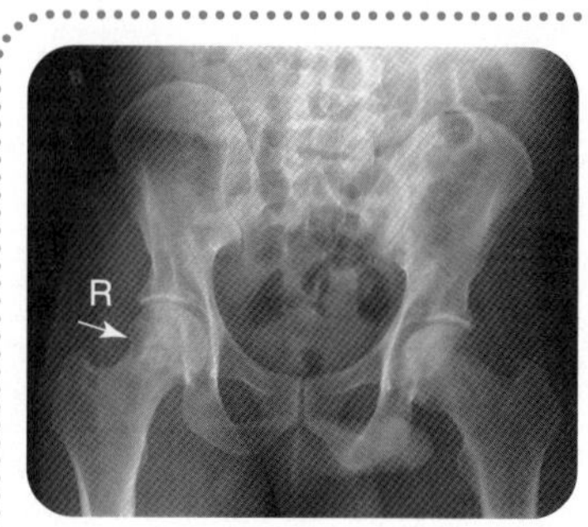

A 41-year-old man who is positive for the human immunodeficiency virus (HIV) is taking antiretroviral therapy. (He is a cocaine and intravenous drug abuser.) He presents to the emergency department with left hip pain that he sustained after a fall.

Clinical Presentation

Avascular necrosis (AVN), which is also known as *osteonecrosis* or *aseptic necrosis*, usually presents with complaints of severe hip or groin pain. Moreover, it is associated with pain-limited range of motion and gait. Initially, radiographs may be negative; findings of AVN appear on standard radiographs several weeks later. AVN may be traumatic, with the risk increasing following severe, acute trauma. Risk factors for atraumatic AVN include alcoholism, steroid use, chronic renal disorders, sickle cell and other hemoglobinopathies, Cushing disease, Gaucher disease, and HIV.

Groin pain may occur with groin strains, lumbar radiculopathies (third lumbar [L3] nerve), or occult hernias. Patients with pulled groin muscles have pain and soreness over the adductor muscles and inguinal region. Moreover, groin strains improve with analgesic medication and cold packs. Severe cases may require physical therapy. Lumbar (L3) radiculopathies are associated with pronounced low back pain that is exacerbated by flexion and positive straight leg raising signs. Moreover, sensory impairment to the upper one-third of the thigh (L3 sensory dermatome) may occur.

CLINICAL POINTS

- Patients may present with hip or groin pain.
- Initial plain radiographs may be negative.
- AVN may take 3 to 4 weeks to appear on standard radiographs.
- Sclerotic and/or cystic changes in the bone with a deformed femoral head may be evident.
- A positive Stinchfield or Faber test indicates intra-articular hip pathology. This may represent degenerative joint disease, acute fracture, metastatic disease, AVN, or a labral tear.

Radiographic Evaluation

Plain radiographs of the hip should be ordered, both anteroposterior (AP) and lateral (frog leg) views. If these are normal, magnetic resonance imaging (MRI) may also be performed (Fig. 12.1). Bone scans are highly sensitive but very nonspecific. An MRI scan produces superior anatomic delineation.

AVN may be classified into four different stages:

Stage 1: Standard radiographs are normal, but early AVN is detectable on MRI.
Stage 2: The femoral head develops cystic and sclerotic changes, which are apparent on standard radiographs. However, the shape of the femoral head remains intact.
Stage 3: The crescent sign is identified as a sclerotic rim along the femoral head. A subchondral radiolucent line runs beneath the rim of the femoral head, which is caused by osteonecrosis and bony reabsorption near the

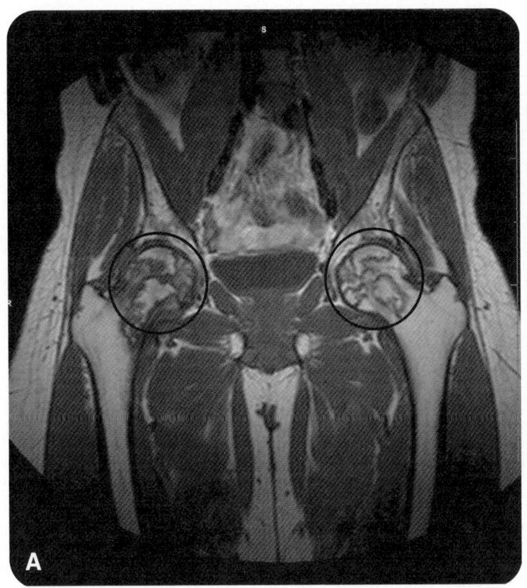

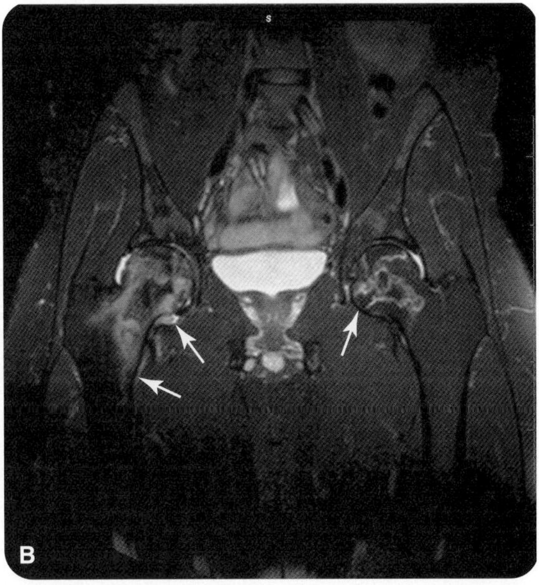

Figure 12.1 Magnetic resonance imaging of the bilateral hips demonstrates abnormal serpiginous signal in the bilateral femoral heads and necks on **(A)** T1-weighted and **(B)** T2-weighted images, consistent with avascular necrosis and bilateral bone infarcts. In addition, there is increased T2-signal in the right femoral head and neck, consistent with bone marrow edema. Compare with the normal T1 and T2 signals in the femoral diaphysis.

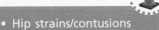

articular surface. The crescent sign is identified with cystic and sclerotic changes in the femoral head. It represents advanced AVN.

Stage 4: There is a collapse with flattening of the femoral head associated with marked sclerosis. As the condition progresses, the sclerosis is caused by necrotic bone that appears more dense, and the necrotic bone diminishes in size and becomes even more sclerotic. Ultimately, the diseased subchondral bone collapses, leading to deformation of the femoral head, and subsequently joint space narrowing and acetabular damage (Fig. 12.2).

PATIENT ASSESSMENT

1. Hip or groin pain
2. Positive Stinchfield (active straight leg raise) test
3. Pain-limited passive range of motion
4. Antalgic gait (limp)

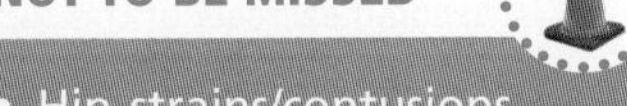

NOT TO BE MISSED

- Hip strains/contusions
- Hip fractures
- Labral tears
- Hip dislocations
- Metastatic disease
- Paget disease
- Greater trochanteric bursitis
- Hematoma
- Abscess
- Osteomyelitis
- Bone tumors

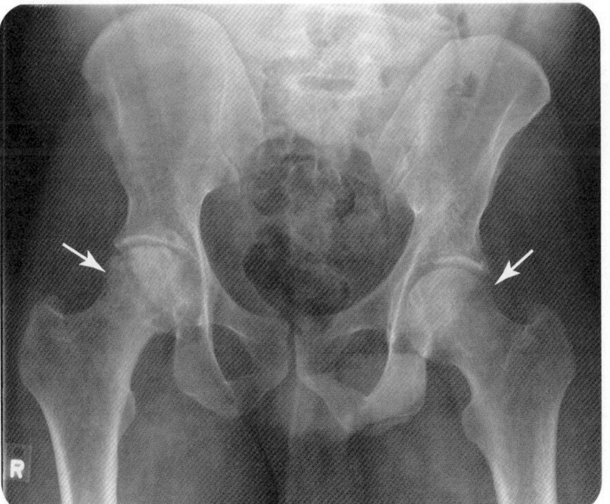

Figure 12.2 Repeat plain radiograph examination of the patient in the initial case approximately 17 months later, demonstrating progression of sclerosis in the right femoral head with subsequent flattening of the subchondral bone. There are subtle focal areas of sclerotic bone in the contralateral femoral neck.

Treatment

On diagnosis of AVN of the hip, the patient should be referred to an orthopedic surgeon for further evaluation. The treatment of AVN is dependent on the stage of the disease process.

For early-stage AVN, management involves serial examinations and radiographs to check for progression of the disease. The slightest amount of progression may warrant surgical treatment. There is no well-established medical management of AVN, although recent studies show promise for the use of bisphosphonates for early-stage AVN. Core decompression is one surgical option for relatively early-stage AVN of the femoral head. The surgery involves drilling a hole through the femoral neck into the femoral head to decrease pressure within the bone. Occasionally, the procedure involves placing a vascularized fibular autograft into the drill hole. During this procedure, the fibula bone is harvested with its blood vessel from the leg and placed into the drill hole and the blood vessel connected to a vessel near the hip. This is thought to increase blood flow to the hip. This treatment is typically reserved for younger patients, and results are mixed.

For advanced stages of AVN, total hip arthroplasty (THA) has been the mainstay of treatment, especially in patients with acetabular cartilage injury. However, it has been shown that more than 75% of patients younger than 50 years who undergo THA for AVN need revision THA 17.8 years after surgery. Outcomes of revision THA are much worse than primary THA, and they are associated with higher rates of complications. Hip resurfacing is a treatment that involves "capping" the femoral head without removing as much bone as in THA. This preservation of femoral bone stock is thought to make revision to a THA at a later age more successful than revision of a primary THA. Although hip resurfacing has a theoretical benefit over THA for patients younger than 50 years with advanced AVN, the procedure has mixed initial short-term results and there is a lack of long-term data. Furthermore, hip resurfacing is contraindicated in patients with AVN who have large (>1 cm) cystic changes in the femoral head. (See Chapter 10 for more information regarding total hip replacement and hip resurfacing.)

Core decompression is ineffective in late-stage AVN because the femoral head deformation associated with well-developed AVN cannot be reversed.

WHEN TO REFER

- Patients with suspected or confirmed AVN warrant referral.

Suggested Readings

Coleman BG, Kressel HY, Dalinka MK, et al. Radiographically negative avascular necrosis: detection with MR imaging. *Radiology.* 1988;168:525–528.

DeSmet AA, Dalinka MK, Alazaki NP, et al. ACR appropriateness criteria: avascular necrosis of the hip. http://www.guideline.gov/summary/summary.aspx?doc_id=8296. Accessed September 15, 2009.

Glickstein MF, Burk DL, Schiebler ML, et al. Avascular necrosis versus other diseases of the hip: sensitivity of MR imaging. *Radiology*. 1998;169:213–215.

Khanna AJ, Yoon TR, Mont MA, et al. Femoral head osteonecrosis: detection and grading by using a rapid MR imaging protocol. *Radiology*. 2000;217:188–192.

Lang P, Jergeseen HE, Mosely ME, et al. Avascular necrosis of the femoral head: high-field strength MR imaging with histologic correlation. *Radiology*. 1988;169:517–524.

McKee MD, Waddell JP, Kudo PA, Schemitsch EH, Richards RR. Osteonecrosis of the femoral head in men following short-course corticosteroid therapy: a report of 15 cases. *CMAJ*. 2001;164(2):205–206.

Mitchell MD, Kundel HL, Steinberg ME, et al. Avascular necrosis of the hip: comparison of MR, CT and scintigraphy. *AJR Am J Roentgen*. 1986;147:67–71.

Molia AC, Strady C, Rouger C, et al. Osteonecrosis in six HIV-infected patients receiving highly active antiretroviral therapy. *Ann Pharmacother*. 2004:38(12):2050–2054.

Teh J. Imaging the hip. *Imaging*. 2007;19(3):234–238.

Zurlo JV. The double-line sign. *Radiology.* 1999;15:541–542.

SECTION 3

Knee and Leg

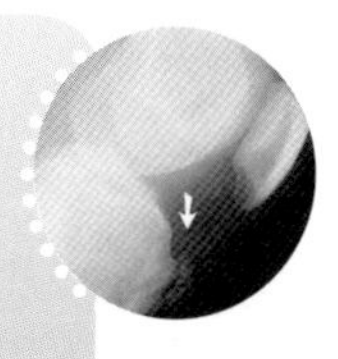

Chapter 18 Osgood–Schlatter Disease

George M. Bridgeforth, Kimberly Shellcroft, and John Cherf

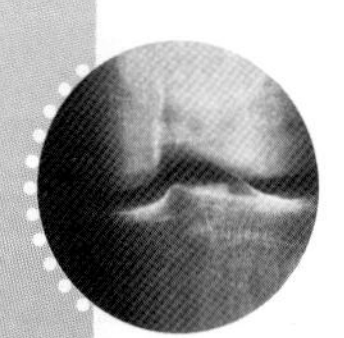

Chapter 19 Bipartite Patella

George M. Bridgeforth and John Cherf

Functional Anatomy

The knee is a complex hinge joint. In addition to flexion and extension, it allows for some rotation of the femur on the articulating tibia. Moreover, when the knee is partially flexed to approximately 30 degrees, there is limited adduction (medial movement) and abduction (lateral movement) as well. The articulation between the distal femur (thigh) and the proximal tibia (shin) forms a saddle joint. The rounded ends of the distal femoral condyles (i.e., articulating bony surfaces) articulate with the slightly depressed concave surfaces (tibial plateau and menisci) of the tibia. The slightly raised bony area that separates the medial and lateral tibia plateau (tibia condyles) is called the tibia spine (or median eminence).

This bony articulation between the distal femur and proximal tibia is cushioned by the medial and the lateral menisci (cartilage). The menisci are about the size of a dollor and are shaped like the letter C. The menisci act as shock absorbers; they are the brake pads of the knee. The menisci prevent the articulating bony surfaces of the saddle joint from rubbing against each other. During flexion, the rounded femoral condyles glide posteriorly over the tibial plateau. During extension, the tibial condyles roll forward in the opposite direction. In addition to providing a cushion that allows for smoother joint flexion and extension, the menisci help prevent the weight of the upper body from damaging the bony articular surfaces. During compression, the menisci provide a more even layer of synovial fluid; this allows for smoother flexion and extension.

The tibia condyles, which comprise the medial and lateral tibia plateau, have slightly different configurations and function. The medial tibia plateau (and its meniscus) is slightly larger and more oblong than the lateral plateau. During the last 30 degrees of knee extension and the first 30 degrees of flexion, there is a slight rotation of the femur. The medial femur rotates internally on the more oblong medial femoral condyle during the final phase of extension (last 30 degrees) and rotates externally during the initial phase of flexion (first 30 degrees). This rotary mechanism is important because it creates a locking mechanism that provides for additional stability of the knee during full extension.

The principal ligaments of the knee are the anterior cruciate ligament (ACL), the posterior cruciate ligament (PCL), the medial collateral ligament (MCL), and the lateral collateral ligament (LCL) (Fig. 1). The cruciate ("crossed") ligaments are located at the center of the knee. They provide additional stabilization by preventing gliding of the femur on the tibia during flexion and extension. The ACL originates between the anterior tibial condyles, and it inserts along the medial surface of the lateral femoral

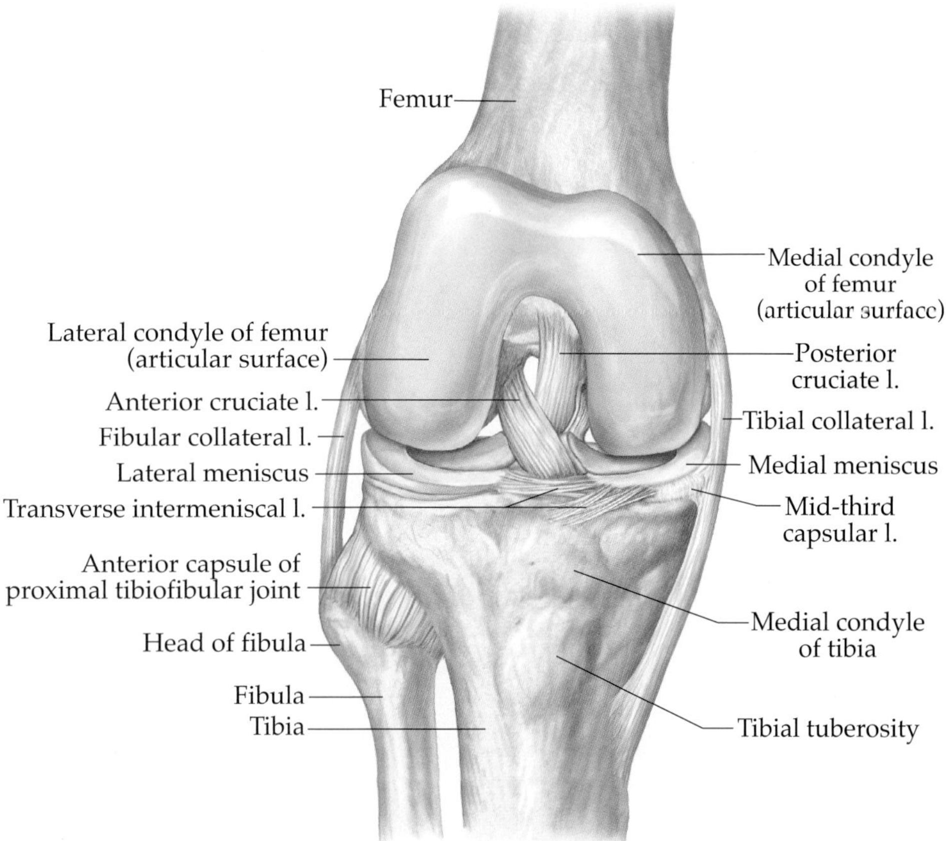

Figure 1 Right knee ligaments anterior labeled. Asset provided by Anatomical Chart Co.

condyle. The PCL originates from the posterior intercondylar region, of the tibia and it attaches to the lateral surface of the medial femoral condyle. The ACL prevents the tibia from excessive sliding (forward) during flexion and extension. The PCL prevents the tibia from excessive sliding in the opposite direction. Complete tears in either or both ligaments may lead to joint instability and degenerative arthritis over time.

Medial and lateral stability of the knee is primary provided by the MCL and LCL. The cord-shaped LCL, which is also called the fibular collateral ligament, lies outside of the joint capsule. It extends from the lateral epicondyle (the nonarticulating rounded section at the end of a bone that serves as an attachment for the ligaments and tendons) of the femur to the head of the fibula. On the opposite side, the MCL is a broad band that is fused with the surrounding joint capsule. Moreover, it is firmly attached to the medial meniscus. This firm attachment helps explain one of the reasons why medial meniscus injuries are more common than lateral meniscus injuries. The MCL extends from the medial epicondyle of the femur to the medial condyle and proximal tibia. The LCL helps stabilize the knee against a varus force. The MCL helps protects the knee against a valgus.

The patella is the largest sesamoid (sesame-shaped) bone in the body. The tendon that extends from the quadriceps to the upper pole of the patella is the quadriceps tendon; the ligament that extends from the lower pole of the patella to the tibia tubercle (a bony prominence on the upper tibia) is the patella tendon. The patella not only works as a shield that protects the internal structures of the knee joint but also increases the length of the lever arm of the quadriceps. During knee extension, the lever arm of the knee is elongated by the quadriceps and the patella tendons. From a biomechanical standpoint, this longer lever arm increases the force of the quadriceps to extend the lower leg (i.e., the longer the lever arm, the greater the force). In addition, the patella serves as a fulcrum (i.e., a bending or tilting point) when knee flexion is initiated by the hamstrings.

CHAPTER 13

Patella Fractures

George M. Bridgeforth and John Cherf

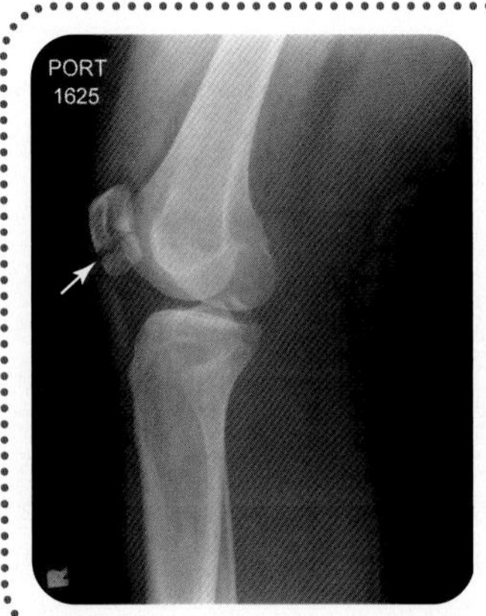

A 24-year-old woman presents with marked swelling, pain, and soreness of the right knee after a motor vehicle accident. She cannot bend or straighten her right knee.

Clinical Presentation

Patella fractures make up approximately 1% of all fractures and are usually seen in active people aged between 20 and 50 years. This injury is nearly twice as likely to occur in men compared with women. The **mechanism of injury** is usually a direct blow to the patella, resulting from a low-energy fall or a high-energy dashboard injury, or it may be indirect, resulting from running or jumping. Direct injuries cause comminuted fractures and indirect injuries, cause avulsion fractures, generally from the sudden contraction of the quadriceps. Fractures are usually characterized by the acute onset of pain, swelling, and tenderness. There may be a large effusion, and patients are often unable to ambulate.

CLINICAL POINTS

- Moderate to severe swelling, usually moderate to severe patella tenderness, is characteristic.
- Patients present with pain, limited range of motion, and antalgic gait (limp).
- Causes include direct impact and indirect blows.

The physical examination of an acute injured knee may be hampered by apprehension and guarding. The initial inspection should check for signs of an effusion, acute inflammation, open wounds (potential portals for serious infections), or structural abnormalities. It should include an inspection of the entire leg for any evidence of a potential compartment syndrome (pallor or a swollen extremity). The presence of a large effusion indicates possible internal derangement from an intra-articular fracture or cruciate ligament tears. It should be noted that most knee fractures and contusions are not characterized by marked inflammation. On the other hand, septic joints have marked erythema, warmth, and tenderness. Untreated, septic joints may cause widespread joint destruction. Therefore, they should be subject to an immediate diagnostic aspiration; treatment is directed toward the underlying cause.

It is important to palpate the entire knee carefully for pain, swelling, and tenderness. Palpation should include not only the patella but also the joint spaces, the distal femoral condyles, the proximal tibia condyles (the epicondylar regions), the quadriceps and patella tendon, the pes anserine bursa, and the medial and collateral ligaments. Pain in the condylar regions may represent a condylar fracture, whereas pain along the medial joint line may be secondary to a meniscus tear. Focal tenderness of the pes anserine bursa about 2.5 cm below the medial joint line may be secondary to pes anserine bursitis.

Although this remains a diagnosis of exclusion, it may be treated with analgesic medication and cold packs—a steroid injection may be reserved for refractory cases. The Ottawa rules concerning radiography (see "Radiographic Evaluation") do not exclude underlying soft tissue injuries (i.e. tears); therefore, a thorough and systematic knee examination is essential.

Although the differential diagnosis for acute knee injuries is long, it is necessary to rule out a soft tissue contusion, an associated knee fracture, or internal derangement. A soft tissue contusion is characterized by pain, swelling, and tenderness. Although range of motion may be affected, stability of the knee is intact. Moreover, radiographs do not reveal any acute fractures. Follow-up studies such as a computed tomography (CT) or magnetic resonance imaging (MRI) should be reserved for patients who do not improve with conservative treatment (analgesics, cold packs, and physical therapy for severe cases). CT is slightly more sensitive for detecting an occult fracture, whereas an MRI is superior for detecting internal derangement (torn menisci, torn cruciate ligaments). However, MRI scans provide excellent sensitivity for detecting occult fractures.

Serious soft tissue injuries of the knee may occur following acute trauma, with or without an associated fracture. Twisting injuries may occur prior to impact, especially with falls and sports injuries. A torn medial meniscus (cartilage) is more common than a torn lateral meniscus. The medial meniscus is responsible for bearing a greater load (i.e., body weight), and it is firmly attached to the medial collateral ligament. Patients often complain of a burning pain along the inside of the knee—at the medial joint line. Associated complaints include trouble bending the knee, locking, clicking, and trouble using the stairs. Patients with torn cartilage have trouble performing and maintaining a full squat.

The following tests may be useful in examining the patient with a possible patella fracture:

- Straight leg raise: This test is used to detect disc injuries in the back (radicular pain past the knee from 30–60 degrees) or hip pathology (pain in the groin or hip at 30 degrees). There is an inability to extend the leg if the patellar tendon or quadriceps tendon is ruptured. If the patient has a torn meniscus, the knee may lock and the examiner cannot fully straighten the leg. But a straightened leg does not rule out a torn meniscus.
- McMurray test: This test is positive in patients with a torn medial meniscus. The knee is flexed and the lower extremity externally rotated with one hand while inward pressure is applied on the knee by the opposite hand. A positive test is characterized by pain or a painful clicking along the medial joint line.
- Apley compression test: This test is used to detect a torn meniscus only. It is performed with the patient lying face down. The knee is flexed to 90 degrees. Pain with compression and rotation along the joint line indicates a possible meniscal tear. Pain with distraction (as the lower leg is pulled upward) relieves the tension on the cartilage (menisci) and places a strain on the medial or collateral ligaments. Soreness with distraction coupled with palpable pain and tenderness along with good stability favors a medial or collateral ligament strain.

In addition to checking for meniscal injuries, it is important to check the structural integrity of the knee by checking for (ligament) instability. Patients with a completely torn medial collateral ligament exhibit valgus laxity. The unstable knee joint opens on the medial side as the examiner stabilizes the though with one hand as the lower extremity is gently pulled outward. Varus instability is caused by lateral collateral ligament injuries. The unstable knee joint opens on the lateral side as the lower extremity is gently brought inward by the examiner. Because the knee has an anatomic stabilization mechanism in full extension (called the "screw home" mechanism), varus and valgus testing should be performed when the knee is unlocked at 30 degrees. Some examiners have recommended repeating the testing when the knee is fully extended as well.

Patients with torn anterior cruciate ligaments (ACLs) often complain of a "pop" followed by knee pain and swelling. ACL tears may be seen with tibial spine or Segond fractures these. Associated fractures may or may not be present. ACL injuries should be suspected in patients with fractures of the tibial spine (median eminence) or with a Segond fracture. A Segond fracture is an avulsion fracture that occurs at the upper aspect of the lateral tibial plateau. It is best appreciated on the anteroposterior (AP) view. Moreover, Segond fractures have a very strong association with ACL or meniscus tears.

Several clinical tests are used to check for ACL tears. A Lachman test is more sensitive than an anterior draw test. With acute knee trauma, it may be difficult for patients to bend their knees, a Lachman test may be easier to perform as well. The patient flexes the knees to approximately 20–30 degrees some examiners perform the test with the knee slightly related externally. The examiner stabilizes the distal femur with one hand while placing the other hand on the proximal tibia. While keeping the knee stabilized, the tibia is pulled in an anterior direction (anterior translational force); the injured knee is compared with the opposite knee for evidence of joint laxity. A positive test is characterized by the anterior displacement of the tibia (>3 mm) that was not present on the opposite side. The anterior draw test is performed in a similar fashion, except that the knee is flexed to 90 degrees. Both hands are cupped firmly around the calf muscles (with both thumbs placed anteriorly over the knee) as the examiner tries to pull the tibia forward. Any detected laxity should be compared with the opposite knee. In addition, posterior cruciate tears may be detected by posterior translation (i.e., posterior laxity) of the tibia when pushing in the opposite (i.e., backward) directions.

PATIENT ASSESSMENT

1. Look for an associated effusion, which may or may not be present.
2. Be sure to palpate the knee carefully.
3. Determine whether any serious soft tissue injuries are present.

The lateral pivot shift test is performed with the patient supine and the hip abducted (the knee is away from the body) by 30 degrees. A valgus (inward pressure) is placed on the knee at the proximal tibia fibula. With an ACL tear, the tibia subluxes anteriorly at approximately 20 to 40 degrees of flexion. It may difficult to perform this test in patients with large effusions because the patient may demonstrate marked apprehension and guarding.

Radiographic Evaluation

In the acute assessment of patella injuries, the Ottawa Knee Rules, which were developed by emergency department physicians in Canada, may be helpful. Radiographs are recommended if any of the following five criteria is present:

- Patient older than 55 years
- Tenderness at the head of the fibula
- Isolated tenderness of the patella
- Inability to flex the knee to 90 degrees
- Inability to walk four steps immediately following the injury and during the clinical examination

The sensitivity of these guidelines is very high; several studies have reported it to be more than 95%. However, the reported specificity varies between 15% and 30%, so if a patient does not meet any of the guidelines, the chances of missing a fracture by not obtaining a radiograph ranges from 15% to 30%. Until there is comprehensive malpractice protection for physicians who adhere strictly to the Ottawa rules, physicians are advised to use their own discretion.

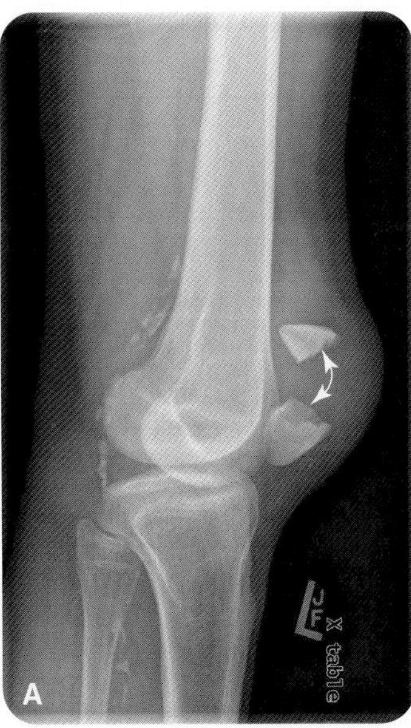

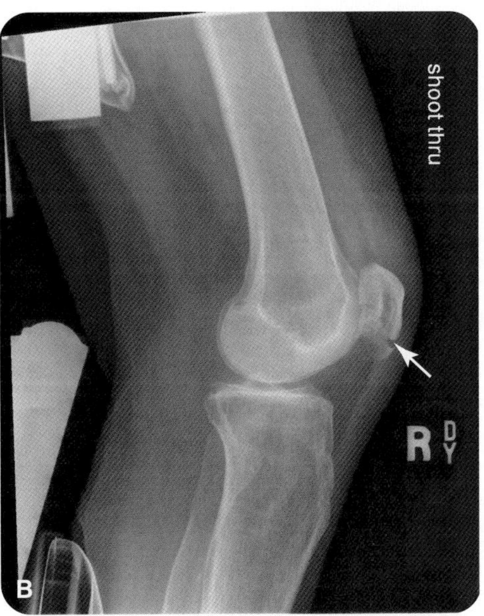

Figure 13.1 **(A)** A lateral radiograph of the knee of a 64-year-old man who fell from his deck demonstrates a gross transverse fracture through the patella with superior distraction of the fractured fragment with a large soft tissue hematoma. Incidentally, there is calcification of the popliteal artery. **(B)** A lateral radiograph of the knee of a 91-year-old woman who has fallen demonstrates an acute fracture of the patella.

Radiographs that should be ordered include the following:

- AP view: may be used as an initial estimate to assess patella fracture separation
- Lateral view: may be used to assess patella fracture displacement (Fig. 13.1)
- Oblique views (two): full trauma series; used to detect tibia plateau fractures. The internal oblique provides a better depiction of the lateral tibial plateau. The external oblique provides a better depiction of the medial tibial plateau.
- Optional views
  - Sunrise (axial) view: used to detect subtle patella fractures and dislocations
  - Merchant view: used to detect subtle patella fractures and dislocations.
  - Intercondylar (tunnel) view: used to evaluate the median eminence for fractures of the tibial spine
  - Cross-table lateral view: used for patients who cannot bend their knee following acute trauma. A large effusion with a fat–fluid level (lipohemarthrosis) indicates an intra-articular fracture or internal derangement.

Patella fractures may be displaced or nondisplaced. If three or more fragments are identified, then the fracture is a comminuted fracture of the patella. The examiner should look for one (solitary fracture) or multiple (comminuted fracture) translucent fracture lines that extend to the cortex. The fracture lines may appear on the AP, lateral, or oblique view. Solitary nondisplaced fractures may be described according to the orientation of their fracture lines as transverse (horizontal), longitudinal (vertical), or slightly oblique (in the case of a patella fracture, actually a slightly slanted vertical fracture). In addition, fractures may be described by their size (centimeters) and location (e.g., upper pole, middle third, lower pole). Fractures at the lower pole are usually avulsion fractures and are associated with an avulsion fracture separation of the patella tendon.

On the lateral view, the examiner should look for a high-riding patella (patella alba) with a separated avulsed bony fragment (or absent patella tendon) distally. The examiner should trace the outline of the patella tendon to the tibial tuberosity. The finding (plus a normal quadriceps extension) indicates that the

NOT TO BE MISSED

- Knee damage
  - Knee (patella) contusion
  - Degenerative arthritis (osteoarthritis)
  - Patella dislocation
  - Traumatic effusion with or without internal derangement
  - Septic joint
  - Patella/quadriceps tendon rupture
  - Torn meniscus injury
  - Prepatella bursitis
  - Patella tendonitis
  - Patella after (high-riding patella)
  - Bipartite patella
- Other joint damage in the knee
  - Rheumatoid arthritis (look for rheumatoid arthritic changes in other joints)
  - Gout (hot, erythematous, and tender)
  - Psoriatic arthritis (look for nail pitting and salmon-colored plaques)
  - Tuberculosis (chronic lymphoid effusion, history of alcoholism)

patella tendon is intact. If the patella tendon is completely disrupted, there is a massive effacement (darkening) of the subpatellar area, which is caused by a traumatic effusion. In addition, the patella tendon is untraceable. For patients with large effusions who cannot bend the knee, a cross-table lateral view is very helpful. A lipohemarthrosis produces a fat–blood interface sign, which resembles an air–fluid level. This indicates probable intra-articular derangement from either torn cruciate ligaments or a fracture inside the joint capsule (i.e., fracture of the median eminence or the femoral or tibial condyles). Further evaluation is warranted. An MRI should be obtained to rule out internal derangement.

On lateral and oblique views, it is important to be able to identify and trace the circumference (i.e., outer rim) of the entire patella. Moreover, the patella should be examined for evidence of displacement (dislocation) as well. Most patella dislocations are laterally displaced. Subtle transverse fracture is only seen on the lateral view (Fig. 13.2). The sunrise and Merchant views are also used to detect subtle fractures.

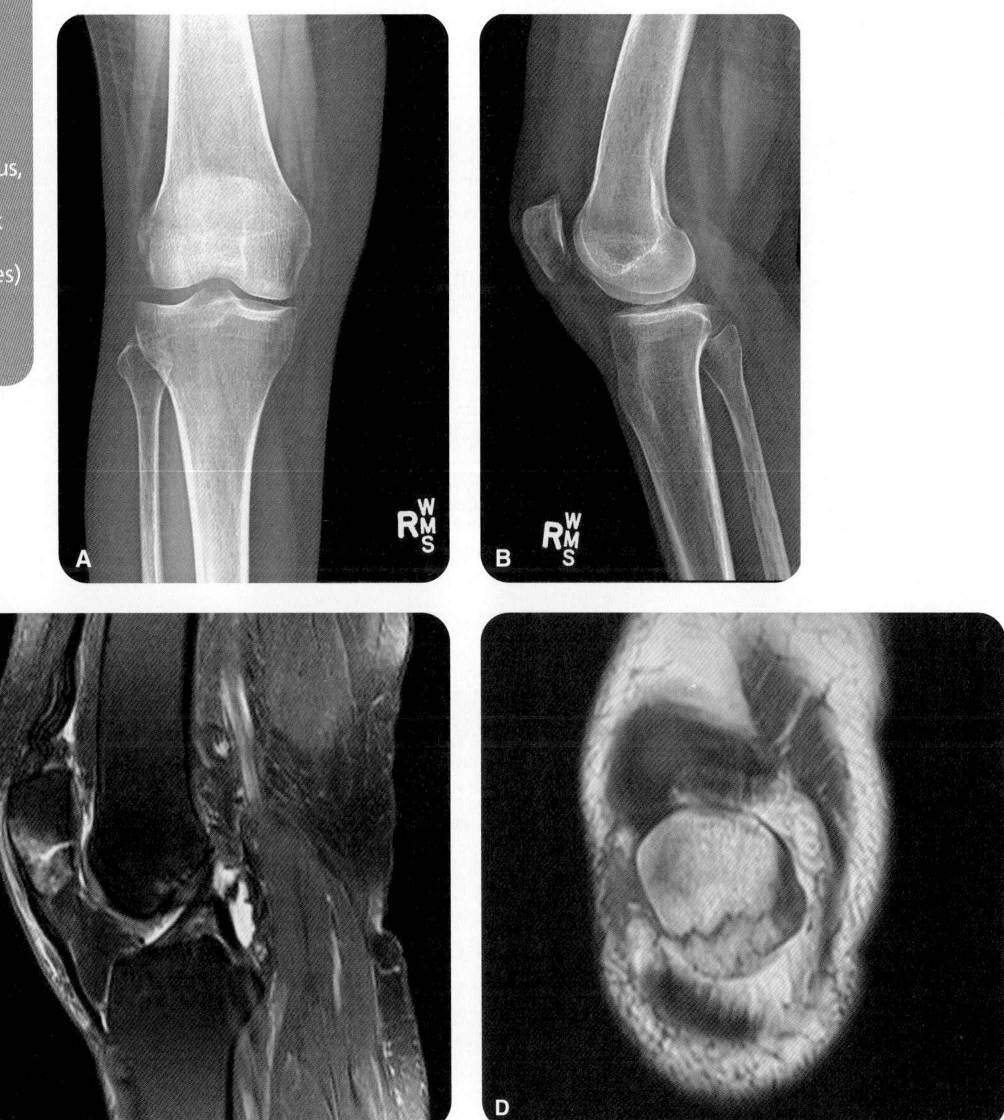

Figure 13.2 **(A, B)** Subtle transverse fracture is seen only on the lateral view. Notice, however, that there is soft tissue density in the suprapatellar space on the lateral radiograph. The fracture is more obvious on the magnetic resonance imaging scan. **(C)** The sagittal proton density fat-saturated sequence shows extensive bone marrow edema, and the coronal **(D)** T1-sequence shows a linear band of low signal in the patella representing the fracture line. (Courtesy of Richard Kim, MD).

If the Ottawa rules are positive but the initial radiographs are unremarkable, close follow-up should be obtained. If the patient is not improving, then an MRI scan (or CT scan) should be obtained. The CT scan has a slightly higher sensitivity for detecting occult fractures. The MRI provides better depiction of the internal architecture of the knee. It is useful for detecting meniscus and cruciate ligament tears.

Treatment

The treatment of patellar fractures is largely based on the type of the fracture. The overall goals of treating fractures of the patella are to preserve patella and knee extensor mechanism function and mitigate complications associated with an articular surface fracture. An irregular articular surface is at risk of developing posttraumatic arthritis. The treatment options for patients with patellar fractures include nonoperative treatment, tension band wiring techniques, partial patellectomy, partial patellectomy combined with tension band wiring, and total excision or patellectomy.

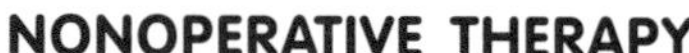

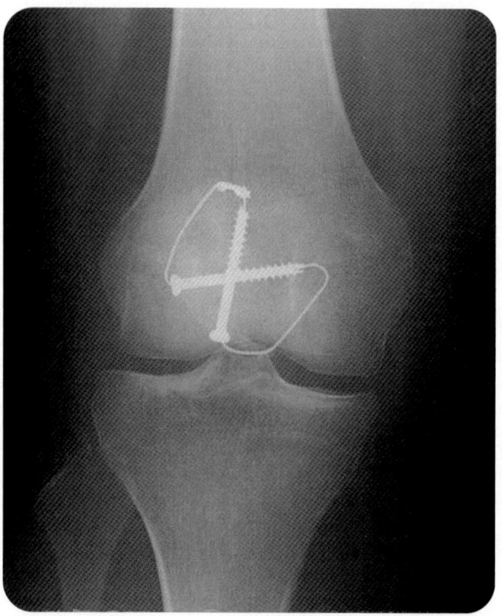

Figure 13.3 Postoperative anteroposterior radiograph of the right knee from the patient from the case presentation demonstrating a fixation wire and screws.

NONOPERATIVE THERAPY

Nonoperative therapy is reserved for nondisplaced fractures with and intact extensor mechanism. Fractures that meet the nonoperative indications have fracture displacement or separation of less than 3 mm and articular step-off of less than 2 mm. The extensor mechanism must also be intact. Therapy includes immobilization and possibly non–weight-bearing ambulation. Immobilization involves splinting in extension. This can be accomplished with a knee immobilizer. This immobilization usually lasts for 4 to 6 weeks. Patients should be encouraged to bear weight as tolerated. Physician therapy may be used to optimize the range of motion and muscle strength.

OPERATIVE THERAPY

Operative therapy is recommended in patients with patella fractures with more than 2 mm of articular displacement or 3 mm of fragment separation. Comminuted fractures, disruption of the articular surface, and the presence of displaced loose bodies in the joint are all indications for surgery. The fracture pattern determines the type of surgical procedure performed. Surgical options range from tension band wiring (Fig. 13.3) to partial patellectomy (excision of part of the fractured patella) to total patellectomy (removal of the entire fractured patella). Displaced fractures may require surgical intervention that includes open reduction and internal fixation. Patients with tense, painful knee effusions (hemarthrosis) may also benefit from arthrocentesis for pain relief.

The ultimate goal for obtaining a healthy joint is to obtain a congruent joint surface. Fractures that heal in a nonanatomic position are a risk factor for developing posttraumatic arthritis.

WHEN TO REFER

- Immediate referral
  - Locked knee with an inability to flex or extend the knee
  - Open fractures or massive effusions
  - Neurovascular impairments (swelling, dusky cyanotic pallor, decreased or diminished pulses, impaired sensation)
  - Septic joints
- Surgical referral
  - Separated fragments (>3 mm) or a step-off fragment displacement greater than 2 mm

Suggested Readings

Hoppenfeld S, Murthy VL, Thomas MA, et al. *Treatment and Rehabilitation of Fractures*. Philadelphia, PA: Lippincott Williams & Wilkins; 1999.

SECTION 3 Knee and Leg

Kaplan PA, Walker CW, Kilcoyne R, et al. Occult fracture patterns of the knee associated with anterior cruciate ligament tears: assessment with MR imaging. *Radiology*. 1992;183:835–838.

Seaberg DC, Yealy MD, Lueknes T, et al. Ottawa and Pittsburgh rules for acute knee injuries. *Ann Emerg Med*. 1998;32:8–13.

Shearman C, El-Khoury GY. Pitfalls in the radiologic evaluation of extremity trauma, II: the lower extremity. *Am Fam Physician*. 1998;57:995–1002.

Tandeter H, Shvartzman P, Stevens MA. Acute knee injuries: use of decision rules for selective radiograph ordering. *Am Fam Physician*. 1999;60:2599–2608.

CHAPTER 14

Patella Dislocations

George M. Bridgeforth and John Cherf

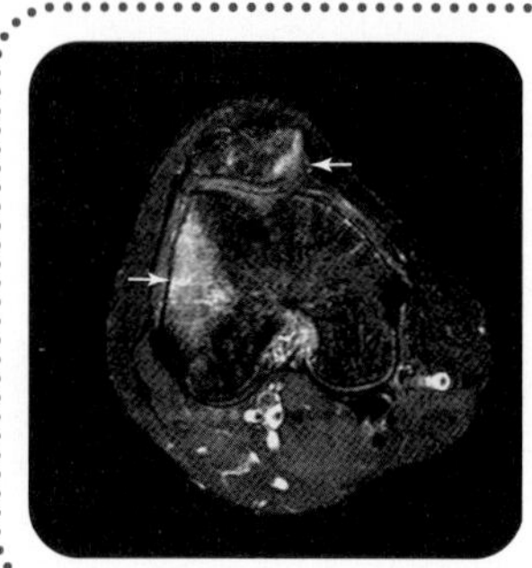

A 21-year-old woman complains of right knee pain, which began after she fell on the sidewalk 1 month ago.

Clinical Presentation

Most patella dislocations are characterized by pain, swelling, and limited weight-bearing. Patients may complain of a "pop," with the knee "popping back into place." There may be mild to moderate swelling. Usually, there is no associated erythema, and the knee is not warm. However, pain-limited range of motion may be present, and the patient may exhibit an antalgic gait (pronounced limp).

Most patella, dislocations occur when the kneecap comes completely out of its groove and rests on the outside of the knee joint. The **mechanism of injury** is a twisting action. This injury common, particularly in adolescent girls and athletes. Sports frequently associated with patella dislocation include soccer, gymnastics, and ice hockey.

When the kneecap goes "out of joint" the first time, ligaments that normally hold the kneecap in position are torn. The structure most often torn is the medial patellofemoral ligament. This ligament secures the patella to the inside (medial) of the knee. When a patella dislocation occurs, the medial patellofemoral ligament is damaged and allows the kneecap to move out of the groove (Fig. 14.1). Once this ligament is torn, it often does not heal properly, and the patella can then dislocate more easily, which is why patella dislocation recurs in some patients with this ligament injury. It should be noted that some subluxations might not be as apparent on examination.

A useful sign for dislocated patella is the presence of patella apprehension. The knee is placed into slight flexion, and both hands are placed across the patella with both thumbs placed on the medial side of the patella. The patella is slowly pushed laterally by the examiner's thumbs. Patients with a patella instability views (barring an acute fracture) complain of pain and apprehension. In response, they try to straighten the knee, which locks the knee preventing further displacement.

CLINICAL POINTS

- Most dislocations are lateral.
- Patients have an antalgic gait.
- Patients with ruptured quadriceps or patella tendons have knee effusions with an inability to extend the knee against gravity.

Radiographic Evaluation

It is necessary to order anteroposterior (AP), lateral. Optional radiographs include the following:

- Sunrise (axial) view: used to detect subtle patella fractures and dislocations

PATIENT ASSESSMENT

1. An effusion, which may or may not be present
2. Pain and limited range of motion
3. Patella apprehension (Fairbanks test). With the knee flexed at 30 degrees, the patella is pushed in a lateral direction.

Patellar dislocation

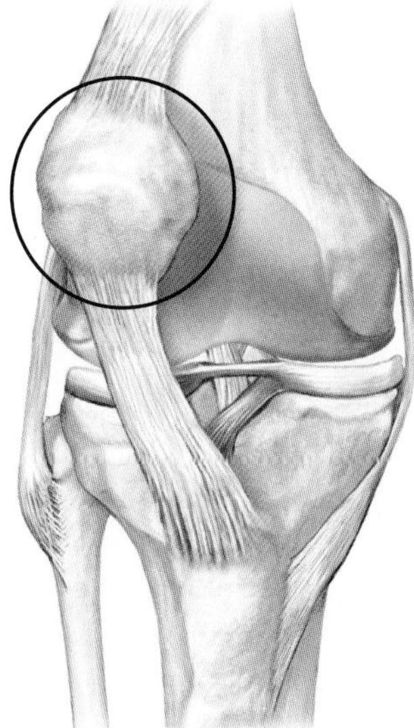

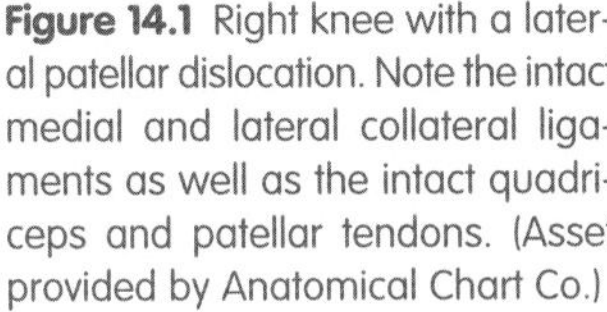

Figure 14.1 Right knee with a lateral patellar dislocation. Note the intact medial and lateral collateral ligaments as well as the intact quadriceps and patellar tendons. (Asset provided by Anatomical Chart Co.)

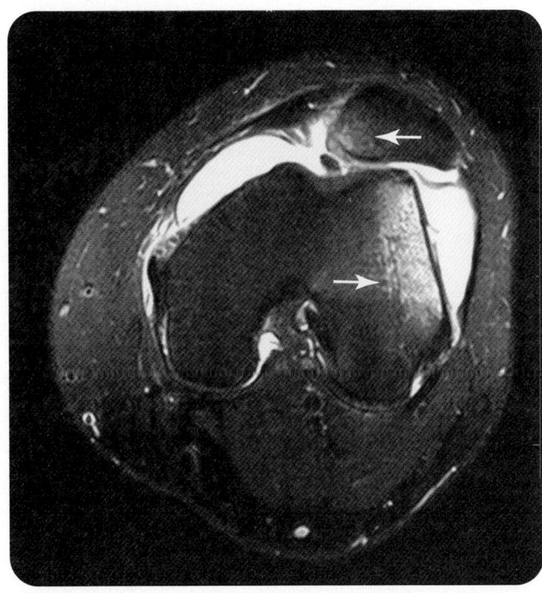

Figure 14.2 An axial T2-weighted image through the left knee of an 18-year-old male rugby player who injured his knee during a match. Demonstrated is a bone marrow edema pattern consistent with transient lateral patellar dislocation-relocation. There is an extensive knee joint effusion with an associated tearing of the anteromedial retinaculum/capsule resulting in lateral positioning of the patella. There is a shallow trochlear groove.

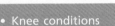

NOT TO BE MISSED

- Knee conditions
- Knee contusion
- Knee strain
- Torn medial meniscus
- Patella fracture
- Anterior (or posterior) cruciate ligament tear
- Prepatellar bursitis
- Patella tendonitis
- Pes anserine bursitis
- Baker cyst
- Ruptured patella/ quadriceps tendon
- Joint conditions that may involve the knee
- Traumatic effusion with or without internal derangement
- Septic joint
- Gout
- Rheumatoid arthritis
- Psoriatic arthritis

- Merchant view (axial view): used to detect subtle patella fractures and subluxations; has better sensitivity than a sunrise view for detecting subtle subluxations. It may be used to measure the sulcus angle. It is the choice of most orthopedic experts.
- Cross-table lateral view: used to detect a fat–blood interface (a lipohemarthrosis), which may indicate an underlying intra-articular fracture or internal derangement. It is particularly useful in patients who have trouble bending their knees.

Most patellar dislocations are laterally displaced (Fig. 14.2). Patella dislocations may be identified on the AP view when the outer rim of the patella lies outside the lateral epicondyles of the distal femur and proximal tibia. Medial dislocations occur but are less common. Subtle patella fractures that are not readily apparent on standard radiographs may be detected by a sunrise or Merchant view. A magnetic resonance imaging (MRI) can aid in the detection of osteochondral fractures or patella subluxations.

If the patient has a high-riding patella associated with an effusion, a ruptured patella tendon should be considered. The outline of the patella tendon is not traceable on the lateral view. It is effaced by a massive effusion.

Patients with high-riding patellas with intact tendons have a congenital condition known as *patella alta*. Normally, the ratio of the patella tendon (measured from the inferior pole of the patella to the tibia tubercle) should be approximately the same length as the patella. If the length of the patella tendon exceeds the length of the patella by a factor of 2 or more, the patient has patella alta. Generally, it is an incidental finding best appreciated on the lateral radiograph. Symptomatic cases are usually treated with pain medications, cold packs, and physical therapy (see Fig. 14.3).

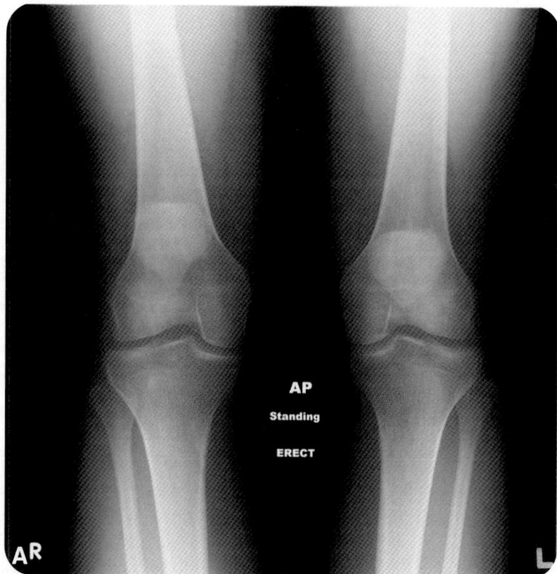

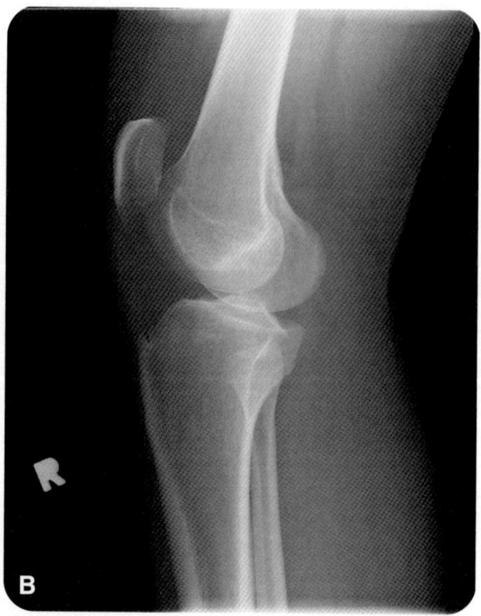

Figure 14.3 A 40-year-old woman has chronic right knee pain with no history of trauma. **(A)** An anteroposterior radiograph of the bilateral knees demonstrates superior position of the right patella compared with the left. **(B)** A lateral view of the right knee demonstrates patella alta.

Treatment

Two types of treatment options are generally available, depending on the degree of dislocation.

NONSURGICAL THERAPY

Patients are initially treated with a compression dressing and immobilization with the knee in extension. Most cases are treated nonsurgically with a closed reduction. This can be accomplished by extending the knee. (Following reduction of acute dislocations, radiographs should be repeated and checked for occult fractures.) Aspiration may be considered for patients with a tense effusion (hemarthrosis). Adjunctive measures include icing, analgesics, and weight-bearing as tolerated. Physical therapy is often initiated to regain the range of motion and muscle strengthening (particularly the quadriceps muscle).

Additional treatment should include exercises that emphasize strengthening the quadriceps tendon and regaining full range of motion. Bracing and taping has been described as additional treatment options; however, their role is questionable.

SURGICAL THERAPY

Patients with chronic recurrent maltracking and instability may require surgery. Surgery for lateral patellar instability may include a lateral retinacular release, proximal realignment (medial quatricplasty), and/or distal realignment (medication of the tibial tubercle). The presence of loose bodies is also an indication for the need of surgery. These are typically the result of a fracture of the patella or trochlea of the femur and can be removed arthroscopically. These procedures are all designed to improve the biomechanics of the extensor mechanism in order to keep the patella stable.

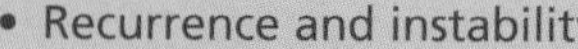

WHEN TO REFER

- Recurrence and instability
- Loose bodies
- Suspected ruptured quadriceps or patella tendon

Suggested Readings

Ballas M, Tyteko J, Mannarino F. Commonly missed orthopedic problems. *Am Fam Physician*. 1998;57(2): 267–274.

Calmbach WL, Hutches M. Evaluation of patients presenting with knee pain, II: differential diagnosis. *Am Fam Physician*. 2003;68:917–922.

Gilley JS, Gelman MI, Edson M, Metcalf RW. Chondral fractures of the knee. *Radiology*. 1981;138:51–54

Harris JH Jr, Harris WH. *The Radiology of Emergency Medicine*. Philadelphia, PA: Lippincott Williams & Wilkins; 1999.

Mink JH, Deutsch A. Occult cartilage and bone injuries of the knee: detection, classification, and assessment with MR imaging. *Radiology*. 1989;170:823–829.

Mink JH, Levy T, Crues JV. Tears of the anterior cruciate ligament and menisci of the knee: MR imaging evaluation. *Radiology*. 1988;167:769–774.

Nance EP, Kay JJ. Injuries of the quadriceps mechanism. *Radiology*. 1982;142:301–307.

Sternbach GL. Evaluation of the knee. *J Emerg Med*. 1986;4:133–143.

Tandeter HB, Shvartzman P, Stevens M. Acute knee injuries: use of decision rules for selective radiograph ordering. *Am Fam Physician*. 1999;60:2599–2608.

CHAPTER 15

Tibial Plateau Fractures

George M. Bridgeforth and John Cherf

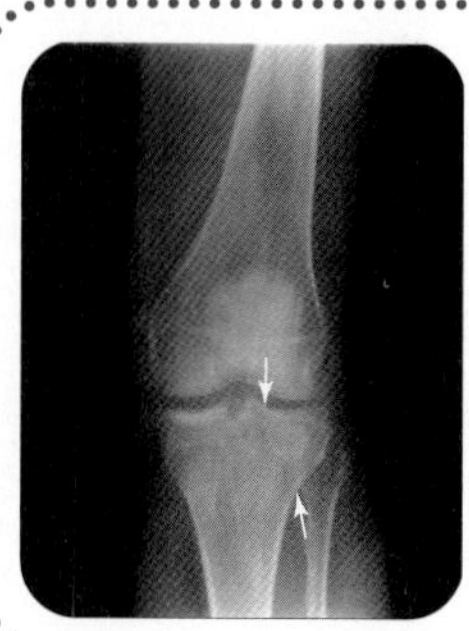

A 49-year-old man slipped and fell on the ice. He now complains of severe right knee pain. He has marked difficulty weight-bearing on the right knee.

Clinical Presentation

Tibial plateau fractures involve the tibial plateau, or the upper surface of the tibia (Fig. 15.1). The most common **mechanism of injury** is axial loading that might result from a fall or a direct blow, usually to the outside of the knee. Sometimes tibial plateau fractures are called "bumper" fractures, because they may result from impact with automobile bumpers. Normally, patients have a recent history of trauma to the knee area. Older people may fall, and younger people may injure themselves playing sports. They may be unable to bear weight on the injured knee. Symptoms include pain, joint stiffness, and swelling. A knee effusion typical.

A knee fracture or a severe knee contusion is characterized by acute swelling, ecchymosis, focal tenderness, and impaired range of motion (especially if the fracture extends to the articular surface of a joint). These signs always point the examiner to the injured area. The differential diagnosis of tibial plateau fractures also includes damage to the collateral ligament, medial or lateral meniscus, or anterior or posterior cruciate ligament. Several tests may be used to determine the actual problem. In an acute setting with high-impact trauma, the patient may have marked swelling, guarding, and apprehension, which may make it difficult to perform these tests.

A medial or collateral ligament tear is characterized by pain, tenderness, and swelling with valgus (medial collateral ligament) or varus (lateral collateral ligament) laxity. Collateral ligament instability should be checked with the knee in slight (30 degrees) flexion. When the knee is fully extended, an anatomic rotation automatically locks the knee in place medical. Collateral ligament instability is tested by stabilizing the knee with one hand and applying inward pressure against the knee while slowing pulling the lower extremity outward away from the body. With a medial collateral ligament tear, the valgus instability is characterized by the inward (medial) deviation of the knee with an outward deviation of the lower extremity. The instability is caused by a torn medial collateral ligament. With a lateral collateral ligament tear, the opposite effect occurs. There is varus instability, which is reflected by outward displacement of the knee when pressure is applied from an inward to outward direction. Moreover, it is associated with inward deviation of the lower extremity (toward the body) as the lower extremity is pulled inward by the examiner.

CLINICAL POINTS

- Trauma to the knee may result in a tibial plateau fracture.
- It is necessary to check for a compartment syndrome (markedly swollen calf with neurovascular impairment).
- Patients may have an associated fibular head fracture (swelling, bruising, pain, and soreness) with or without a peroneal nerve palsy.

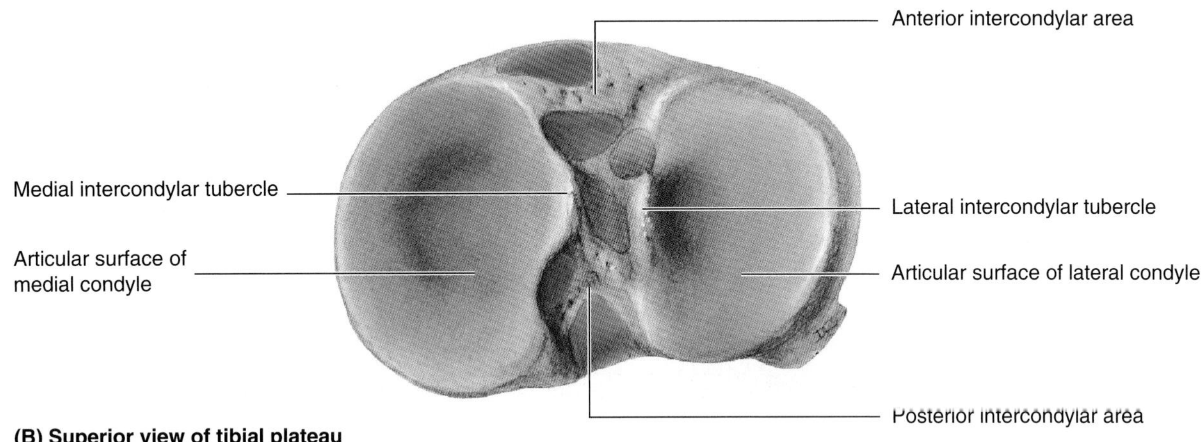

Figure 15.1 The anterior cruciate ligament (ACL) extends from the anterior intercondylar region of the tibia to the medical surface of the lateral condyle of the femur. The posterior cruciate ligament (PCL) extends from the posterior intercondylar region to the lateral medial condyle of the femur. Fractures of the tibial plateau may result in associated injuries to the ACL, PCL, and the menisci. (From Moore, Dalley AF II. *Clinical Oriented Anatomy.* 4th ed. Baltimore, MD: Lippincott Williams & Wilkins; 1999.)

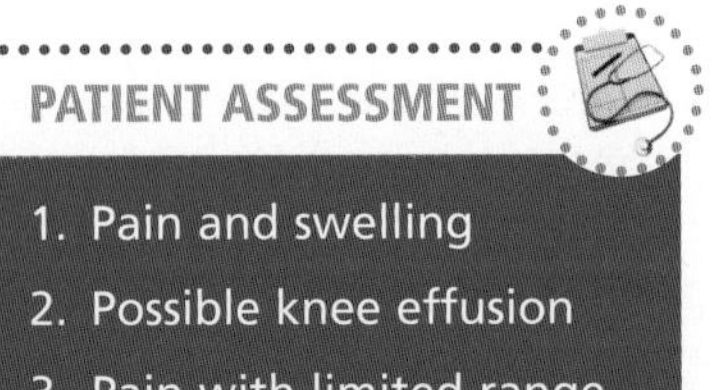

PATIENT ASSESSMENT

1. Pain and swelling
2. Possible knee effusion
3. Pain with limited range of motion
4. Antalgic gait

NOT TO BE MISSED

- Knee contusion
- Patella fracture
- Terrible triad: ACL, medial meniscus tear, and medial collateral ligament instability
- Segond fracture
- Septic joint (warm, red, and tender)
- Gout
- Rheumatoid arthritis
- Psoriatic arthritis

Standard tests for a medial or lateral menisci tear may be pain limited. A McMurray test is performed by stabilizing the knee with one hand and the lower extremity with the other. The knee is flexed and then externally rotated. Next, the knee is gradually straightened. Pain at the medial joint line that occurs either with external rotation or while the externally rotated leg is straightened is considered positive for a medial meniscus tear. Pain at the lateral joint line with internal rotation indicates a lateral meniscus tear. In addition, the Apley compression test may be positive. The patient lies face down, and the examiner places both hands around the ankle region and applies downward pressure. Pain with compression indicates a torn meniscus. (Patients with a torn meniscus also have trouble squatting.) It should be noted that in a patient with a large effusion with a tibial plateau fracture, the standard stability tests are limited by marked swelling, pain-limited range of motion, apprehension, and guarding. In these instances, cross-table lateral radiographs may be helpful. If there is a large effusion or if the patient exhibits a fat-blood interface (looks like an air–fluid level), then the examiner should suspect intra-articular pathology such as a condylar fracture, a fracture of the median eminence, or a torn cruciate ligament.

Anterior or posterior cruciate tears are assessed by performing a Lachman or an anterior posterior drawer test. A Lachman test is performed with the patient supine with the knee flexed to 20–30 degrees. One hand is placed above the knee, and the other hand is placed below the knee. An anterior translation of the tibial plateau indicates an acute ACL tear, whereas a posterior translation of the tibial plateau indicates a posterior cruciate ligament tear. An anterior and posterior drawer test, which is less sensitive, is similar to a Lachman test except that it is performed with the knee flexed to 90 degrees. The examiner sits near the patient's foot and grasps the upper calf muscles with both hands. With the thumbs placed over the knee, the examiner checks for anterior or posterior translation of the tibial plateau. A positive test should always be compared with the opposite side.

To evaluate an ACL injury, a pivot shift test can also be used. It is performed with the patient supine. First, the examiner applies inward pressure at the knee. Second, he or she flexes the knee. With an acute ACL tear, there is an anterior translation (i.e., forward displacement) of the tibial plateau between 20 and 40 degrees of flexion. The displaced tibia should snap back into place past 40 degrees.

In addition, it is vital to check the popliteal, dorsal pedis, and posterior pulses, as well as the extremity for coldness or pallor. It should be noted that in darker-skinned patients, pallor may not be exhibited. Sensation should also be evaluated and be documented. Compartment syndromes may follow and are characterized by marked swelling of the knee or the lower extremity. Careful and thorough documentation is essential. Finally, a serious injury to the lateral tibial condyle may be associated with a fibular head fracture. Damage to this region may result in a peroneal palsy. Patients have trouble dorsiflexing the ankle (lifting the ankle upward against gravity).

Radiographic Evaluation

It is necessary to obtain anteroposterior (AP), lateral (frog leg) (Fig. 15.2), and oblique views (two). Optional radiographic views include the following:

- Sunrise view
- Merchant view
- Intercondylar (tunnel) view (allows for better visualization of the intercondylar fossa)

Most bumper fractures are caused by an outside force that is directed inward. The valgus force (from outside inward) causes the fracture of the lateral tibial plateau. Severe forces may result in disruption of the medial collateral ligament and the ACL as well as a torn lateral meniscus. The lateral meniscus tear is caused by a disrupted tibia plateau from the valgus force. Valgus forces may produce the "unhappy triad of O'Donoghue." This second type of injury is characterized by a disrupted medial collateral ligament, a torn ACL, and a torn medial meniscus. The medial meniscus is closely attached to the medial collateral ligament. A large valgus force can disrupt both the closely attached structures.

The examiner should look for Segond fractures. A Segond fracture is a small displaced fracture (like a small fleck) of the lateral tibia condyle. It is usually identified on the AP view. Unless an examiner is specifically looking for Segond fractures, he or she may easily miss them. They are associated with ACL tears in many cases.

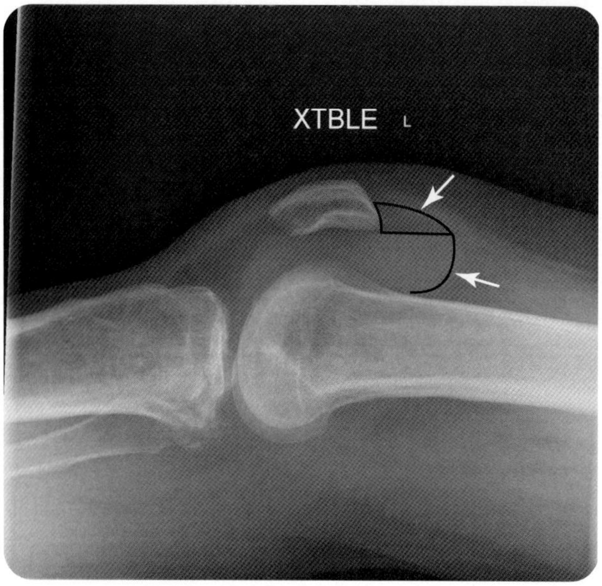

In most patients, computed tomography (CT) reveals what is seen on conventional radiography. However, CT is critical for formulating a plan for surgical treatment of some fractures (Fig. 15.3). The role of magnetic resonance imaging (MRI) is currently being studied. MRI is an excellent technique for the evaluation of soft tissue injuries that may accompany a tibial plateau fracture, especially the unhappy triad.

XTBLE L

Figure 15.2 A lipohemarthrtosis layers in the suprapatellar knee joint on the cross-table lateral view of the left knee related to an acute, comminuted fracture through the lateral tibial plateau extending to the articular surface. ⊕: A fat blood interface.

Treatment

Initial treatment for tibial plateau fractures includes immobilization of the injured knee and limb in a brace and application of a soft compression dressing. Nonoperative treatment is often indicated for nondisplaced or minimally displaced fractures and includes immobilization and non–weight-bearing ambulation. Patients should not put any weight on the knee for several weeks. Partial weight-bearing is often initiated 8 to 12 weeks after the fracture. When the fracture becomes more stable, physical therapy is begun to optimize the range of motion and strengthen the muscles in the injured limb. How quickly

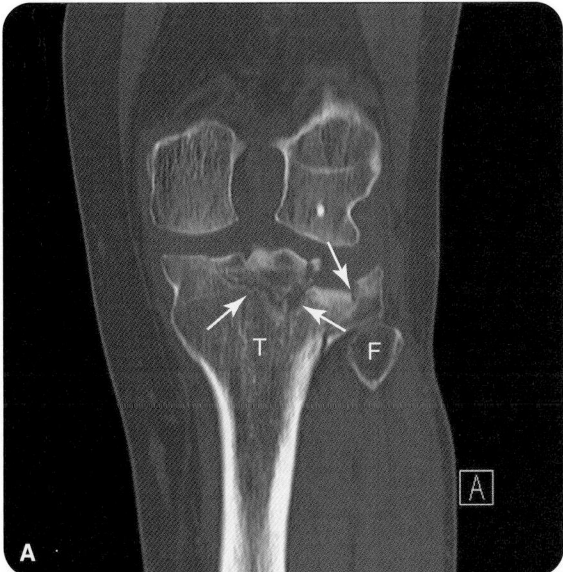

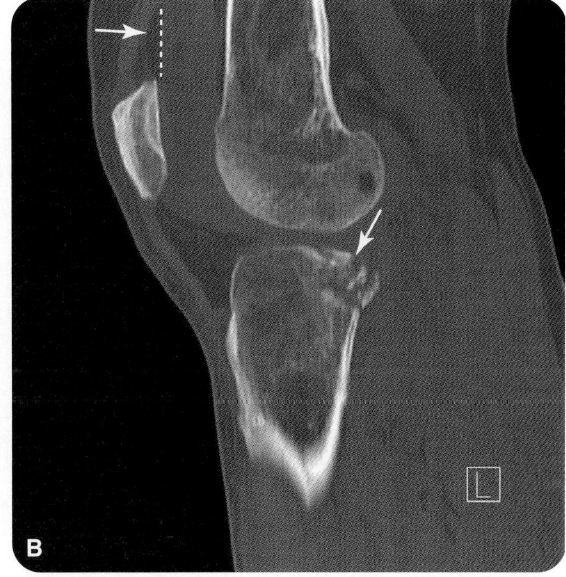

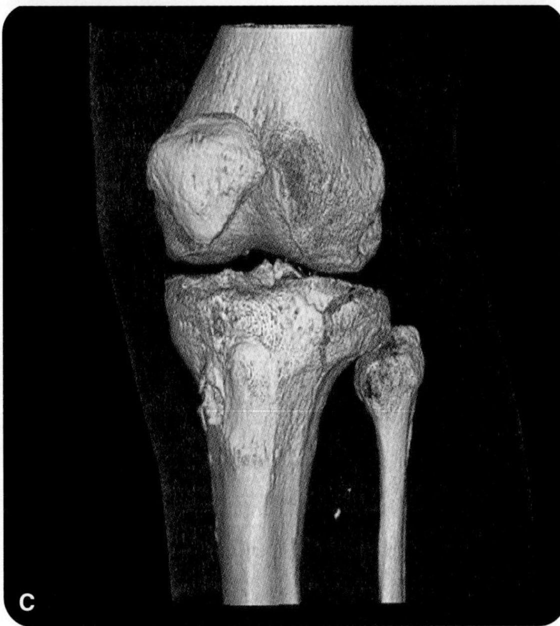

Figure 15.3 **(A)** Coronal and **(B)** sagittal reformatted images and **(C)** three-dimensional reconstructed image from the patient in the introductory case. The computed tomography scan enables the clinician to appreciate the complexity and relationship of the fracture fragments in multiple planes. This allows for accurate surgical planning without surprises in the operating room.

nonoperative healing may progress depends on the fracture pattern. Patients with tense, painful knee effusions (hemarthrosis) may also benefit from arthrocentesis.

Displaced fractures and depressions of the joint surface may require surgical intervention that includes open reduction, internal fixation, with possible bone grafting, followed by early range-of-motion exercises. Many studies address the cutoff between nonoperative and operative treatment. The range of articular depression that can be accepted ranges from 2 mm to 1 cm. The ultimate goal for obtaining a healthy joint is to obtain a congruent joint surface and is why the surgeons obtain a CT. The basic principles for operative treatment of tibial plateau fractures are restoration of the articular surface and reestablishment of tibial alignment. Surgery often involves buttressing of the elevated articular segments and bone grafting. Fracture fixation can be achieved with screws alone, plates and screws, or external fixation devices.

WHEN TO REFER

- Open fractures, massive effusions, locked knees, compartment syndromes, or neurovascular compromise (immediate referral)
- Acute peroneal palsy (immediate referral)

Numerous complications can occur as a result of nonoperative and as well as operative treatment. These complication rates range from 10% to 54%. Most nonoperative complications are related to immobilization and recumbency. These complications include thromboembolic disease, pneumonia and a stiff knee. Patients with fractured knees that heal in a nonanatomic position are at risk for posttraumatic arthritis.

Suggested Readings

Barrow BA, Fagan WA, Parker L, Albert MJ. Tibial plateau fractures: evaluation with MR imaging. *Radiographics.* 1994;14:553–557.

Berkson EM, Virkus WW. High-energy tibial plateau fractures. *J Am Acad Orthop Surg.* 2006;14:20–23

Capps GW, Hayes CW. Easily missed injuries around the knee. *Radiographics.* 1994;14:1191–1210.

Colletti P, Greenberg H, Terk MR. MR findings in patients with acute tibial plateau fractures. *Comput Med Imaging Graph.* 1996;20(5):389–394.

Jensen DB, Rude C, Daas B, Bjerg-Nielson A. Tibial plateau fractures: a comparison of conservative and surgical treatment. *J Bone Joint Surg Br.* 1990;72(1):49–52.

Kode L, Lieberman JM, Motta AV, et al. Evaluation of tibial plateau fractures: efficacy of MRI imaging compared to CT. *AJR Am J Roentgenol.* 1994;163:141–147

Koval KJ, Helfet DL. Tibial plateau fractures: evaluation and treatments. *J Am Acad Orthop Surg.* 1995;3:86–94.

Musahl I, Tarkin P, Kobbe C, Trioupis C, Siska PA, Pape HC. Trends and techniques in open reduction and internal fixation of fractures of the tibial plateau. *J Bone Joint Surg Br.* 2009;91(4):426–433.

Mustonven AO, Koivikko M, Lindahl J, Koskiven SK. MRI of acute meniscal injury associated with tibial plateau fractures: prevalence, type, and location. *AJR Am J Roentgenol.* 2008;191(4):1002–1009.

Newberg AH, Greenstein R. Radiographic evaluation of tibial plateau fractures. *Radiology.* 1978;126:319–323.

Raffii M, Firooznia H, Golimbu C, Bonano J. Computed tomography of tibial plateau fractures. *AJR Am J Roentgenol.* 1984;142(6):1181–1186.

CHAPTER 16

Tibial Spine Fractures

George M. Bridgeforth and John Cherf

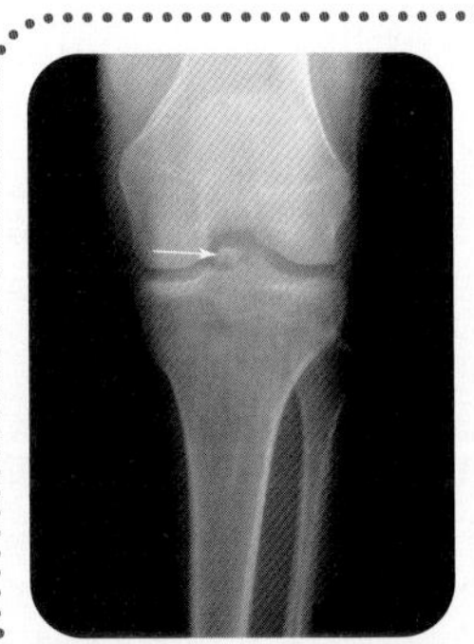

A 20-year-old intoxicated woman complains of marked pain, swelling, and tenderness after her left knee strikes the dashboard in a motor vehicle accident. She has trouble flexing this knee and complains of marked pain on standing and walking.

Clinical Presentation

Tibial spine (intercondylar) fracture is a fracture of the median eminence, which is one of two bony moundlike elevations at the proximal surface of the tibia. Structural damage to the tibial spine is commonly associated with cruciate ligament injuries. These fractures are generally caused by an anterior-to-posterior, high-impact, forces that are directed against a flexed knee, such as motor vehicle accidents and contact sports injuries. Symptoms include pain-limited range of motion, with an inability to flex or extend the knee, and reluctance to bear weight. Marked swelling of the affected knee is also evident.

Like all traumatic knee injuries it is essential that a thorough neurovascular examination of the extremity be conducted. The extremity should be examined carefully for pallor, although this feature may not be readily apparent in dark-skinned individuals. However, if the patient is coherent, he or she may complain of coldness or numbness. In addition, it is essential to check the popliteal, dorsalis pedis, and posterior tibial pulses. The popliteal pulse may be checked by placing the four fingers of each hand and palpating firmly at the center of popliteal fossa (i.e., back of the knee). The dorsal pedis pulse is located with four fingers by palpation along the medial border of the extensor hallucis longus tendon in the forefoot. The posterior tibial pulses are located by placing four fingers behind the medial malleolus near its base.

Marked swelling of the knee or lower extremity, coupled with diminished (or absent) pulses, diffuse motor weakness, and sensory impairment represents either severe neurovascular damage or secondary damage from a compartment syndrome. With a compartment syndrome, there is markedly elevated pressure and swelling inside the lower extremity, which impairs the vascular supply to the muscles and the nerves. Untreated, it can cause permanent neurological damage and, in severe cases, result in amputation of the extremity.

Septic joints that are very warm, erythematous (red), and tender do not usually follow acute traumatic injuries. However, they may be caused by open wounds in patients seen for the first time 1 or 2 days after the injury. Septic joints, with or without open wounds, should undergo an immediate diagnostic aspiration.

CLINICAL POINTS

- High-impact injuries are the usual cause of these fractures.
- With a large effusion, guarding and apprehension, which may make stability tests difficult to perform, are common.
- Associated internal derangement, especially tears of the anterior or posterior cruciate ligaments, may occur (Fig. 16.1).

PATIENT ASSESSMENT

1. Pain, with limited range of motion
2. Marked tenderness
3. Swelling
4. Antalgic gait (limp)

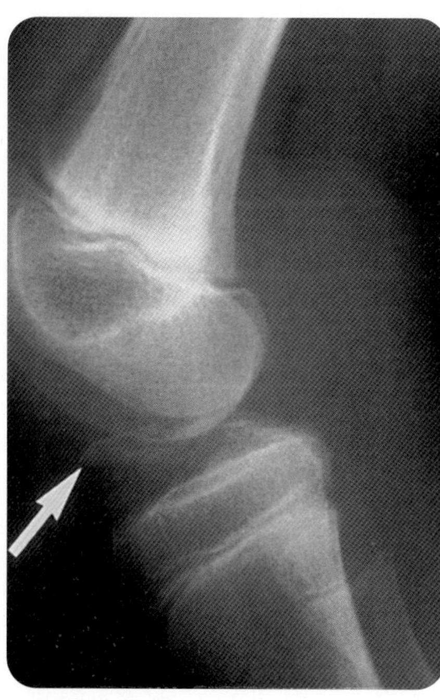

Figure 16.1 Avulsion fracture of the tibial spine in a 9-year-old girl. A significant hemarthrosis was present and was aspirated. In an adult, the same mechanism of injury would have resulted in a tear of the anterior cruciate ligament. (From Fleisher GR. *Textbook of Pediatric Emergency Medicine.* 5th ed. Philadelphia, PA: Lippincott Williams & Wilkins; 2005.)

Radiographic Evaluation

Tests to order include anteroposterior, lateral, and (two) oblique views (Figs. 16.2a and 2b). (Two oblique radiographs may be used as part of a full trauma series, especially with high-impact injuries, to check for condylar fractures.) Optional tests include the following:

- Sunrise view: used to detect subtle fractures and dislocations of the patella
- Merchant view: used to detect subtle fractures and dislocations of the patella. It is more sensitive than a sunrise view. It is preferred by many orthopedic specialists.
- Intercondylar view: allows for better visualization of the tibia spine for the detection of tibial spine fractures

According to the Harris classification system, there are three types of tibial spine (intercondylar) fractures (Fig. 16.3). Type I fractures are nondisplaced or demonstrate minimal displacement. Type II fractures show a "hinge"-like elevation, which is generally seen in the anterior compartment on the lateral view. Type III fractures are characterized by a displacement of the tibial spine. With a suspected injury to the tibial spine, an intercondylar view allows for better visualization of the tibial spine. Internal and external oblique radiographs may help detect a neighboring condylar fracture.

With tibial spine injuries, where patients usually have trouble bending the markedly swollen knee, the addition of a cross-table lateral radiograph may be extremely useful. The presence of a fat–blood interface or lipohemarthrosis (i.e., it looks like an air–fluid level) inside the knee is strongly associated with intra-articular fractures or an internal

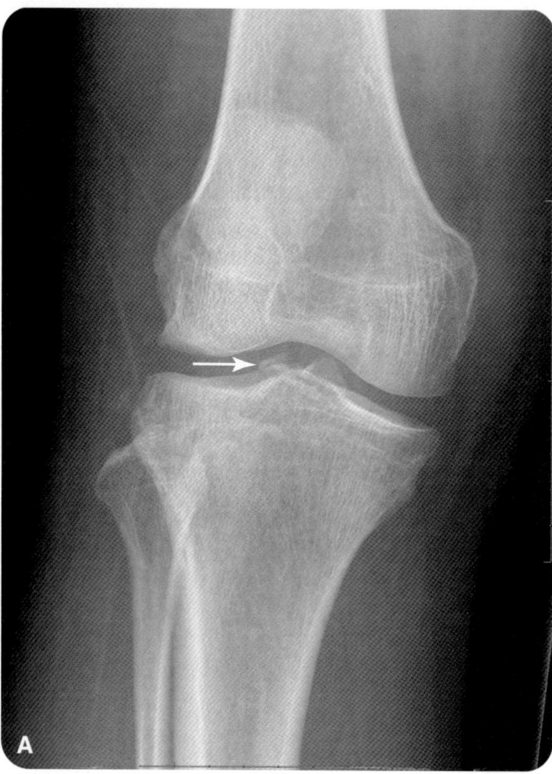

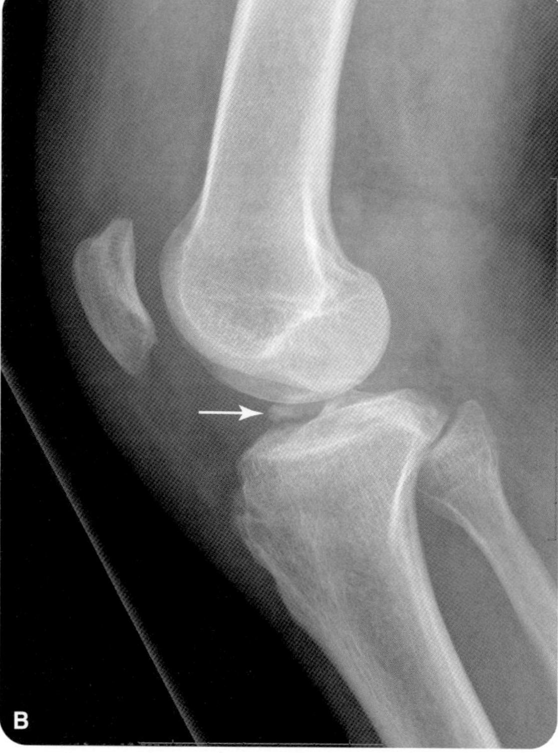

Figure 16.2 **(A)** Anteroposterior and **(B)** lateral radiographs of the left knee, demonstrating an acute fracture of the lateral tibial spine.

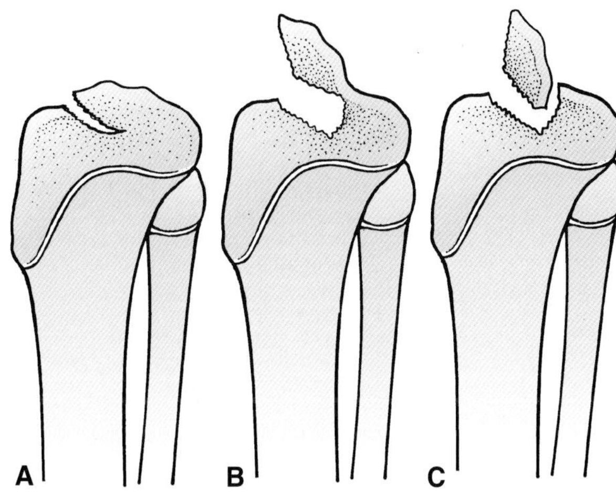

Figure 16.3 Classification of tibial spine fractures. **(A)** Type I, minimal displacement. **(B)** Type II, hinged posteriorly. **(C)** Type III, complete separation. (From Bucholz RW, Heckman JD, Court-Brown C, et al., eds. *Rockwood and Green's Fractures in Adults*. 6th ed. Philadelphia, PA: Lippincott Williams & Wilkins; 2006.)

NOT TO BE MISSED

- Knee contusion
- Knee fracture with or without internal derangement
- Acute anterior cruciate ligament tear
- Quadriceps (or patella) ligament tear
- Cellulitis
- Septic arthritis

derangement in approximately 75% of cases. It should prompt further evaluation of the knee. Although a computed tomography scan provides slightly better sensitivity for occult fractures, a magnetic resonance imaging scan may be used to detect occult fractures as well as internal derangement to the cruciate ligaments, the menisci (cartilage), or the surrounding collateral ligaments.

Treatment

The treatment of tibial spine fractures is largely determined by the degree of fracture displacement. Immobilization is used for undisplaced and minimally displaced fractures. Immobilization with a cast or brace or closed reduction may be sufficient. Knee extension may reduce anterior tibial spine fractures that are hinged posteriorly. With nonoperative techniques, repeat radiographs are necessary to ensure that there is no progressive fracture displacement. Completely separated fractures and posteriorly hinged fractures that are not reduced require surgical intervention, which involves reducing the fracture and may necessitate fixation. Operative techniques include open reduction with immobilization, open reduction with internal fixation, arthroscopic reduction with immobilization, and arthroscopic reduction with wire or screw fixation.

The prognosis with effective treatment is very good. Most fractures heal with an excellent functional outcome despite the presence of possible subtle residual knee laxity.

When tibial spine fractures occur in children, care must be taken to ensure patient compliance with all treatment options. Potential complications in children include nonunion, malunion, arthrofibrosis, and growth disturbances.

WHEN TO REFER

All patients should be referred, especially those with the following conditions:

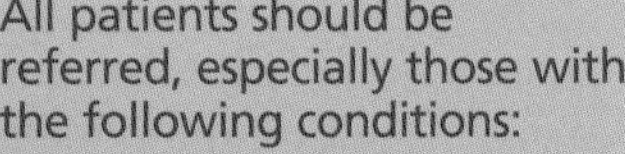

- Massive effusions
- Open fractures
- Locked knee joints
- Neurovascular compromise (damage to the popliteal, dorsal pedis, or posterior tibial arteries).

Suggested Readings

Ahmad CS, Shubin Stein BE, Jeshuran W, Nercessian OR, Henry JH. Anterior cruciate ligament function after tibial eminence fracture in skeletally mature patients. *Am J Sports Med*. 2001;29:339–345.

Johnson MW. Acute knee effusions: a systematic approach to diagnosis. *Am Fam Physician*. 2000;61: 2391–2400.

Kaplan PA, Walker CW, Kilcoyne RF, et al. Occult fracture patterns of the knee associated with anterior cruciate ligament tears: assessment with MR imaging. *Radiology*. 1992;183:835–838.

Kogan M, Marks P, Amendola A. Technique for arthroscopic suture fixation of displaced tibial intercondylar eminence fractures. *Arthroscopy*. 1997;13(3):301–306.

Meyers M, McKever F. Fracture of the intercondylar eminence of the tibia. *J Bone Joint Surg.* 1959;41:209–222.
Palmer WE, Levine SM, Dupuy DE. Knee and shoulder fractures: association of fracture detection and marrow edema on MR images with mechanism of injury. *Radiology.* 1997;204:395–401.
Prince JS, Laor T, Bean JA. MRI of anterior cruciate ligament injuries and associated findings in the pediatric knee: changes with skeletal maturation. *AJR Am J Roentgenol.* 2005;185:756–762.
Rademaker MV, Kerkhuffs GM, Kager J, et al. Tibial spine fractures: a long-term follow-up study of open reduction and internal fixation. *J Orthop Trauma.* 2009;23(3):203–207.
Shearman C, El-Khoury GY. Pitfalls in the radiologic evaluation of extremity trauma, II: the lower extremity. *Am Fam Physician.* 1998;57:995–1002.
Toyhyama H, Kutsumi K, Yasuda K. Avulsion fracture at the femoral attachment of the anterior cruciate ligament after intercondylar eminence fracture of the tibia. *Am J Sports Med.* 2002;30(2)279–282.

CHAPTER 

Degenerative Joint Disease (Osteoarthritis)

George M. Bridgeforth and John Cherf

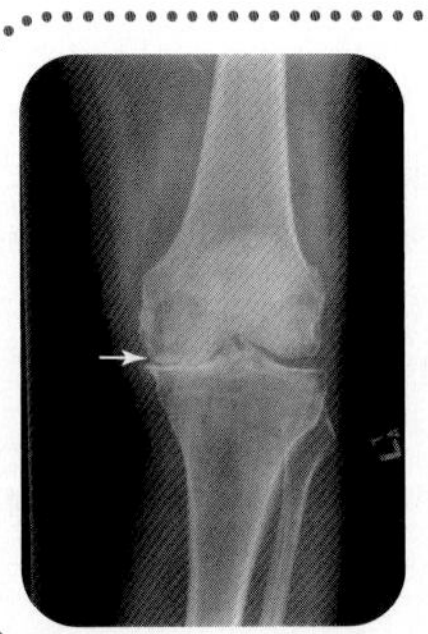

A 87-year-old man presents with left knee swelling and pain, which he has had for several months.

Clinical Presentation

The clinical hallmark of degenerative joint disease, or osteoarthritis (OA), is hypertrophy with decreased range of motion. Mild swelling is common, and stiffness and soreness may be present. Patients sometimes describe the pain as an intense ache, and they may also complain that their knees creak or even "lock." Degenerative joint disease has a predilection for the knees, hips, spine, and the small joints of the hands. The presence of other joint deformities characteristic of OA, such as Heberden nodes (hypertrophy of the distal interphalangeal joints) in some of the fingers, may be a helpful associated finding. The most common form of arthritis, degenerative joint disease, is the leading cause of chronic disability in the United States. It predominantly affects older individuals. The **mechanism of injury** is a degenerative process, and the condition develops our time.

The historical presence of locking or clicking inside of the knee is suspicious for a meniscus tear. However, locking may be caused by loose bodies or torn cartilage. The medial meniscus bears a greater load (i.e., more of the body weight), and a medial meniscus tear is more common than a lateral meniscus tear. Moreover, the medial meniscus is less mobile because it is firmly attached to the medial collateral ligaments and therefore more prone to damage from twisting injuries. Elderly patients with degenerative arthritis after develop a degenerative medial meniscus tear.

The presence of joint "mice" inside the knee may present floating loose bodies. This condition is characterized by the separation of small osteochondral body (i.e., small, usually rounded section of bone and cartilage). On a radiograph, it appears as a very small saucer-shaped defect inside the knee.

As previously stated, OA may be associated with mild to moderate swelling (Fig. 17.1). If the affected joint appears acutely warm, swollen, and tender, a diagnostic aspiration should be performed immediately. The differential diagnosis includes acute cellulitis (a neighboring open wound may serve as a portal for infection), gonorrhea, gout, rheumatoid arthritis, and psoriatic arthritis. OA is generally a bilateral condition; septic joints are usually unilateral. Treatment is directed at the underlying cause.

CLINICAL POINTS

- Swelling is often characteristic.
- Morning aching and stiffness.
- Older people are often affected.

PATIENT ASSESSMENT

1. Limited range of motion
2. Mild swelling and stiffness
3. Pain, especially with weight-bearing
4. Joint hypertrophy in later stages

NOT TO BE MISSED

- Knee contusion or fracture
- Rheumatoid arthritis (usually bilateral)
- Gout (unilateral but may be bilateral)
- Psoriatic arthritis (oligoarticular)
- Septic joint (unilateral)

Radiographic Evaluation

Radiographs that should be ordered include anteroposterior (AP), lateral, and oblique views (two). Two oblique views are used in a full trauma series to evaluate for condylar fractures of the tibial plateau. Optional views include the following:

- Sunrise view: used to check for subtle fractures and dislocations
- Merchant view: used to check for subtle fractures and dislocations. The preferred choice of many specialists, the Merchant view is superior to a sunrise view when checking for subtle fractures and dislocations.
- Cross-table lateral view: used as part of a trauma series. It is particularly useful when the patient has trouble bending the knee fully. The presence of a lipohemarthrosis indicates either an intra-articular fracture or derangement (i.e., cruciate ligament tear).
- Intercondylar view: used to better visualize the tibia spine. It is used to detect fractures of the median eminence (tibia spine).

Degenerative joint disease is frequently characterized by narrowing of the joint space (Fig. 17.2). On the AP view, it is necessary to look for narrowing of the medial joint space initially followed by early osteophyte formation at the epicondyles (i.e., the outer joint margins). Additional features may include subchondral sclerosis (sclerotic changes in the bony regions beneath the articulating cartilage). Moreover, there may be small subchondral cysts.

There are four radiographic hallmarks of degenerative joint disease. However, all of these characteristics do not have to be present in order to make a diagnosis.

- Narrowing of the joint space
- Subchondral sclerosis
- Osteophytic bone formation
- Subchondral cyst formation

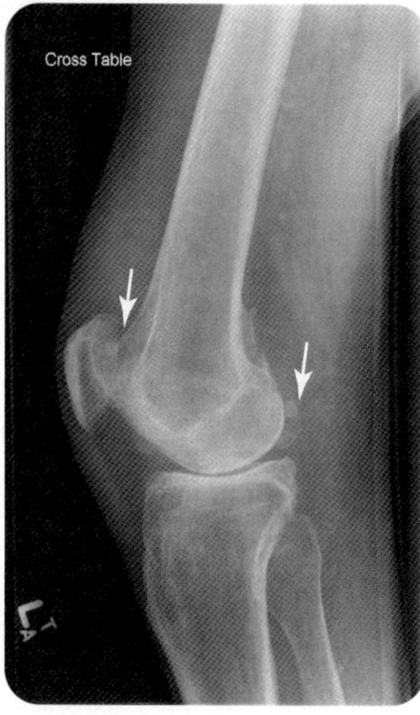

Figure 17.1 A lateral projection of the left knee, demonstrating moderate medial compartment narrowing with osteophyte formation and patellar joint space narrowing, in the patient in the introductory case. There is a suprapatellar knee joint effusion.

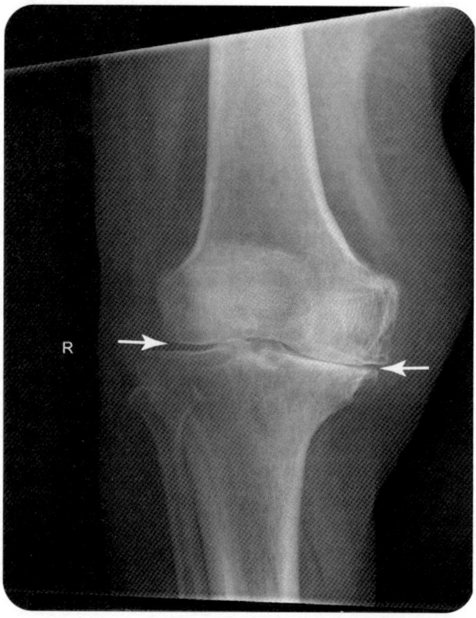

Figure 17.2 A single anteroposterior view of the right knee in a 72-year-old woman with generalized pain. There is medial and lateral knee joint compartment narrowing with spurring of the medial compartment.

Treatment

The goals of all types of treatment are pain relief and improved function. Treatment of OA varies depending on severity. It may involve exercise, manual therapy, lifestyle modification, medication, and surgical interventions. Many patients can be managed for years with conservative therapeutic methods before they undergo surgery. The timing of surgery is determined by pain, loss of function, age, body habitus, and overall health.

- Patients with early OA of the knee should be treated with conservative care, including weight loss (possible nutrition referral), soft cushioned footwear, over-the-counter nonsteroidal anti-inflammatory drugs (NSAIDs), a home exercise program (often with physical therapy referral), icing, and activity modification. Individuals who cannot tolerate NSAIDs may be treated with acetaminophen.
- Patients with moderate OA may require prescription analgesics and prescription NSAIDs, intra-articular steroid injections, and possible arthroscopy (when meniscal tears or loose bodies are present with mechanical symptoms).

Some patients with moderate to severe OA of the knee may require an osteotomy around the knee to correct deformity of the limb. This may include a proximal tibial osteotomy for a varus arthritic knee and a distal femoral osteotomy for a valgus arthritic knee. Patients with advanced OA of the knee often require some type of arthroplasty or knee replacement surgery. These reconstructive procedures require replacing all three components of the knee (total knee replacement) (Fig. 17.3). However, some patients may be candidates for a partial replacement (unicompartmental knee replacement or bicompartmental knee replacement).

Ambulatory aids are important for many patients. It should be noted that some of the many over-the-counter treatments are not backed by sound clinical research. Two recently marketed treatment modalities include viscosupplementation (joint fluid therapy) and OA bracing. Both of these methods can be expensive, and their long-term efficacy is uncertain.

WHEN TO REFER 

- Patients should be evaluated for a knee replacement when there is radiographic evidence of marked degeneration (i.e., bone on bone) and the patient has pain limited ambulation that has failed to improve with conservative care.

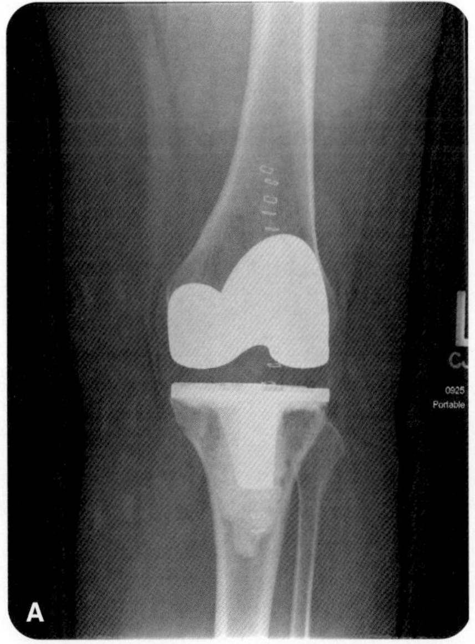

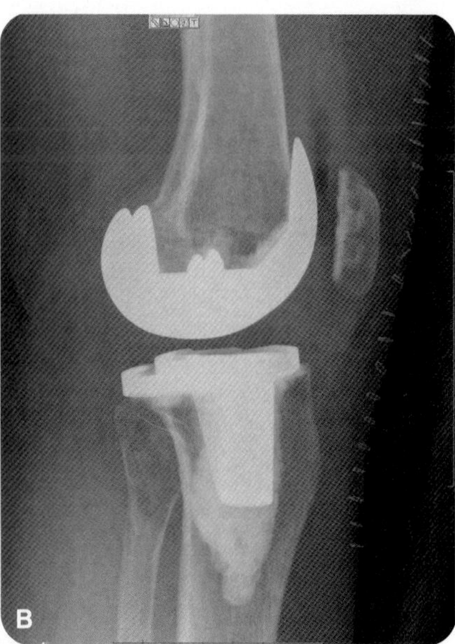

Figure 17.3 **(A)** Anteroposterior and **(B)** lateral radiographs of the left knee in a 60-year-old man with osteoarthritis of the left knee status post–total knee arthroplasty.

Suggested Readings

Buckland-Wright JC. Quantitative radiography of osteoarthritis. *Ann Rheum Dis*. 1994;53:268–275.

Calmbach WL, Hutchens M. Evaluation of patients presenting with knee pain, II: differential diagnosis. *Am Fam Physician*. 2003;68:917–922.

Chan WD, Stevens MR, Sack K, et al. Osteoarthritis of the knee: comparison of radiography, CT, and MR imaging to assess extent of severity. *AJR Am J Roentgenol*. 1991;157:799–806.

Deyle GD, Henderson NE, Matekel RL, et al. Effectiveness of manual physical therapy and exercises in osteoarthritis of the knee: a randomized, controlled trial. *Ann Intern Med*. 200;132:173–181.

Dleppe P, Basler HP, Chard J, et al. Knee replacement surgery from osteoarthritis: effectiveness practice variations, indications and possible determinants of utilization. *Rheumatology*. 1999;38:73–83.

Hunter DJ, Niu JB, Zhang Y, et al. Premorbid knee osteoarthritis is not characterised by diffuse thinness: the Framingham Osteoarthritis Study. *Ann Rheum Dis*. 2008;67(11):1545–1549.

Hunter DT, LeGraverand MP, Eckstein F. Radiologic markers of osteoarthritis progression. *Medscape Today*. http://www.medscape.com. Accessed July 9, 2009.

Kornaat P, Bloem JL, Ceulman R, et al. Osteoarthritis of the knee: association between clinical features and MR imaging findings. *Radiology*. 2006;239:811-817.

Manke NJ, Lane NE. Osteoarthritis: current concepts in diagnosis and management. *Am Fam Physician*. 2000;61:1795–1804.

Swagerty DC, Hellinger D. Radiographic assessment of osteoarthritis. *Am Fam Physician*. 2001;64:279–286.

CHAPTER 18

Osgood–Schlatter Disease

George M. Bridgeforth, Kimberly Shellcroft, and John Cherf

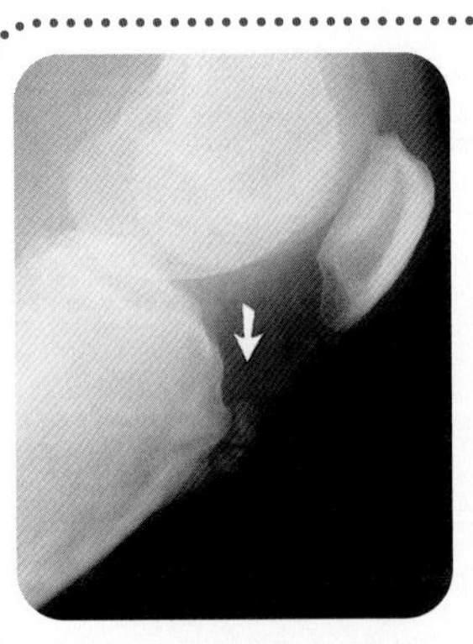

An 18-year-old man complains of pain, swelling, and soreness of the right upper tibia. The pain is worse after playing basketball and climbing stairs. (Reprinted with permission from Yochum TR, Rowe LJ. Essentials of Skeletal Radiology. *2nd ed. Baltimore, MD: Lippincott Williams & Wilkins; 1996:1291, Fig. 13.59B.)*

Clinical Presentation

Osgood–Schlatter disease is a common cause of knee pain in physically active adolescents. The disease is characterized by inflammation—pain, swelling, and tenderness—at the tibial tubercle. It is a nontraumatic condition. Patients commonly complain of pain and soreness at the tibial tubercle while climbing stairs. The tibial tubercle is the bony prominence below the patella; it is where the patella tendon is anchored. Clinical findings consist of pain, swelling, and tenderness of the tibia tubercle in an adolescent (or young adult) with normal stability tests. It is not uncommon for patients with chronic Osgood–Schlatter disease to develop a prominent tibia tubercle on one or both sides (Fig. 18.1). Approximately 25% of cases are bilateral.

CLINICAL POINTS

- The tibia tubercle(s) may appear prominent in long-standing cases.
- The disease usually begins in adolescence and resolves by adulthood.
- Symptoms may develop in association with growth spurts.

Usually, Osgood–Schlatter disease resolves by early adulthood. The condition may be aggravated by sports that involve an extensive amount of running and jumping. Traditionally, the disease was thought to be more common in adolescent boys. However, it has been increasing in adolescent girls as well since athletic programs for girls have expanded.

The differential diagnosis of Osgood–Schlatter disease includes patellar tendonitis, prepatellar bursitis, infrapatellar bursitis, torn meniscus, torn cruciate ligament, torn patellar tendon, and pes anserine bursitis. Patellar tendonitis is characterized by pain and soreness of the patellar tendon with normal stability tests. Prepatellar bursitis is characterized by spongy swelling, tenderness, and soreness over the lower patella. Infrapatellar bursitis is seen as spongy swelling, tenderness, and soreness below the inferior pole of the patella. Pes anserine bursitis, is seen as focal tenderness of the pes anserine bursa. It is approximately 2 cm below the medial joint line.

Most patients with a torn medial meniscus have trouble squatting and are not able to duckwalk (walk in a squatting position). McMurray test can be used to confirm the presence of a meniscus tear; however, the sensitivity of the test is on the order of 50% to 60%. This test is performed with the patient supine by flexing the knee and then rotating the lower leg externally. Pain occurring along the medial joint line with external rotation that follows gradually straightening of the knee is positive for a medial meniscus tear. Pain that occurs along the lateral joint line with internal rotation followed

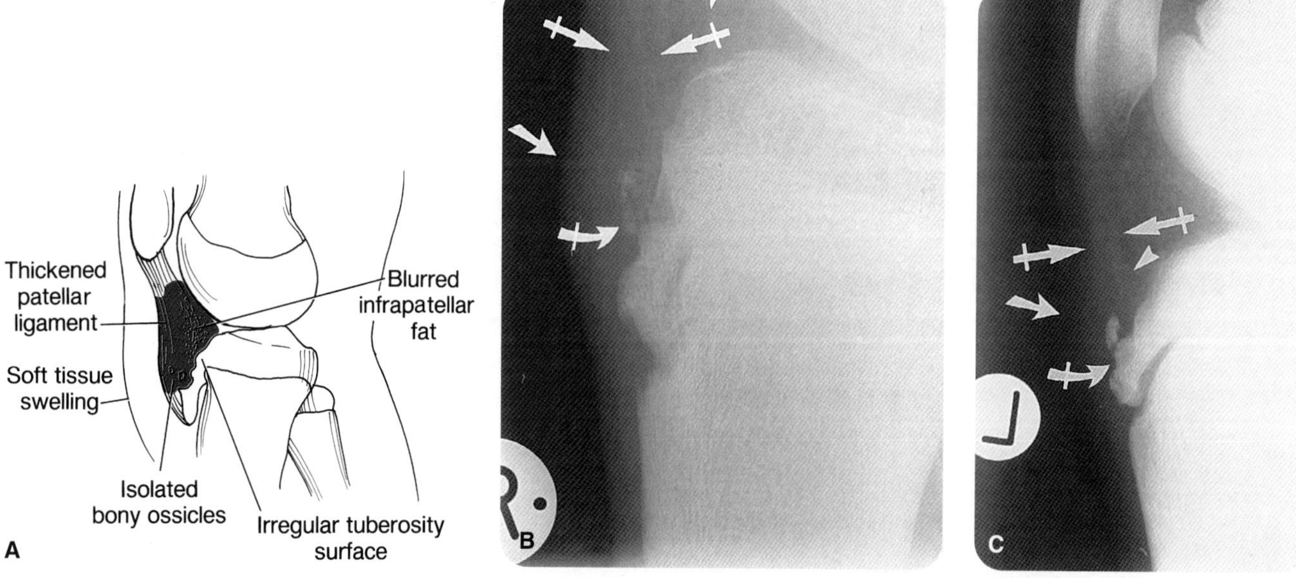

Figure 18.1 Characteristic features of Osgood–Schlatter disease. **(A)** Diagram. **(B** and **C)** Lateral knee. Observe the edema over the tibial tuberosity (*arrows*), blurred infrapatellar fat (*arrowhead*), thickened patellar ligament (*crossed arrows*), and fragmentation of the tuberosity (*curved crossed arrows*). (From Yochum TR, Rowe LJ. *Yochum and Rowe's Essentials of Skeletal Radiology*. 3rd ed. Philadelphia, PA: Lippincott Williams & Wilkins; 2004.)

by gradually straightening the knee is consistent with a lateral meniscus tear.

Patients with a torn anterior cruciate ligament (ACL) may have a positive Lachman test. This is characterized by anterior–posterior instability of the tibial plateau with knee flexed to approximately 30 degrees. It is more sensitive than an anterior–posterior drawer test, which checks for anterior–posterior instability of the tibial plateau; the examiner places both thumbs on the knee and cups the upper calf muscles with both hands. ACL tears have an anterior translation of the tibia, whereas posterior cruciate ligament tears have a posterior glide. Ligaments strains are less severe but still bothersome. Medial or collateral ligament strains are characterized by pain and soreness along the collateral ligament. Collateral ligament tears are accompanied by valgus (inward displacement of the knee) or varus (outward displacement of the knee). Valgus instability is caused by a complete tear in the medial collateral ligament, whereas varus instability is caused by a complete tear in the lateral collateral ligament.

A positive finding on either McMurray test or Lachman test should be checked by repeating the test on the opposite, normal knee. A pivot shift test (for ACL instability) is performed by applying valgus (inward pressure) at the knee with one hand while rotating the ankle medially (i.e., rotating the ankle inward toward the body. At approximately 20 degrees of flexion, the tibial plateau subluxes forward. The tibial plateau slides back into place past 40 degrees of knee flexion. A patient with a completely torn patella tendon has pain, swelling, and tenderness beneath the patella. However, there is an inability to extend the knee against gravity.

PATIENT ASSESSMENT

1. Visible lump over the tibial tuberosities
2. Knee pain that increases during activities such as running and jumping and while ascending or descending stairs
3. Pain in affected area on impact with any object

Radiographic Evaluation

Tests that should be ordered include anteroposterior, lateral, and oblique views (Fig. 18.2). Optional tests include the following:

NOT TO BE MISSED

- Knee contusion (pain, swelling, and tenderness)
- Tibial fracture (pain, swelling, and focal tenderness)
- Knee strain (swelling, collateral ligament soreness)
- Patella tendonitis (pain and tenderness of the patella tendon)
- Patellar tendon rupture (inability to extend the knee against gravity)
- Infrapatellar bursitis (swelling and tenderness of the bursa directly below the inferior pole of the patella)
- Pes anserine bursitis (focal tenderness 2.5 cm below the medial joint line)
- Sinding–Larsen–Johansson disease (a similar disorder but at the proximal patella attachment)
- Torn ACL
- Chondromalacia (grinding of the posterior surface of the patella)

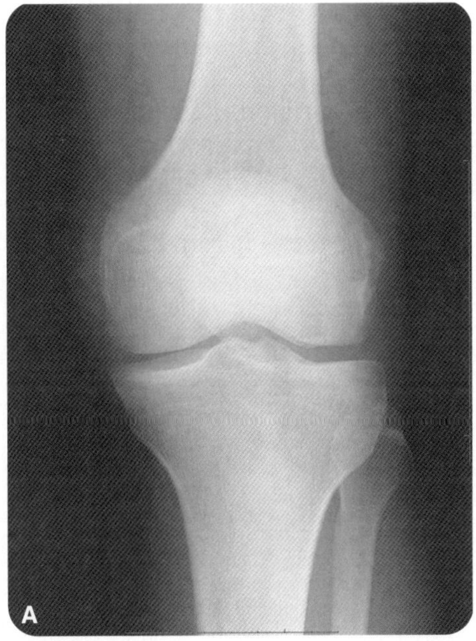

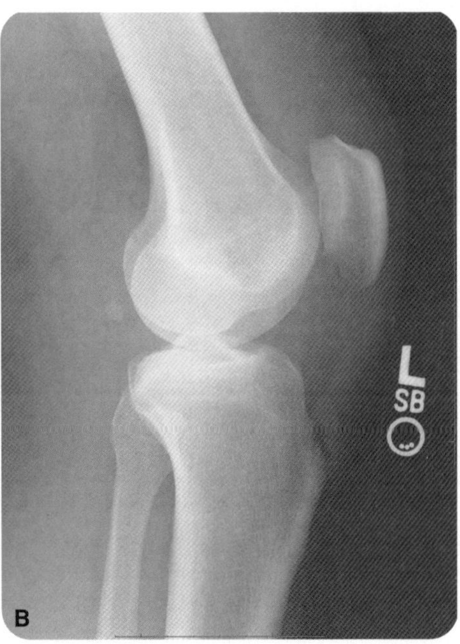

Figure 18.2 **(A)** Anteroposterior and **(B)** lateral radiographs of the knee, demonstrating Osgood–Schlatter disease.

- Full trauma series
  - Two oblique views: may be used as part of a full trauma series following high-impact collisions. The oblique views are examined to detect tibial plateau fractures.
  - Sunrise or Merchant view: for patellar dislocations and subtle fractures. A Merchant view is used by specialists and has better sensitivity for detecting subtle patella dislocations.
- Intercondylar view: used to examine the tibial spine for fractures of the median eminence

It is important to note the fragmentation and the splintering of the tibia tubercle, which is usually best appreciated on the lateral view (see Fig. 18.1). The tibia tubercles may be prominent in patients with long-standing disease. Soft tissue swelling looks like a faint haze on a radiograph. It is one way to differentiate between acute and chronic conditions. However, soft tissue swelling may be seen in other conditions as well, including contusions, fractures, and other inflammatory arthritic conditions. Generally, the absence of prominent soft tissue swelling rules out an acute fracture.

Treatment

Key elements of treatment include the following:

- Rest, ice, compression, elevation (RICE)
- Nonsteroidal anti-inflammatory drugs (NSAIDs) for pain
- Strengthening and stretching exercises for quadriceps and hamstrings
- Soft cushion insoles and knee pads

WHEN TO REFER

- Most cases improve with conservative treatment.
- Referral may be considered for cases that do not improve after 4 to 6 weeks of physical therapy.

In many cases, Osgood–Schlatter disease is a self-limiting condition that can be managed with conservative treatment. Rest is essential to provide pain relief and allow for proper healing. Mild cases require the patient to limit activities that cause pain, ice the affected area, and take an NSAID for pain relief. Severe symptoms unrelieved by conservative measures may require more extended breaks from activity, with gradual return to activity over several

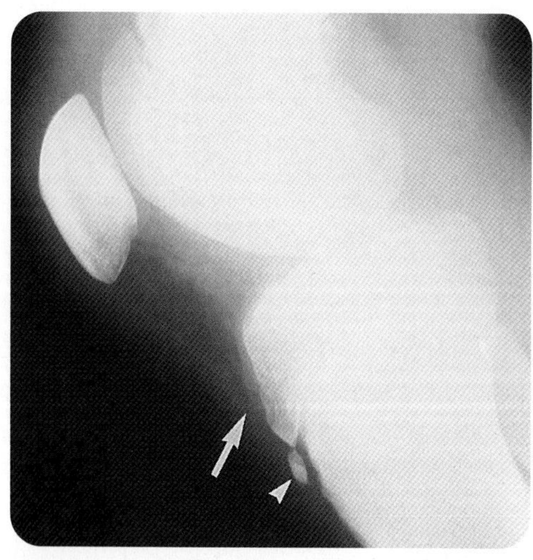

Figure 18.3 Osgood–Schlatter disease: inactive phase. Lateral knee. Note the ossicle at the tibial tuberosity (*arrowhead*), which may coalesce and disappear in adulthood, in this 12-year-old patient with previous Osgood–Schlatter disease. The sharp infrapatellar inferior angle is normal and indicates a lack of adjacent soft tissue edema (*arrow*). (From Yochum TR, Rowe LJ. *Yochum and Rowe's Essentials of Skeletal Radiology*. 3rd ed. Philadelphia, PA: Lippincott Williams & Wilkins; 2004.)

months thereafter. Soft cushion insoles and knee pads can be used when the patient returns to activity to decrease stress on the knee and protect the affected area. Physical therapy (e.g., quadriceps-strengthening exercises) may be necessary. Rarely, patients with Osgood–Schlatter disease may require bracing or casting if they are unwilling to follow activity restrictions. Symptoms that are chronic and refractory to conservative management may require referral for surgical treatment.

Preventive measures include stretching and strengthening exercises of the quadriceps and hamstrings. Strengthening exercises should primarily focus on maintaining strength rather than increasing strength. Symptoms can wax and wane over 12 to 24 months and commonly resolve when bones mature (Fig. 18.3).

Suggested Readings

Bowers KD. Patellar tendon avulsion as a complication of Osgood-Schlatter's disease. *Am J Sports Med*. 1981;9(6):356–359.

Kujula U. Osgood–Schlatter's disease in adolescent athletes. *Am J Sports Med*. 1985;13(4):236–241.

Ogden JA, Tross RB, Murphy MJ. *J Bone Joint Surg*. 1980;62:205–215.

Scotti DM, Sadhu V, Helmberg F, O'Hara AE. Osgood-Schlatter's disease: an emphasis on tissue changes in roentgen diagnosis. *Skeletal Radiol*. 1979;4(1):21–25.

Woolfrey BF, Chandler ET. Manifestations of Osgood-Schlatter's disease in late teenagers and early adulthood. *J Bone Joint Surg*. 1960;42:327–369.

CHAPTER 19

Bipartite Patella

George M. Bridgeforth and John Cherf

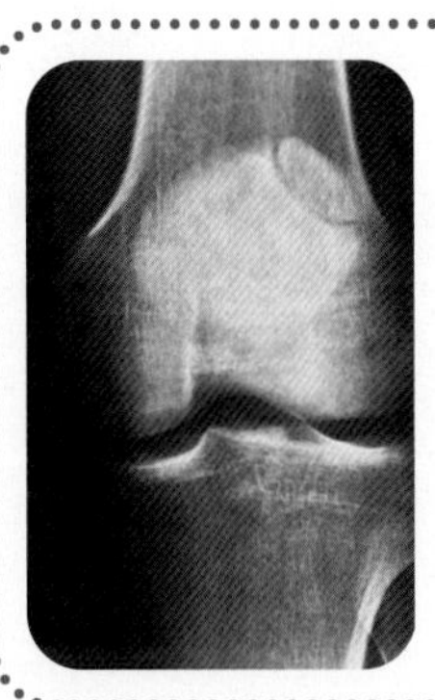

A 26-year-old man fell and bruised his right knee. He now complains of pain, swelling, and tenderness. (From Bucholz RW, Heckman JD. Rockwood & Green's Fractures in Adults. *5th ed. Philadelphia, PA: Lippincott Williams & Wilkins; 2001.)*

Clinical Presentation

Bipartite patella is a congenital condition in which the patella is actually two separate bones, not one, as is usually the case. The cause is incomplete fusion of the ossification centers of the patella. Generally, individuals do not know that they have the disorder. Most cases are asymptomatic; incidental findings on radiographs confirm the presence of the condition. At least 1% of people are affected, and the reported incidence may be as high as 6%. The condition is nine times more common in men than in women and is usually unilateral.

A bipartite patella rarely causes pain and functional limitations that require treatment. Direct trauma to the patella or repetitive injury may trigger symptoms. Common manifestations include pain directly over the patella, swelling at the synchondrosis, and pain-limited range of motion of the knee.

CLINICAL POINTS

- The reported incidence of bipartite patella may be as high as 6%.
- The condition occurs more often in men.
- Most cases are bilateral.

PATIENT ASSESSMENT

1. Usually asymptomatic
2. Radiographic finding
3. Knee pain following trauma or overuse

Radiographic Evaluation

It is necessary to order anteroposterior (AP), lateral, and oblique views. Optional radiographs include the following:

- Full trauma series (for serious traumatic injuries)
- Oblique views (two): used on a full trauma series to assess for condylar fractures
- Sunrise or Merchant view: used to check for subtle patella dislocations and vertical patella fractures (Fig. 19.1). A Merchant view is more sensitive for detecting patella subluxations.
- Intercondylar view: used to check for tibial spine and tibial plateau fractures

Usually, a bipartite patella appears as a large rounded bone fragment, which is generally located in the upper outer quadrant. It is best seen on the AP view (Fig. 19.2). Occasionally, it may be misdiagnosed as a fracture. This confusion may be important for medicolegal reasons (see "Treatment"). However, unlike an acute fracture, a bipartite patella usually has smooth but parallel margins. One researcher has noted that when a bipartite patella appears as a separate bony island, it may have sclerotic margins. Another has pointed out that the pieces of a bipartite patella do not fit together exactly, like a puzzle, but that the separate bone fragments from a fracture do appear to fit together like the pieces of a puzzle.

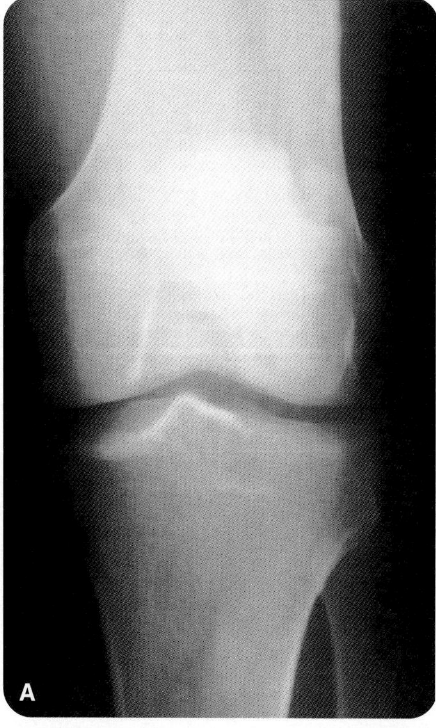

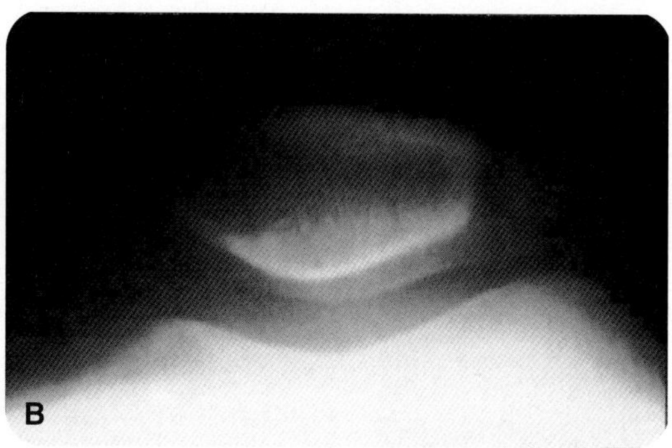

Figure 19.1 Radiographic appearance of a bipartite patella on anteroposterior **(A)** and Merchant **(B)** views of the knee. (Courtesy of Dr. Rebecca Loredo.) (From Bucholz RW, Heckman JD. *Rockwood & Green's Fractures in Adults*. 5th ed. Philadelphia, PA: Lippincott Williams & Wilkins; 2001.)

NOT TO BE MISSED

- Patella fracture
- Knee contusion
- Degenerative osteoarthritis
- Septic joint (marked inflammation)
- Prepatellar bursitis (mild swelling, tenderness patella bursa)
- Patellar tendonitis (soreness of the patella tendon, antalgic gait)
- Ruptured patella/ quadriceps tendon (inability to extend the knee against gravity)
- Chondromalacia (grinding of the posterior surface of the patella)

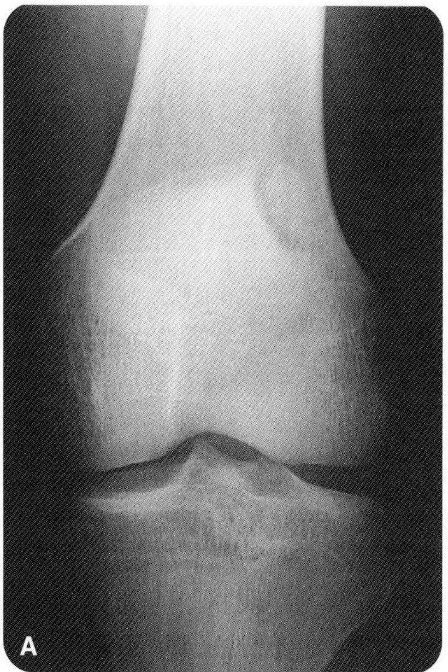

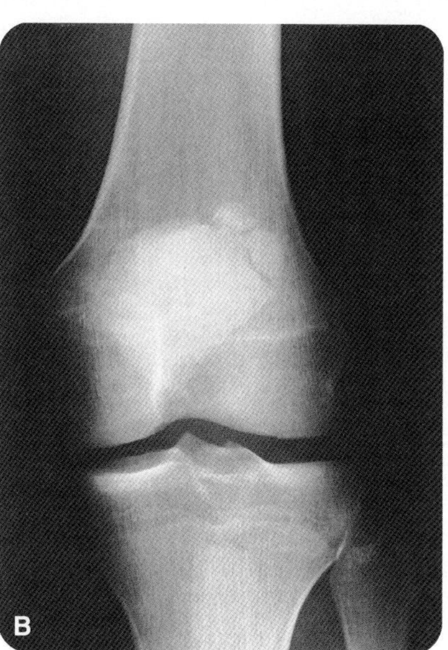

Figure 19.2 Patella, ossification abnormalities. **(A)** Bipartite patella, anteroposterior knee. Observe the smoothly marginated separated segment at the upper outer pole of the patella. **(B)** Tripartite patella, anteroposterior knee. Note the two separated fragments in the same location. Bipartite and tripartite patellae almost always occur on the superolateral margin of the patella. They should not be confused with patellar fracture because fractures usually occur through the waist of the patella and do not have smooth, often sclerotic, margins. (Courtesy of Kenneth E. Yochum, DC, St. Louis, Missouri.) (From Yochum TR, Rowe LJ. *Yochum And Rowe's Essentials of Skeletal Radiology*. 3rd ed. Philadelphia, PA: Lippincott Williams & Wilkins; 2004.)

The fabella sign, another congenital finding that is also asymptomatic, involves displacement of the fabella. It is a normal variant seen in approximately 15% of the population. This sesamoid-shaped bone is found in the lateral hamstring muscle. Best appreciated on the lateral view, the bone is usually located behind the knee in the upper calf (lateral gastrocnemius). Inexperienced primary practitioners sometimes misdiagnose a displaced fabella as a fracture. It does not require treatment.

Treatment

Most patients with bipartite patella are asymptomatic and require no particular treatment. Those with symptomatic conditions usually respond to a short period of conservative, nonoperative treatment. The goal of treatment is to decrease the stress across the fibrous union of the patella. Use of rest, ice, analgesics, and sometimes anti-inflammatory medications and physical therapy are often successful. Immobilization with a knee brace may also help reduce symptoms.

Surgery is indicated in rare cases when pain persists despite a comprehensive course of conservative treatment. It involves excising the nonossified fragment or rigid fixation with bone grafting. The surgical procedure depends on the location of the fragment. If the symptomatic lesion is large, it may be treated with bone graft and open reduction and rigid internal fixation. A lateral release or detachment of the vastus lateralis insertion has also been described as a surgical option.

WHEN TO REFER

- Referral is necessary only in rare cases that do not respond to conservative treatment.

Suggested Readings

Atesok K, Doral MN, Lower J, Finsterbush A. Symptomatic bipartite patella: treatment alternatives. *J Am Acad Orthop Surg*. 2008;16(8):455–461.

Erkonen WE, Smith WL. *Radiology 101: The Basics and Fundamentals of Imaging*. Philadelphia, PA: Lippincott Williams & Wilkins; 2005:191–193.

Greenspan A. *Orthopedic Imaging*. 4th ed. Philadelphia, PA: Lippincott Williams & Wilkins; 2004:264–265.

Harris J, Harris W, Noveline R. *The Radiology of Emergency Medicine*. 3rd ed. Baltimore, MD: Lippincott Williams & Wilkins; 1993:940–943.

Mettler F. *Essentials of Radiology*. Philadelphia, PA: WB Saunders; 1996:352.

Moore KL, Dalley A. *Clinically Oriented Anatomy*. 4th ed. Philadelphia, PA: Lippincott Williams & Wilkins; 1999:537.

Rosen P, Doris PE, Barkin RM, Barkin SZ, Markovchick VJ. *Diagnostic Radiology in Emergency Medicine*. St Louis, MO: Mosby; 1992:196.

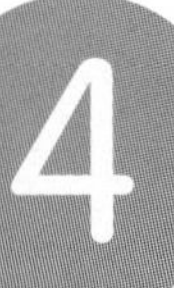

SECTION 4

Ankle

Functional Anatomy

The ankle is fascinating structure that comprises two joints, the talocrural joint and the subtalar joint. The talocrural joint is a hinge joint that is formed by the articulations of the distal fibula and tibia with the rounded dome of the talus. The dome of the talus forms a mortise-like structure with the concave surface of the distal tibia (Fig. 1). This weight-bearing structure forms a mortise joint that is supported laterally by a stirrup-like extension of the non–weight-bearing distal fibula and medially by the distal tibia.

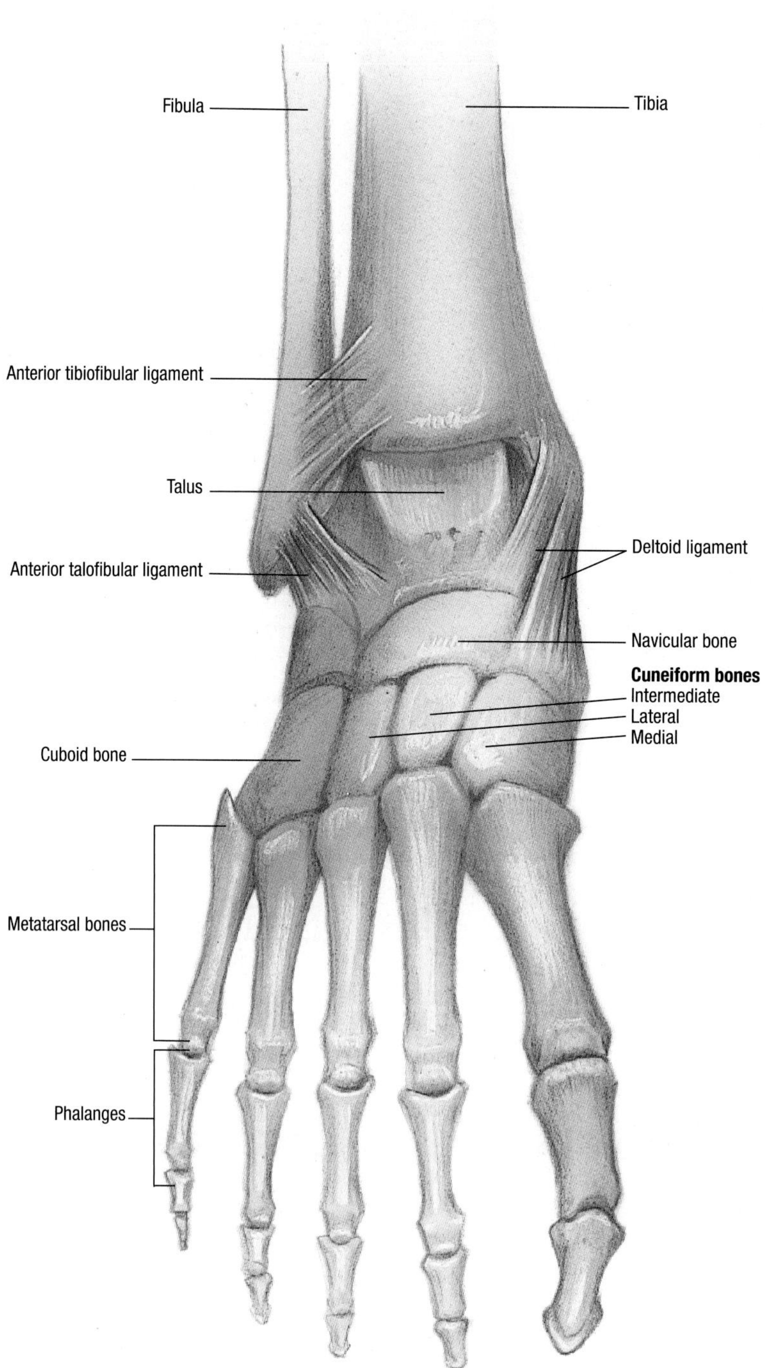

Figure 1 Ankle and foot. Frontal view. Asset provided by Anatomical Chart Co.

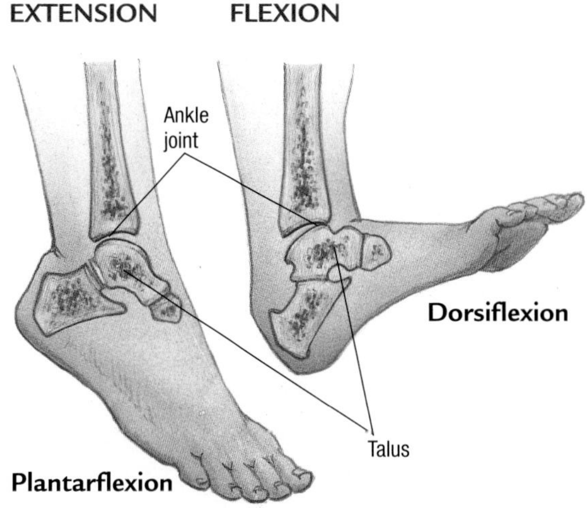

Figure 2 Extension and flexion. The muscles and tendons of the ankle joint are responsible for dorsiflexion (upward motion) and plantarflexion (downward motion) of the foot. Inversion (inward motion) and eversion (outward motion) of the foot take place in the joints below the talus. Asset provided by Anatomical Chart Co.

The distal fibula and its surrounding supporting structures form the lateral malleolus, and the distal tibia and its surrounding supporting structures form the medial malleolus. The hinge joint of the talocrural ankle mortis allows for dorsiflexion (elevation of the foot in a sagittal [i.e., up-down plane] and plantar flexion [depression of the foot in the opposite direction]) (Fig. 2). The subtalar joint is principally responsible for inversion, which is characterized by the inward movement of the forefoot in the medial direction, and eversion, which is characterized by the outward movement of the forefoot in a lateral direction.

The subtalar joint is the articulation of the base of the talus and the rostral calcaneus. Movement of the sole in an inward (medial direction) is supination, whereas movement of the sole of the foot in an outward (lateral direction) is pronation. Supination is combination of plantar flexion and ankle inversion, with medial adduction (inward motion) of the forefoot. On the other hand, pronation is a combination of dorsiflexion and ankle eversion, with lateral abduction (outward motion) of the forefoot. Supination and pronation require the joint actions of the talocrural and the subtalar joint. The subtalar joint allows the ankle to shift on uneven ground.

The surrounding supporting structures consist not only of the medial (distal tibia) and lateral (malleolus) but also of the supporting ligaments and joint capsule. The anterior talofibular ligament, the posterior talofibular ligament, and the calcaneofibular ligament form the lateral collateral ligament, which prevent excessive eversion of the ankle and joint dislocation. A very strong fanlike deltoid ligament constitutes the medial collateral ligament. The deltoid ligament actually comprises four ligaments—the anterior tibiotalar ligament, the tibionavicular ligament, the tibiocalcaneal ligament, and the posterior tibiotalar ligament. The medial collateral ligament helps prevent excessive inversion and ankle dislocations.

The distal tibiofibular syndesmotic complex, which comprises the anterior tibiofibular ligament, the posterior tibiofibular ligament, and the interosseous membrane, provides further support to anchor the distal tibia and fibula. Rotational injuries to the ankle may cause disruption of this complex and result in ankle instability.

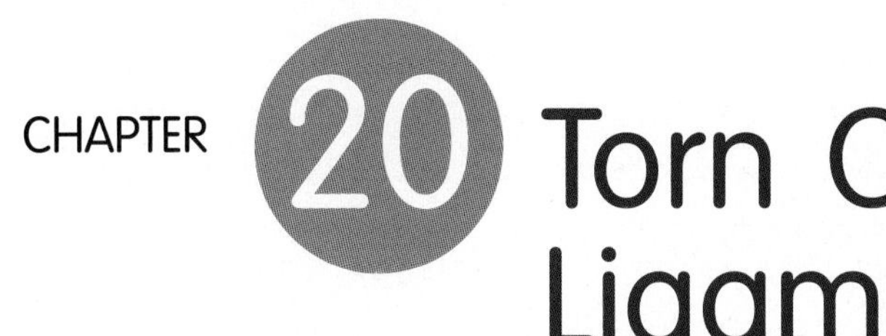

Torn Collateral Ligaments

George M. Bridgeforth and George Holmes

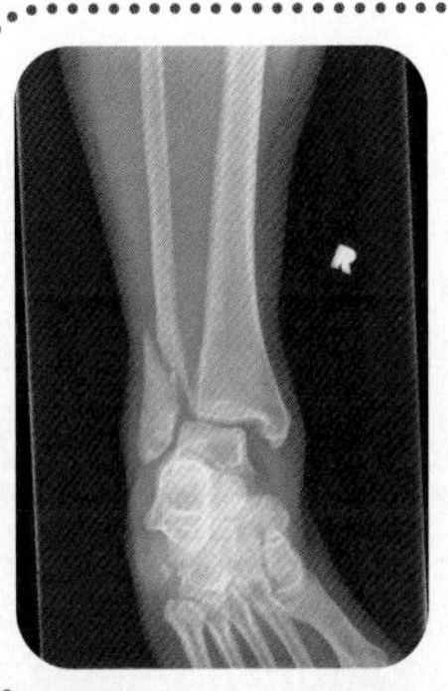

A 45-year-old woman fell. On physical examination, she has medial and lateral right ankle pain and swelling.

Clinical Presentation

Tears of the collateral ligaments of the ankle result in ankle sprains. Such tears are classified on the basis of severity. Clinically, there are three grades of ankle sprains, depending on the degree of the ligament tear (Table 20.1). Ankle ligaments are grouped into two categories—lateral collateral ligaments and medial collateral ligaments. The **mechanisms of injury** involved in tearing of collateral ligaments are as follows:

- Medial collateral ligament: ankle eversion with impact (valgus force) (Fig. 20.1)
- Lateral collateral ligament: ankle inversion with impact (varus force) (Fig. 20.2)

Patients with torn ankle ligaments complain of pain, swelling and bruising, and tenderness. Loss of functional ability, including weight-bearing, is high. Pain-limited range of motion is characteristic.

The Ottawa rules were developed by a group of Canadian emergency physicians as a set of guidelines that assist physicians in assessing ankle injuries. A concise synopsis of the Ottawa rules for foot and ankle injuries recommends that radiographs should be obtained in the following circumstances:

- There is point tenderness anywhere along the posterior aspect of the distal 6 cm of the medial or lateral malleolus.
- There is an inability to take four steps during an examination.
- There is tenderness over the navicular bone at the base of the fifth metatarsal.

The Ottawa rules have excellent sensitivity. According to many studies, the sensitivity is well more than 90% (perhaps even 100%). However, the specificity varies between 15% and 30%. In other words, if any one of the previously mentioned criteria is met, the physician should obtain radiographs. However, the complete absence of any of the Ottawa findings may not rule out an ankle fracture in selected cases. Until there is malpractice legislation to protect physicians who adhere strictly to the Ottawa rules, the individual physician is advised to use his or her own discretion.

When assessing an acute ankle injury, it is always necessary to check for tenderness of the talus and the fifth metatarsal. If there is tenderness of the

CLINICAL POINTS

- Pain-limited ambulation is characteristic.
- Heel pain (calcaneal fracture) may be present.
- Tears of collateral ligaments vary in severity.
- There may be an associated talar or fifth metatarsal (Jones vs. styloid) fracture.

Table 20.1 Acute Ankle Sprains

GRADE	DEGREE OF TEAR OF COLLATERAL LIGAMENT	CHARACTERISTICS
1	Microscopic tear(s)	Mild swelling Stable Weight-bearing
2	Partial tear	Moderate swelling Stable Limited weight-bearing
3	Complete tear	Marked swelling Unstable No weight-bearing

talus (especially with dorsiflexion) or the fifth metatarsal, then radiographs of the foot should be ordered as well. Fifth metatarsal fractures are often missed because the examiner looks only at the ankle injury. Also, the talus should be palpated, to check for talar pain with ankle dorsiflexion, which may indicate an associated talar fracture. In addition, the proximal fibula should be checked for pain and tenderness (Maisonneuve fracture or spiral fracture of the fibula that extends to the proximal fibula). This is associated with a torn distal tibiofibular syndesmotic complex. Heel pain (calcaneal fracture) is also a possibility.

The examiner should use the anterior–posterior drawer test to check for ankle instability (torn anterior tibiofibular ligament). The examiner stabilizes the ankle with one hand and cups the heel with the opposite hand, checking for forward movement of the subtalar joint. A positive test indicates a torn anterior tibiofibular ligament.

PATIENT ASSESSMENT

1. Pain, swelling, and tenderness
2. Possible fracture sites: malleolus, proximal fifth metatarsal posterior tibia, talus, proximal fibula, heel
3. Possible instability
4. Possible neurovascular impairment (cold limb with diminished or absent pulses or sensation)

Right foot — Medial view

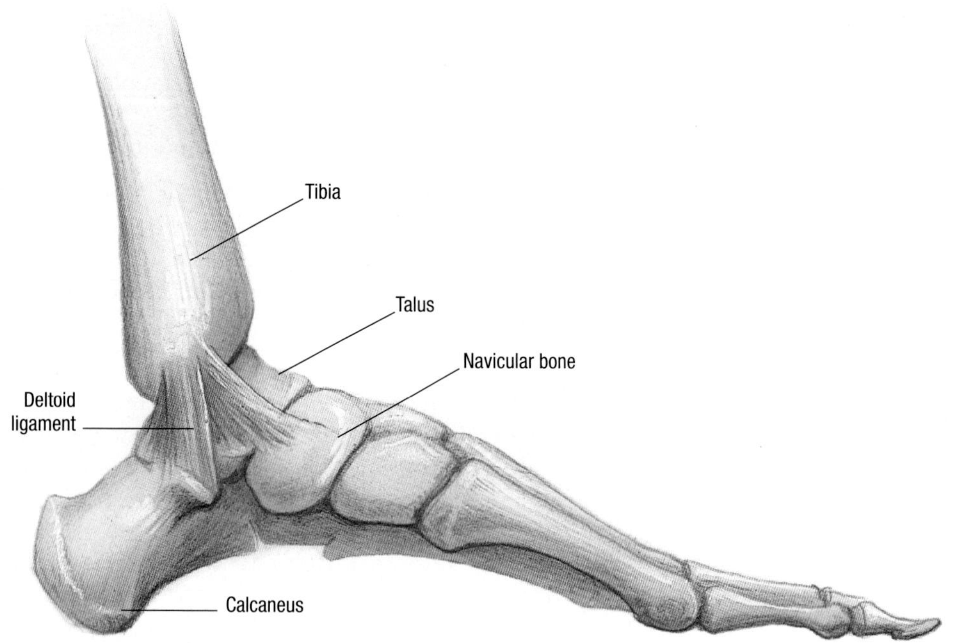

Figure 20.1 The medial collateral ligament is formed by the broad-shaped deltoid ligament. It helps prevent subluxations of the ankle during eversion. (Courtesy of the Anatomical Chart Co.)

Right foot — Lateral view

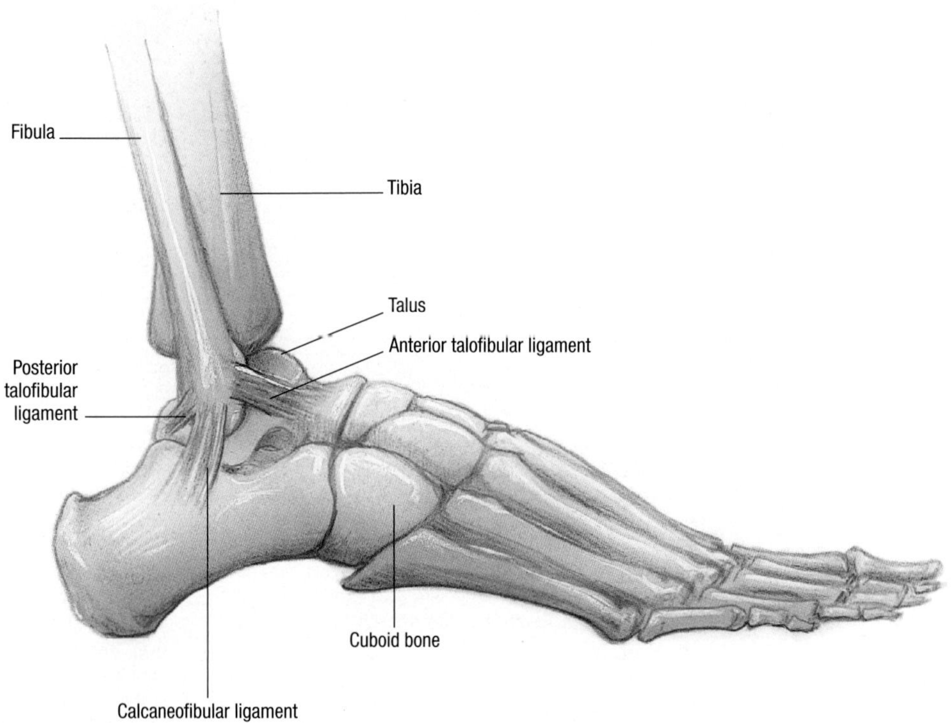

Figure 20.2 Lateral collateral ligaments of the ankle: the anterior talofibular ligament, the posterior talofibular ligament, and the calcaneofibular ligament. They prevent subluxation of the ankle during inversion. (Courtesy of the Anatomical Chart Co.)

NOT TO BE MISSED

- Ankle fracture (open vs. closed)
- Ankle contusion versus sprain
- Associated fifth metatarsal fracture (Jones vs. styloid)
- Associated talar fracture
- Gout
- Psoriatic arthritis
- Septic joint

Radiographic Evaluation

Radiographs to order include anteroposterior (AP), lateral, and oblique views. Optional radiographs include the following:

- Stress views, which are usually obtained by specialists. They are used to check for ankle instability from ruptured lateral ligaments. The examiner holds the ankle in a varus (inward) or valgus (outward) position during the radiographic process. An increase in the joint space is compatible with a collateral ligament tear.
- Mortise view, which is obtained with the ankle rotated internally by 10 degrees. A mortise view eliminates the overlap of the distal fibular and tibia seen on the routine AP projections. It allows for better visualization of the talar dome and the distal tibia (plafond). It may be ordered as part of the acute trauma series for suspected ankle fractures, especially in cases involving high-impact trauma.

If there is tenderness of the talus, the examiner should consider a mortise view. Fractures of the talus or navicular may not be present on initial radiographs. If the patient has persistent pain and soreness that is not resolving, a magnetic resonance imaging (MRI) scan may be warranted. A computed tomography scan is useful in detecting occult fractures, and it has excellent sensitivity. However, an MRI provides an image of the surrounding ligaments and may be more useful in detecting a tear in the distal tibiofibular syndesmotic complex. If there is tenderness of the navicular or the fifth metatarsal, foot radiographs (in addition to ankle radiographs) should be evaluated. Standard ankle radiographs may allow for limited evaluation of the navicular and the fifth metatarsal, and there is better delineation of the navicular

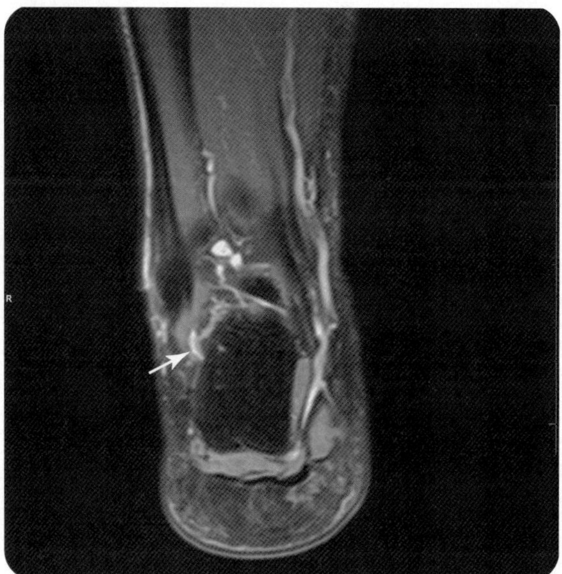

Figure 20.3 A selected coronal view from magnetic resonance imaging of the right ankle from a 28-year-old man who rolled his ankle in a hole in the ground. This demonstrates a tear of the distal fibulocalcaneal ligament (*arrow*) with adjacent soft tissue edema.

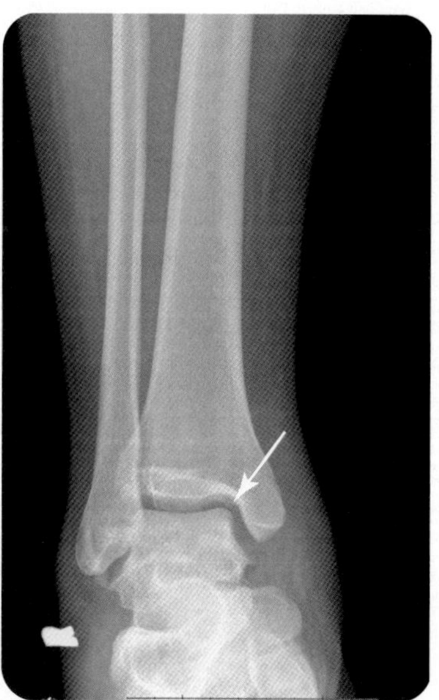

Figure 20.4 A frontal radiograph of the right ankle from an 18-year-old man involved in a motor vehicle collision. This demonstrates marked soft tissue swelling over the medial malleolus, widening of the medial clear space, and possible small avulsion fracture overlying the medial tibial plafond (*arrow*).

and the fifth metatarsal with foot radiographs. In addition, MRI is also used to detect occult fractures.

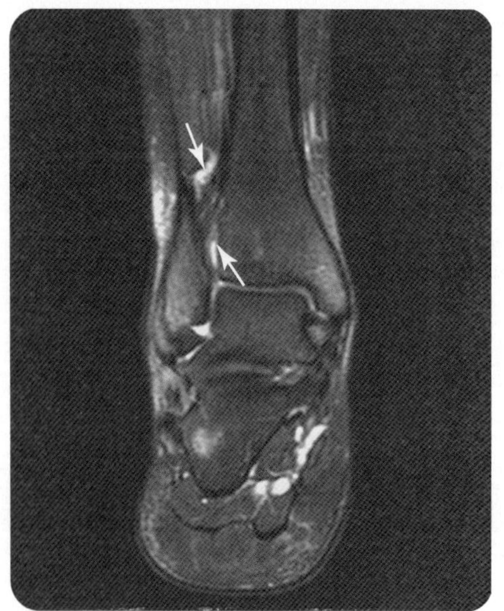

Figure 20.5 A 37-year-old woman presents with right ankle pain after a twisting injury 1 month prior. A selected coronal T2-weighted, fat-saturated image of the right ankle demonstrates edema within the anterior tibiofibular ligament (*arrow*) consistent with a mild sprain.

TORN LATERAL COLLATERAL LIGAMENTS (FIG. 20.3)

Physicians should look for marked soft tissue swelling, with an increase in the talar–fibular joint space more than 5 mm. These findings are suspicious for torn lateral collateral ligaments. In addition, the examiner should compare the distance between the talus and the fibula as well with the distance between the talus and the tibia. A marked separation on one or both sides may be secondary to unilateral or bilateral torn ligaments.

TORN MEDIAL COLLATERAL LIGAMENTS (FIG. 20.4)

Purely isolated injuries of the medial collateral (deltoid) ligament are uncommon, because the deltoid (medial collateral) ligament is very strong and very broad. Usually, such injuries are eversion injuries. When there is marked swelling and soreness of the medial collateral ligament, the clinician should examine the patient carefully for an associated distal fibular fracture, a tear of the tibiofibular syndesmotic complex (ankle pain in the distal interosseous space with dorsiflexion), or a Maisonneuve fracture (proximal fibula).

DISTAL TIBIOFIBULAR SYNDESMOTIC COMPLEX TEARS (FIG. 20.5)

The distal tibiofibular syndesmotic complex is composed of the interosseous membrane, the anterior tibiofibular ligament, and the

WHEN TO REFER

- Immediate referral is necessary for patients with grade 3 sprains with neurovascular compromise.
- Referral should be considered for patients with grade 2 sprains that do not improve after 4 to 6 weeks of conservative care.
- Referral to orthopedic surgery is necessary for patients with grade 3 sprains, who should be kept non–weight-bearing status.

posterior tibiofibular ligament. It is a key stabilizer of the ankle mortise. Clinically, tears in this area may be identified by pronounced pain in this region with palpation and with dorsiflexion. Radiographically, tears in this complex may be identified by an increased separation between the distal tibia and the distal fibula. On a normal AP view, the distal fibula and tibia should cross slightly.

Treatment

Grade 1 and grade 2 ankle sprains can generally be treated conservatively in the primary care setting. Grade 1 sprains usually resolve after 4 to 6 weeks of conservative care (analgesic medication; rest, ice, compression, and elevation [RICE]). Grade 2 sprains may require an ankle (stirrup) brace, or an ankle support, and physical therapy. The patient pain limited weight bearing may require canes or crutches for additional support. Grade 3 sprains, which are by definition unstable, should be referred to orthopedics. In general, the majority of grade 3 sprains can be treated with casting for approximately 6 weeks. Ankle sprains with neurovascular compromise must be referred immediately.

Suggested Readings

Bachmann LM, Kolb E, Koller MT, et al. Accuracy of Ottawa ankle rules to exclude fractures of the ankle and mid-foot: a systemic review. *BMJ*. 2003;326:417.

Ebell MH. Point of care guides: evaluating the patient with an ankle or foot injury. *Am Fam Physician*. 2004;70:1535–1536.

Ivins D. Acute ankle sprain: an update. *Am Fam Physician*. 2006;74:1714–1720.

Kannus P, Renstrom P. Treatment for acute tears of the lateral ligaments of the ankle. *J Bone Joint Surg*. 1991;73:305–312.

Koehler SC, Eiff P. Overview of ankle fractures. *UpToDate*. http://www.uptodate.com. Accessed July 2, 2009.

Mainwaring BL, Daffner RH, Riemer B. Pylon fractures of the ankle: a distinct clinical and radiologic entity. *Radiology*. 1988;168:215–218.

Mazzone MF, McCue T. Common conditions of the Achilles tendon. *Am Fam Physician*. 2002;65:1805–1810.

Rosenberg Z, Beltran J, Bencardino JT. MR imaging of the ankle and foot. *Radiographics*. 2000;20:S153–S179.

Stiell IG, McKnight RD, Wells GA, et al. Implementation of the Ottawa knee rule for the use of radiology in acute knee injuries. *JAMA*. 1997;278:2075–2078.

Vander Griend R, Michelson JD, Bone LB. Instructional course lectures: fractures of the ankle and the distal part of the tibia. *J Bone Joint Surg*. 1996;78:1772–1783.

Wexler RK. The injured ankle. *Am Fam Physician*. 1998;57(3):474–480.

Wolfe MW, Uhl TL, McCluskey LC. Management of ankle sprains. *Am Fam Physician*. 2001;63:93–104.

CHAPTER 21

Unimalleolar Fractures

George M. Bridgeforth and George Holmes

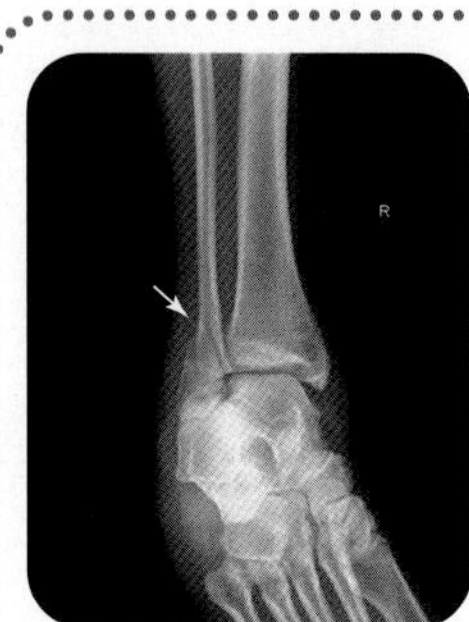

A 39-year-old man with schizophrenia presents with right ankle pain and swelling 10 days after a fall. He is unable to take four steps.

Clinical Presentation

Ankle fractures are becoming increasingly common, and they account for approximately 10% of all fractures. About two-thirds of these injuries are unimalleolar fractures, which affect the distal fibula, or less commonly, the distal tibia (Fig. 21.1). Most unimalleolar fractures affect the distal fibula, but it is important to note that fractures below the distal tibial plafond (ceiling) are generally stable. This region is sometimes called the *tibiotalar line*. The talar dome is a curved structure supported on either side by two bony stirrups (the distal fibula and tibia) and surrounding collateral ligaments. Most fractures below the tibial plafond have sufficient surrounding structural support.

The surrounding supporting structures consist not only of the medial (distal tibia) and lateral malleolus (distal fibula) but also the supporting ligaments and joint capsule. The lateral collateral ligaments, which prevent excessive eversion of the ankle and joint dislocation, are formed by the anterior talofibular ligament, the posterior talofibular ligament, and the calcaneofibular ligament. The fan-shaped deltoid ligament is actually made up of four ligaments (the anterior tibiotalar ligament, the tibionavicular ligament, the tibiocalcaneal ligament, and the posterior tibiotalar ligament). The medial collateral ligaments help prevent excessive inversion and ankle dislocations.

The **mechanism of injury** is direct trauma. Inversion injuries involve the distal fibula, and eversion injuries involve the distal tibia.

In the introductory case, the patient has marked tenderness of the distal fibula and an inability to take four steps, thus meeting at least two of the Ottawa rules for the evaluation of ankle injuries (see Chapter 20). However, there is no tenderness of the navicular or fifth metatarsal, the third Ottawa criterion. The Ottawa rules have excellent sensitivity (well more than 90%) for the detection of acute fractures. For physicians who adhere strictly to the Ottawa rules, it is recommended that radiographs be obtained within 7 days if the patient does not show any signs of improvement; this may allow detection of a missed occult fracture. The absence of the Ottawa criteria may not completely rule out an acute fracture. Therefore, the examiner is advised to use his or her own discretion.

All patients with ankle injuries should be evaluated for more extensive and serious conditions depending on the history. Details about the causal incident, such as the direction of torque force applied to the ankle and the foot's position,

CLINICAL POINTS

- The majority of ankle fractures are unimalleolar.
- A unimalleolar fracture involves either the distal fibula (more common) or the distal tibia.
- Most oblique and spiral fractures (above the tibial plafond) are unstable.

PATIENT ASSESSMENT

1. Pain, swelling, tenderness, and bruising
2. Limited weight-bearing ability
3. Limited range of motion
4. Possible associated fractures

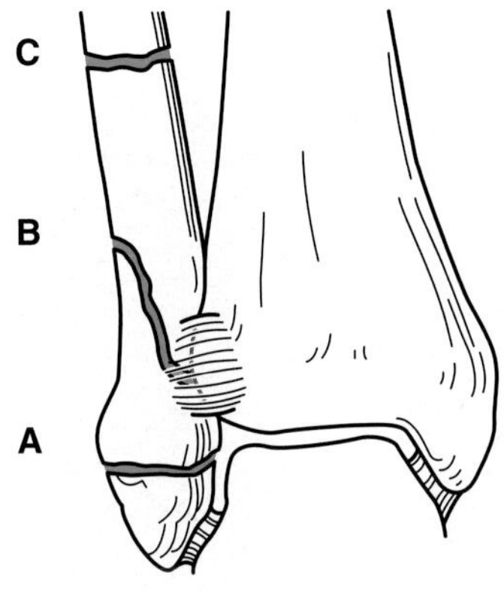

Figure 21.1 Schematic diagram of the AO/OTA classification of ankle fractures. **(A)** There are three types of ankle fractures in the AO/OTA classification: type A, type B, and type C. Each type is further subdivided into three groups. (From Bucholz RW, Heckman JD. *Rockwood & Green's Fractures in Adults*. 5th ed. Philadelphia, PA: Lippincott Williams & Wilkins; 2001.)

help predict the nature and severity of the ankle fracture. Patients do tend to remember the event, but they often cannot recall exactly how the fracture occurred. A thorough examination of the involved ankle is necessary. Symptoms and signs of fracture include pain, swelling, and tenderness of the medial and lateral malleolus, with possibly bruising and discoloration. Inability to bear weight indicates a fracture. There is pain-limited range of motion—dorsiflexion, plantar flexion, inversion, or eversion.

To check for instability, the physician should use the anterior–posterior drawer test for instability. In addition, the physician should

- check varus (inversion) and valgus (eversion) strain for collateral ligament instability
- palpate the navicular and the fifth metatarsal should be palpated for associated foot fractures. Talar pain with dorsiflexion indicates a possible associated talar fracture.
- check the posterior tibia for a fracture of the posterior tibial lip for possible fracture.
- check for heel pain and tenderness, which may be signs of a fracture
- perform a neurovascular examination to check for coldness, pallor, diminished or absent pulses, and diminished or absent pinprick.

Patients with septic joints should have radiographs taken followed by a diagnostic aspiration. The treatment for septic joints is directed toward the underlying cause.

NOT TO BE MISSED

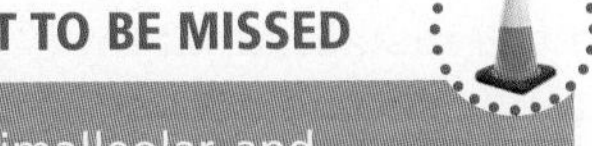

- Bimalleolar and trimalleolar fractures
- Ankle sprains and contusions
- Collateral ligament tears
- Ankle cellulitis (soft tissue infection of the ankle not involving the joint space)
- Septic joint
- Gout
- Rheumatoid arthritis (rheumatoid changes in other joints, especially the wrists and the fingers; usually symmetrical)
- Psoriatic arthritis (often salmon-colored plaques over the knees, elbows, gluteal folds, and nail pitting)
- Associated fifth metatarsal fractures (Jones vs. styloid)
- Associated talar fractures (uncommon)
- Maisonneuve fracture (extends to the upper fibula)
- Bone tumors (rare)

Radiographic Evaluation

Anteroposterior (AP), lateral, and oblique radiographs should be ordered (Fig. 21.2). Optional radiographs that may be necessary include the following:

- Stress views: usually obtained by specialists (however, many specialists prefer weight-bearing views)
- Mortise view (for talar dome fractures, pylon fractures and distal torn interosseous complex injuries): obtained with the ankle rotated internally by 10 to 15 degrees

Magnetic resonance imaging may be necessary for occult fractures and torn ligaments.

The examiner should use the AP view to check for fractures of the distal fibula or tibia. The AP view may be used to check for torn collateral ligaments as well. If there is a 5 mm (or greater) separation between the talus and the surrounding fibula or tibia or if there is pronounced swelling and tenderness on one or both sides, the examiner should suspect a torn collateral ligament.

If the distal tibia or fibula is fractured (and the collateral ligaments on the opposite side are stable), then the patient has a unimalleolar fracture (Fig. 21.3). However, if both the distal tibia and fibula are fractured, then the patient has a bimalleolar fracture. (A unimalleolar fracture with torn collateral ligaments on the opposite side is equivalent to a bimalleolar fracture.)

The lateral view is used to check for fractures of the posterior lip of the tibia. A fracture of the posterior lip of the tibia is caused by a shifting rotating talus. Moreover, the unstable talar rotation would be caused by fractures of the distal fibula and tibia. Therefore, its presence would constitute a trimalleolar fracture. A trimalleolar fracture is characterized by a fracture of the distal fibula, the distal tibia, and the posterior lip of the talus.

The lateral view should be used to check the tuberosity and the proximal shaft of the fifth metatarsal for an associated fifth metatarsal fracture. If the proximal fifth metatarsal is not visualized on the lateral view, then foot radiographs should be obtained or the lateral view should be repeated

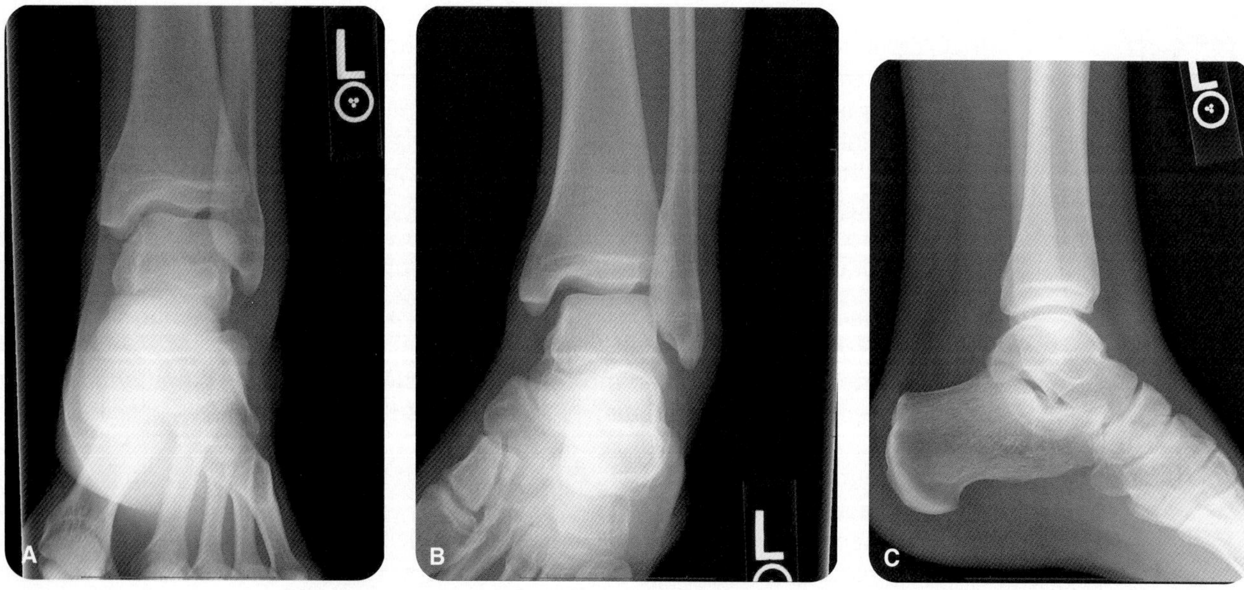

Figure 21.2 **(A)** Anteroposterior, **(B)** lateral, and **(C)** oblique radiographs of a normal ankle.

(Fig. 21.4). In addition, the oblique view and the AP view are helpful in checking tears in the distal tibiofibular syndesmosis. Normally, the distal portions of the fibula and tibia should cross on an AP view or a standard oblique view (but not on a mortise view). If there is a separation between the distal fibular and tibia on an AP view (or standard oblique view), the examiner should suspect a tear of the distal tibiofibular syndesmosis.

The axial load on the ankle mortise produced by the body's weight may demonstrate misalignments in the anatomical structures. The examiner should look for a separation in the medial or lateral ankle mortise equal to or greater than 5 mm (medial or lateral collateral ligament rupture). Acute fractures usually have surrounding soft tissue swelling with dark lines that extend to and break the cortex. Old fractures have sclerotic margins.

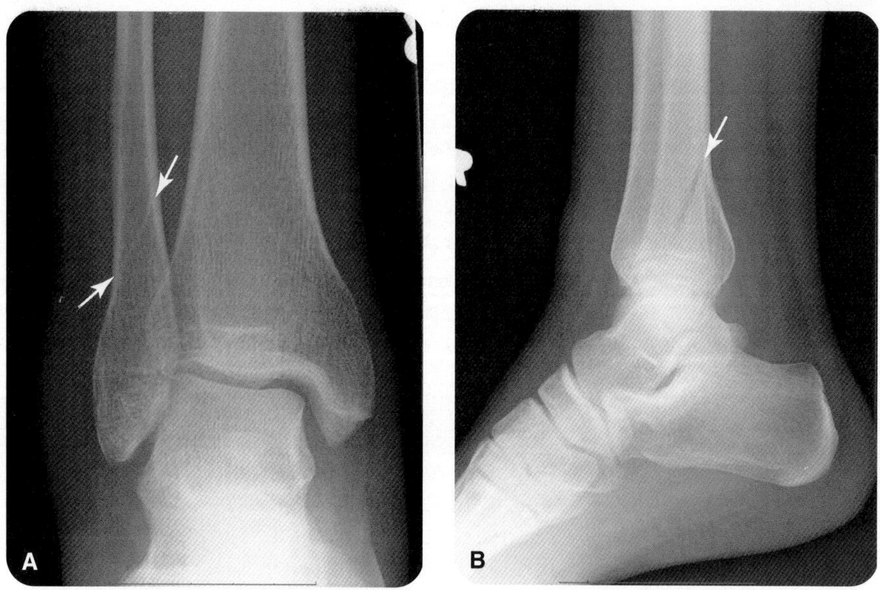

Figure 21.3 A 25-year-old man has injured his ankle while walking the previous night. **(A)** The anteroposterior radiograph demonstrates an oblique sclerotic line through the right distal fibular diaphysis (*arrows*); however, the cortex appears intact. **(B)** The lateral projection better demonstrates that the fibula is fractured and minimally displaced posteriorly.

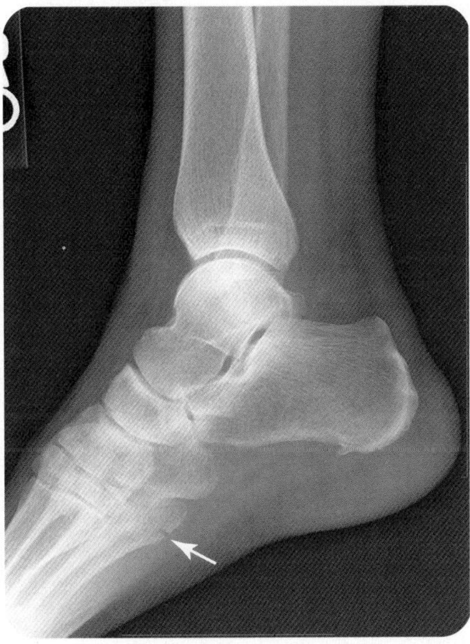

Figure 21.4 A 48-year-old woman steps off a curb and injures her right ankle. The lateral radiograph of the right ankle illustrates an acute fracture of the base of the fifth metatarsal.

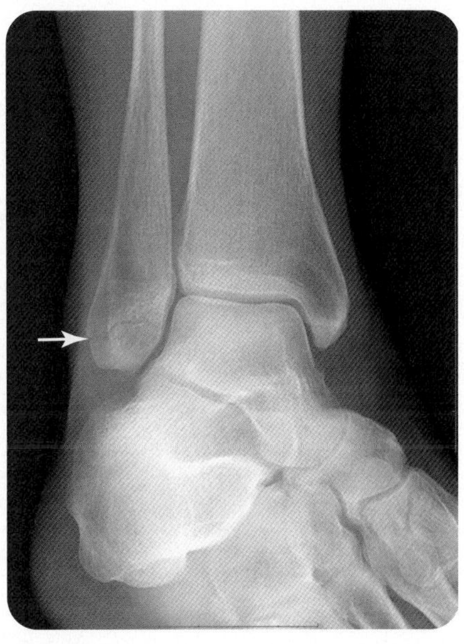

Figure 21.5 A 62-year-old woman who fell presents with lateral right ankle pain. The oblique radiograph demonstrates a transverse fracture of the right distal fibula.

A mortise view eliminates the overlap of the distal fibular and tibia seen on routine AP projections. It allows for better visualization of the talar dome and the distal tibia (plafond). It may be used as part of the acute trauma series, especially for high-impact trauma to detect pylon fractures of the distal tibia or talar dome fractures.

Transverse fractures of the distal fibula below the tibial plafond are sometimes called *Weber A fractures* (Fig. 21.5). These stable fractures do not demonstrate displacement with an axial load (i.e., weight-bearing). Small oblique fibular fractures at the level of the distal tibiofibular complex are sometimes referred to as *Weber B fractures*. Because these fractures are above the tibial plafond, physicians consider these fractures to be unstable. In other words, they manifest displacement with weight-bearing. Spiral fractures, above the distal tibiofibular complex, are unstable. They may extend into the upper fibular (Maisonneuve fracture). They are associated with tears in the distal tibiofibular complex.

It is important to note the following points:

- An unstable fracture should be suspected if the fracture is either displaced or above the tibial plafond. This is best appreciated on the AP view.
- Small avulsion fractures may be associated with ligament disruption.
- An unstable fracture should be suspected if there is a fracture opposite a ligament tear (increased talar space).

WHEN TO REFER

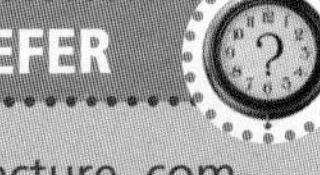

- Any open fracture, compartment syndrome (acute swelling with neurovascular compromise), or displacement should be referred immediately.
- Unstable fractures should be discussed with orthopedics and then referred.
- Stable fractures should be referred if the primary care physician is not experienced with fracture management.

Treatment

Small, stable fractures of the fibula require a stirrup splint, the use of a short leg or walking cast for several weeks. Physical therapy may then be necessary to help restore the normal range of motion. Unstable fractures require a posterior mold and the use of crutches, and no weight-bearing is permissible. Surgery, with open reduction and internal fixation—a fixation plate and fixation screws—is necessary. Until patients have been evaluated by a specialist, patients should be maintained on non–weight-bearing status.

Suggested Readings

Branderser EA, Berbaum KS, Doraman DD, et al. Contribution of individual projections along and in combination for radiographic detection of ankle fractures. *AJR Am J Roentgenol*. 2000;174(6):1691–1697.

Fields KB. Stress fractures of the tibia and fibula. *UpToDate*. http://www.uptodate.com/online/content/topic.do?topicKey=ad-onth/203848view=print. Accessed July 7, 2009.

Haraguchi N, Armiger RS. A new interpretation of the mechanism of ankle fracture. *J Bone Joint Surg*. 2009;91(4):821–829.

Herscovici D, Scaduto JM, Infante A. Conservative treatment of isolated fractures of the medial malleolus. *J Bone Joint Surg Br* 2007;89(10):89–93.

Leeds HC, Ehlrich MG. Instability of the distal tibiofibular syndesmosis after bimalleolar and trimalleolar ankle fractures. *J Bone Joint Surg*. 1984;66:490–503.

Marder RA. Current methods for the evaluation of ankle ligament injuries. *J Bone Joint Surg*. 1994;76:1103–1111.

McConnell T, Creevy W, Tornetta P. Stress examination of supination external rotation-type fibular fractures. *J Bone Joint Surg*. 2004;86:2171–2178.

Micheslon JD. Fractures about the ankle. *J Bone Joint Surg*. 1995;77:142–152.

Pankovich AM. Maisonneuve fracture of the fibula. *J Bone Joint Surg*. 1976;58:337–342.

Vander Griend R, Michelson JD, Bone LB. Instructional course lectures, the American Academy of Orthopedic Surgeons—fractures of the ankle and the distal part of the tibia. *J Bone Joint Surg*. 1996;78:1772–1783.

Bimalleolar (Trimalleolar) Fractures

George M. Bridgeforth and George Holmes

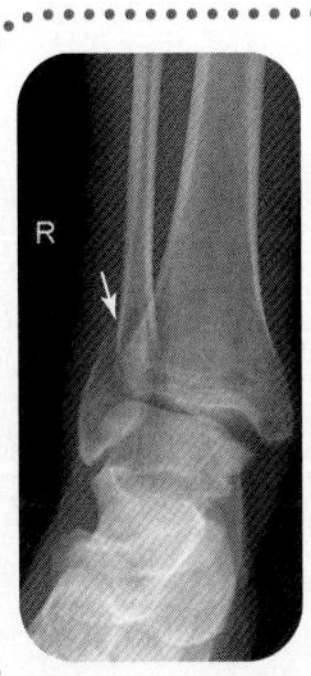

A 46-year-old woman falls on her right ankle while ice-skating.

Clinical Presentation

Bimalleolar and trimalleolar fractures account for more than 30% of all ankle fractures. Patients complain of marked pain, swelling, and tenderness associated with an inability to bear weight or ambulate. The **mechanism of injury** is direct impact caused by inversion or eversion injuries. Inversion injuries occur more often. The non–weight-bearing distal fibula is thinner than the distal tibia. In addition, the lateral collateral ligaments (the anterior and posterior talofibular ligaments and the posterior talofibular ligament) are thinner than the stronger broad-based medial collateral (deltoid) ligament. Eversion injuries are less common, but they are more likely to result in unstable fractures.

Pain, swelling, and tenderness along either or both malleoli may be secondary to an acute fracture or a severe ankle sprain. However, the presence of a distal tibial fracture or a disrupted deltoid ligament (marked swelling 5 mm or greater between the talus and the distal tibia) should prompt the examiner to search for a fracture of the distal fibula or torn lateral collateral ligaments. The physician should

- Perform the anterior and posterior drawer tests to check for ankle instability
- Check for varus and valgus instability
- Check for tenderness along the posterior edge of the tibia posterior tibia (posterior tibial fracture)
- Palpate the fifth metatarsal for an associated metatarsal fracture, the navicular for focal tenderness for possible fracture, and the talus (check for talar pain with ankle dorsiflexion) for an associated talar fracture
- Inspect for heel pain (calcaneal fracture)
- Determine whether there is neurovascular impairment (cold, cyanotic limb with diminished or absent pulses, impaired sensation). **It is essential to document the neurovascular examination carefully.**

CLINICAL POINTS

- Bimalleolar fractures are fractures of the distal fibula and tibia.
- Trimalleolar fractures are fractures of the distal fibula, tibia, and the posterior lip of the distal tibia.
- About one-third of all ankle fractures are bimalleolar and trimalleolar fractures.

PATIENT ASSESSMENT

1. Marked pain, swelling, and tenderness
2. Limited range of motion
3. Difficulty weight-bearing with an inability to take four steps.

Radiographic Evaluation

Anteroposterior (AP), lateral, and oblique views should be ordered. Additional tests to order include the following:

- Mortise view: the ankle is rotated internally 10 to 15 degrees. A mortise view eliminates the overlap of the distal fibula and tibia seen on routine AP

NOT TO BE MISSED

- Open ankle fractures
- Ankle contusion
- Associated fifth metatarsal fracture (Jones vs. styloid)
- Associated talar fracture
- Septic joint
- Gout
- Psoriatic arthritis

projections and allows for better visualization of the talar dome and the distal tibia (plafond). It may be used as part of acute trauma series for high-impact injuries. Uses include detection of pilon fractures of the distal tibia or fractures of the talar dome as well as osteochondritis dissecans of the tibiotalar joint. This latter condition appears as a minute semioval (saucer-shaped) bite mark along the joint line. Osteochondritis dissecans should be suspected in any patient who complains of joint locking or joint mice.

- Stress views: usually obtained by specialists. These views place an anatomical load on the ankle mortise. An increase in the space between the talus and the surrounding fibula or tibia 5 mm or more is suspicious for a complete disruption of the lateral or medial collateral ligament. In addition, a malunion in the anatomical relationship may indicate an old fracture (it is also necessary to look for bony sclerosis). Many specialists prefer weight-bearing views, which may be very useful; however, patients with severe foot and ankle injuries may have problems weight-bearing.

BIMALLEOLAR FRACTURE

A bimalleolar fracture involves the distal fibula and the distal tibia. Bimalleolar fractures are usually appreciated best on the AP view. It is advised to always check the lateral view carefully for a fracture involving the posterior lip of the tibia as well. If there is a third fracture involving the posterior lip of the tibia, then the injury is a trimalleolar fracture. Moreover, if the AP view shows a fracture of the distal fibula or tibia with disrupted collateral ligament on the opposite side is the biomechanical equivalent of a bimalleolar fracture. A bimalleolar fracture should be considered an unstable injury.

The fan-shaped deltoid ligament is stronger than the lateral collateral ligaments. So, if the examiner recognizes an oblique fracture of the distal tibia or a disruption of the deltoid ligament, he or she should suspect either a distal fibular fracture or torn lateral collateral ligaments. With any ankle injury, it is always important to carefully examine the lateral radiograph for talar neck fractures. It is necessary to check the talar dome and neck on the lateral view for an associated talar fracture. Although talar fractures are less common, they can be difficult to identify on standard radiographs and are easily missed.

In addition, the examiner should check the lateral ankle radiograph for a proximal fifth metatarsal for a styloid fracture or Jones fracture. Jones fractures are uncommon but are also easily missed.

TRIMALLEOLAR FRACTURE

A trimalleolar fracture consists of a fracture of the distal fibula and tibia (a bimalleolar fracture) and a fracture of the posterior lip of the tibia as well (Fig. 22.1). When screening for trimalleolar fractures, the lateral radiographs should be examined carefully for an associated trimalleolar (third fracture) of the posterior lip (edge) of the tibia. Damage to the deltoid ligament or an oblique fracture of the medial tibia or a fracture of the distal posterior tibia may be secondary to a shifting rotating talus. An unstable injury should be suspected. Nondisplaced fractures appear as a thin lucent line that generally extends to and breaks the cortex. Fractures involving any of the aforementioned areas may appear as displaced or nondisplaced.

TORN DISTAL TIBIOFIBULAR SYNDESMOTIC COMPLEX

The examiner should note the oblique angularity of the distal fibula on the AP view. The increased interosseous space between the distal fibula and the distal tibia is indicative of a tear in the distal tibiofibular syndesmotic complex.

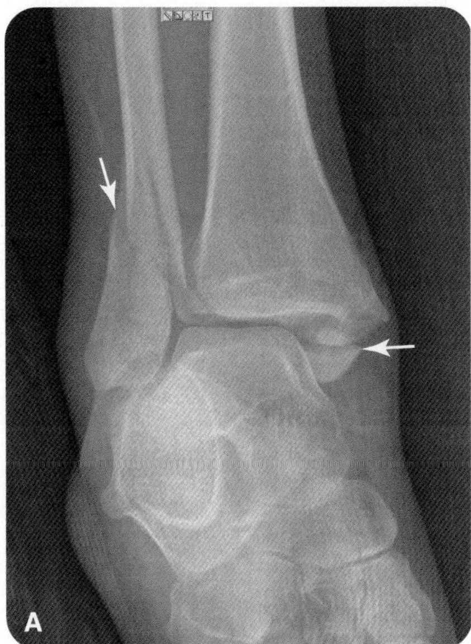

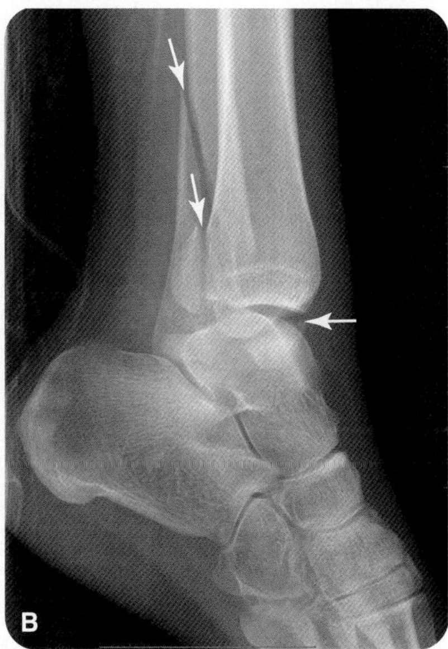

Figure 22.1 **(A)** Anteroposterior and **(B)** lateral radiographs of the right ankle demonstrate a trimalleolar fracture.

This complex is formed by the anterior and posterior tibiofibular ligaments and the interosseous membrane (Fig. 22.2). In addition, the increase in the talofibular joint space is suspicious for torn lateral collateral ligaments as well.

INVERSION INJURY

Inversion injuries to the ankle may sprain the lateral collateral ligaments. Avulsions fractures of the distal fibula may be characterized as tiny chip fractures or transverse (horizontal) fractures. If there is associated talar instability, then the shifting talus may cause an impaction fracture of the distal tibia. Generally, impaction ankle fractures have an oblique configuration. If the examiner identifies an oblique (impaction) fracture of the medial malleolus (distal tibia) without a fibula fracture, then torn lateral collateral ligaments should be suspected. In the absence of a distal fibular avulsion fracture, the torn lateral collateral ligaments result in the talar instability. The shifting talus causes the impaction (oblique) fracture of the medial malleolus (distal tibia).

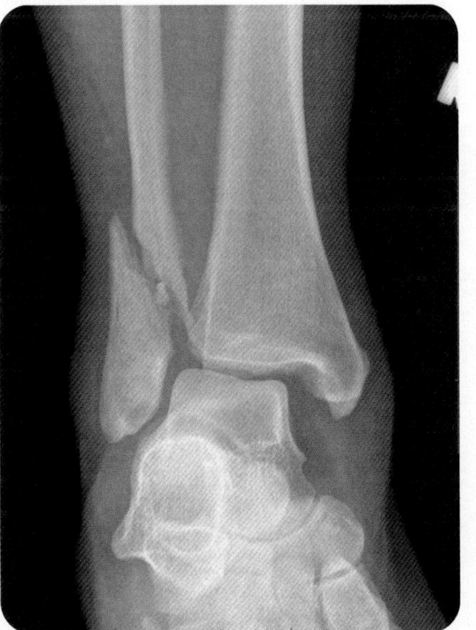

Figure 22.2 Acute, comminuted, oblique fracture of the distal right fibula with widening of the tibiofibular relationship in a 45-year-old woman who has fallen.

EVERSION INJURY

Eversion injuries have the opposite effect. Eversion injuries may cause sprains of the deltoid ligament, but severe forces cause an avulsion fracture of the distal tibia. If there is associated talar instability, the shifting talus may cause an oblique fracture of the distal tibia as well. It is essential to check the lateral view. If the examiner identifies an oblique fracture of the distal fibula without an avulsion fracture of the medial malleolus, then a torn deltoid ligament should be suspected. A magnetic resonance imaging scan or stress views taken by a specialist may detect torn collateral ligaments.

PILON FRACTURES

Pilon fractures, which affect the distal tibia, are commonly seen with falls. In these comminuted fractures, the fracture lines extend to the distal articular surface. They may occur as the result of axial loading (i.e., from high falls). After such falls, the examiner should always inspect the heels for associated calcaneal fractures and the lower thoracic–upper lumbar spine for associated burst fractures. Pilon fractures are unstable (fractures above the talar plafond [dome] are unstable).

Treatment

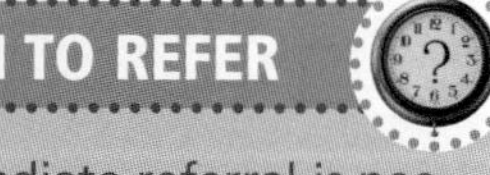

WHEN TO REFER

- Immediate referral is necessary for open fractures, displaced fractures, or neurovascular impairment.

Bimalleolar and trimalleolar fractures are unstable, and until patients are evaluated by an orthopedic specialist, they should put no weight on the affected leg. Generally, a posterior mold, crutches, and pain medication are necessary for most patients. However, some patients with small, nondisplaced fractures may be placed in an air stirrup type of brace. Most patients with minimal displacement require casting for a 4- to 6-week period. For pilon fractures, no weight-bearing on the affected limb is recommended.

Suggested Readings

Branderser EA, Berbaum KS, Doraman DD, et al. Contribution of individual projections along and in combination for radiographic detection of ankle fractures. *AJR Am J Roentgenol*. 2000;174(6):1691–1697.

Fields KB. Stress fractures of the tibia and fibula. *UpToDate*. http://www.uptodate.com. Accessed July 7, 2009.

Haraguchi N, Armiger RS. A new interpretation of the mechanism of ankle fracture. *Journal of Bone and Joint Surg*. 2009;91(4):821–829.

Herscovici D, Scaduto JM, Infante A. Conservative treatment of isolated fractures of the medial malleolus. *J Bone Joint Surg (Br)*. 2007;89(10):89–93.

Leeds HC, Ehlrich MG. Instability of the distal tibiofibular syndesmosis after bimalleolar and trimalleolar ankle fractures. *J Bone Joint Surg*. 1984;66:490–503.

Marder RA. Current methods for the evaluation of ankle ligament injuries. *J Bone Joint Surg*. 1994;76:1103–1111.

McConnell T, Creevy W, Tornetta P. Stress examination of supination external rotation-type fibular fractures. *J Bone Joint Surg*. 2004;86:2171–2178.

Micheslon JD. Fractures about the ankle. *J Bone Joint Surg*. 1995;77:142–152.

Pankovich AM. Maisonneuve fracture of the fibula. *J Bone Joint Surg*. 1976;58:337–342.

Vander Griend R, Michelson JD, Bone LB. Instructional course lectures, the American Academy of Orthopedic Surgeons—fractures of the ankle and the distal part of the tibia. *J Bone Joint Surg*. 1996;78:1772–1783.

CHAPTER 23

Spiral Fractures

George M. Bridgeforth and George Holmes

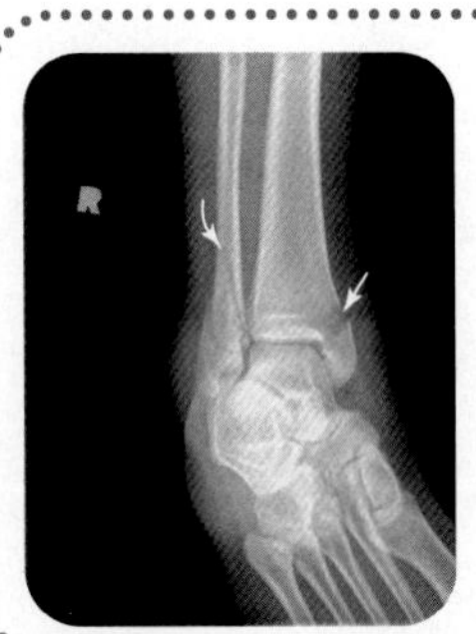

A 26-year-old man who slipped on an icy street presents with pain, swelling, and gross deformity of his right ankle.

Clinical Presentation

A spiral fracture is caused by supination of the foot with external rotation force (torsion injuries). Spiral fractures may occur in downhill skiers, who put their feet into rigid boots that fit firmly onto skis. If a ski breaks or changes direction abruptly, an acutely twisted leg may result.

The fracture in the introductory case is known as a *Weber B fracture* by some orthopedic specialists (see subsequent discussion). It is an oblique fracture of the lateral malleolus that is commonly associated with rupture of the tibiofibular syndesmosis. A more severe fracture is the Maisonneuve fracture (Weber C fracture), a spiral fracture of the distal fibula that extends to the proximal fibula. Fracture of the proximal fibula associated with a torn interosseous ligaments and membrane. These injuries are associated with a disruption of the distal tibiofibular complex.

Pronation is a complex triplanar motion of the foot and ankle consisting of dorsiflexion, ankle eversion, and lateral abduction of the forefoot.* With pronation, the foot and ankle roll outward. Supination is a complex triplanar motion of the foot and ankle consisting of plantar flexion, ankle inversion, and medial adduction of the forefoot. With supination, the foot and ankle roll inward.

Evaluation of the patient is essential. The physician should always check for tenderness of the fibular head and the interosseous region between the distal tibia and fibula and the opposite side for an avulsion fracture of the distal tibia (medial malleolus) or a complete avulsion of the deltoid ligament. Physicians should also inspect the base of the fifth metatarsal for (associated) fractures. In addition, it is always necessary to conduct a thorough neurovascular examination. Signs of pallor, coldness of the foot and ankle (cold dusky limb), diminished or absent dorsalis pedis or posterior tibial pulses, and diminished

CLINICAL POINTS

- Torsion may lead to spiral ankle fractures.
- Marked tenderness, pain, and swelling occur at the fracture site.
- Pain-limited ambulation with an inability to take four steps is characteristic.

PATIENT ASSESSMENT

1. Marked pain and swelling over the distal fibula
2. Pain-limited range of motion
3. Limited weight-bearing

*The gait cycle consists of a stance phase and a swing-through phase. The stance phase accounts for approximately 60% of the gait cycle, and the swing-through phase accounts for the other 40%. The stance phase is subdivided into three phases: heel strike, midstance, and push-off ("toe-off"). Heel strike occurs when the foot first hits the ground when walking or jogging. During heel strike, the foot begins to pronate. Pronation is a complex triplanar motion in which the foot and ankle dorsiflex and roll outward. It accounts for approximately 25% of the stance phase. During the early part of midstance, the foot begins to supinate. Supination is a complex triplanar motion during which foot and ankle show plantar flexion and roll inward. This primes the foot as a lever for the push-off phase.

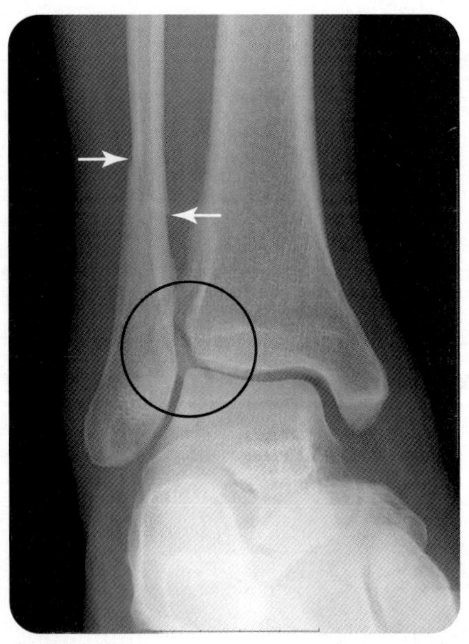

Figure 23.1 Tillaux fracture. A 46-year-old man has right ankle pain after playing volleyball. An oblique radiograph demonstrates an acute spiral fracture of the distal right fibula (*arrows*) and an avulsion of the lateral aspect of the distal tibia (circled).

or absent sensation are important findings. Careful documentation of neurovascular status is essential.

The broad-based medial collateral ligament is made up of the deltoid ligament. The lateral collateral ligaments are composed of the anterior and posterior talofibular ligaments and the posterior calcaneofibular. The broad, thick deltoid ligament is stronger than the lateral collateral ligaments. However, if there is a complete avulsion of either the medial or lateral collateral ligaments associated with a (impaction) fracture of the opposite side, the injury is the equivalent of bimalleolar fracture type of injury. From a biomechanical standpoint, there are now two breaks in the structural support on each side of the ankle. Therefore, these injuries are unstable.

Fractures above the tibia plafond (a horizontal line drawn across the distal tibia) are unstable fractures. There is not enough bony stirrup support for ankle stability. These fractures may be associated with tears in the posterior talofibular ligament, which adds to the lack of surrounding structural support.

A Tillaux fracture is a fracture of the anterolateral process of the tibia. This injury, which usually occurs in adolescent skate boarders or snow boarders, rarely occurs in adults because the ligaments give way first. It appears as a small avulsion fracture along the lateral border of the tibia and is appreciated best on an oblique view (Fig. 23.1).

Classification Systems

LAUGE–HANSEN CLASSIFICATION

Generally, according to the Lauge–Hansen classification, supination and external rotation are the causes of spiral fractures of the fibula. This classification system resulted from a cadaver study conducted in 1950. During this study, scientists applied a directional force either rotational (internal vs. external) or linear (abduction vs. adduction) to a cadaver ankle placed in either supination or pronation. They made an attempt to classify the resulting fracture patterns. Although this complex classification has limited clinical applications, it is a landmark biomechanical study of ankle fractures.

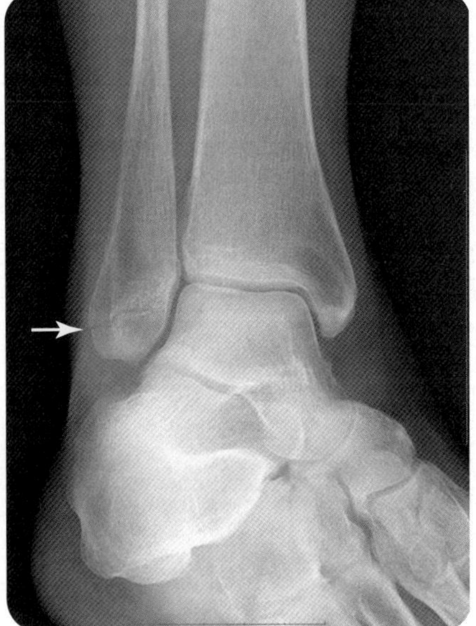

Figure 23.2 A 62-year-old woman who fell presents with lateral right ankle pain. The oblique radiograph demonstrates a transverse fracture of the right distal tibia.

WEBER CLASSIFICATION

- Type A fractures: These are transverse avulsion (or chip) fractures of the distal fibula. Weber A fractures occur below the level of the tibial plafond. Therefore, these are stable fractures in which the deltoid ligament, the distal tibiofibular complex, and the medial malleolus are intact. However, if the medial malleolus is fractured, then these injuries can be unstable. Generally, these are inversion injuries (see Fig. 23.2).
- Type B fractures: These are oblique fractures of the distal fibula. Weber B fractures are caused by an external rotation force to a supinated foot. They usually occur at the level of the distal tibiofibular complex. They may be associated with an avulsion chip fracture, a transverse fracture of the medial malleolus, or a disrupted deltoid ligament (increased in the tibiotalar space). An associated fracture of the medial malleolus or a disrupted deltoid ligament constitutes a bimalleolar fracture. If there is an associated third fracture of the posterior lip of the tibia, then the injury is a trimalleolar fracture. Weber B (oblique) fractures are above the tibial plafond and should be considered unstable fracture unless proven otherwise (see Fig. 23.3).

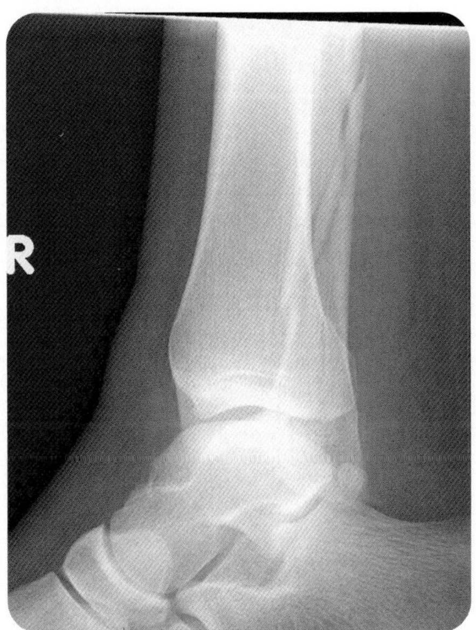

Figure 23.3 Lateral radiograph of the right ankle demonstrates an oblique fracture of the right distal fibular diaphysis well above the tibial plafond.

- Type C fractures: These are spiral fractures of the distal fibula. They are unstable fractures that extend above the level of the tibial plafond. The external rotation force applied to a supinated foot causes a disruption of distal tibiofibular complex. Moreover, it is associated with a disruption of the distal tibiofibular complex. The spiral fracture of the fibula may extend to the upper fibula (Maisonneuve fracture) (Fig. 23.4). These fractures may be associated with fractures of the distal tibia or disruptions of the deltoid ligament (bimalleolar fractures). If there is an associated third fracture involving the posterior lip of the tibia, then the injury is a trimalleolar fracture.

Radiographic Evaluation

Anteroposterior (AP), lateral, and oblique views should be ordered. Optional views include the mortise view and stress views.

The mortise view is taken with the foot internally rotated by approximately 10 or 15 degrees. It allows for better visualization of the talar dome and distal tibia because there is no overlap of the distal tibia and fibula; this makes it especially useful for viewing suspected pilon fractures of the distal tibia or talar dome. Some examiners consider the mortise view to be part of an acute trauma series for high-impact injuries. In addition, this view may be used to detect osteochondritis dissecans. This latter condition appears as a minute semioval (saucer-shaped) bite mark along the joint space. Loose bodies may cause complaints of joint mice or joint locking, especially if the loose body becomes lodged inside the joint.

Stress views are usually obtained by specialists. However, many specialist prefer weight-bearing views. Weight-bearing views allow the examiner to check for collateral ligament disruption or malunion in the normal anatomical relationships. Acute fractures have surrounding soft tissue swelling with clean fracture lines (i.e., dark lines that extend to and break the cortex). Old fractures usually manifest sclerotic margins. However, patients with severe ankle and foot injuries may have trouble weight-bearing.

NOT TO BE MISSED

- Ankle sprain (stable vs. unstable) or contusion
- Nonspiral ankle fracture (open vs. closed)
- Gout
- Psoriatic arthritis
- Septic joint
- Bone tumor (very rare)

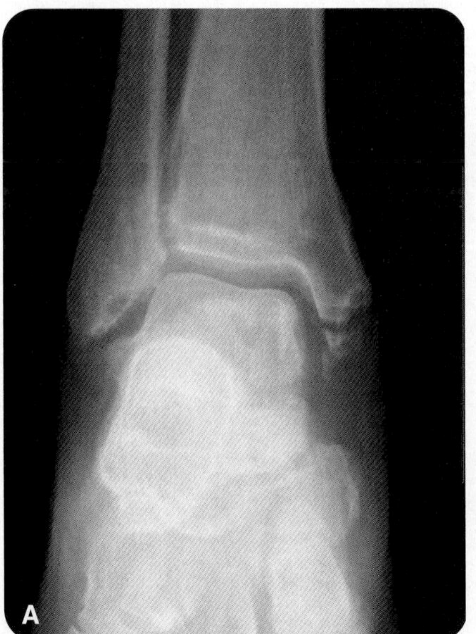

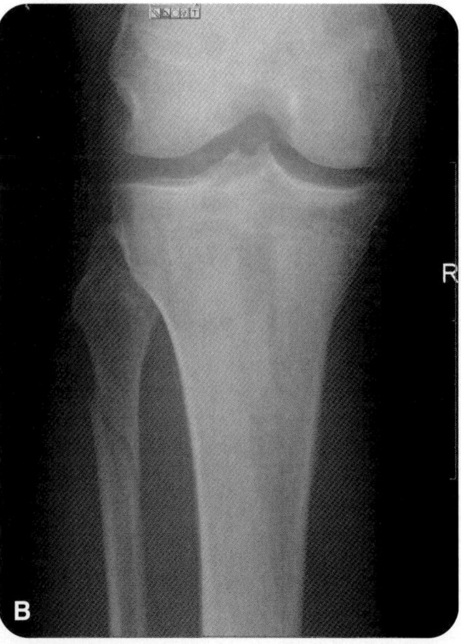

Figure 23.4 Maisonneuve fracture. (A) Anteroposterior radiograph of the right ankle demonstrates an acute avulsion fracture of the medial malleolus. (B) Anteroposterior radiograph (more superior) demonstrates an associated spiral fracture of the proximal fibular diaphysis.

WHEN TO REFER

- Open fractures, fractures with neurovascular impairment, and displaced spiral fractures require immediate referral.
- Nondisplaced spiral fractures that are not referred immediately necessitate discussion with orthopedics and evaluation as quickly as possible.

As previously stated, Maisonneuve fractures are unstable spiral fractures of the distal fibula that extend upward to the proximal fibular. With a Maisonneuve fracture, there are interosseous tears (between the distal tibia and distal fibula) and extend to the level of the proximal fibula. So, additional radiographs of the upper tibiofibular area depicting the fibular head are helpful. In addition, these tears result in a disruption of the distal tibiofibular complex. Normally, on an AP or oblique radiograph, the distal tibia and fibula should cross. The examiner should look for an open space between the distal tibia and fibula. Furthermore, it is important to look for a spiral fracture with lateral displacement of the distal fibula. It is necessary to check the lateral view for (trimalleolar) fractures of the posterior tibial rim (lip) as well. In addition, these fractures may be associated with an avulsion fracture of the medial malleolus (tibia) or a torn deltoid ligament. A torn deltoid ligament may not always be apparent on standard views, but it should be suspected if there is a tibiotalar separation of 5 mm or more.

Treatment

Use of a posterior mold is necessary. Patients should receive pain medication and use crutches to achieve non–weight-bearing status (of the affected limb). Patients with minimally displaced fractures are candidates for closed reduction. Those with displaced fractures usually require surgery. It is critical to achieve and maintain alignment of a fractured ankle.

Suggested Readings

Branderser EA, Berbaum KS, Doraman DD, et al. Contribution of individual projections along and in combination for radiographic detection of ankle fractures. *AJR Am J Roentgenol.* 2000;174(6):1691–1697.

Fields KB. Stress fractures of the tibia and fibula. *UpToDate.* http://www.uptodate.com/patients/content/topicKey=~/5zYKgZUCQB8wz. Accessed July 7, 2009.

Haraguchi N, Armiger RS. A new interpretation of the mechanism of ankle fracture. *J Bone Joint Surg.* 2009:821–829.

Herscovici D, Scaduto JM, Infante A. Conservative treatment of isolated fractures of the medial malleolus. *J Bone Joint Surg Br.* 2007;89(10):89–93.

Leeds HC, Ehlrich MG. Instability of the distal tibiofibular syndesmosis after bimalleolar and trimalleolar ankle fractures. *J Bone Joint Surg.* 1984;66:490–503.

Marder RA. Current methods for the evaluation of ankle ligament injuries. *J Bone Joint Surg.* 1994;76:1103–1111.

McConnell T, Creevy W, Tornetta P. Stress examination of supination external rotation-type fibular fractures. *J Bone Joint Surg.* 2004;86:2171–2178.

Micheslon JD. Fractures about the ankle. *J Bone Joint Surg.* 1995;77:142–152.

Pankovich AM. Maisonneuve fracture of the fibula. *J Bone Joint Surg.* 1976;58:337–342.

Vander Griend R, Michelson JD, Bone LB. Instructional course lectures, the American Academy of Orthopedic Surgeons—fractures of the ankle and the distal part of the tibia. *J Bone Joint Surg.* 1996;78:1772–1783.

CHAPTER 

Accessory Ossification Centers

George M. Bridgeforth and George Holmes

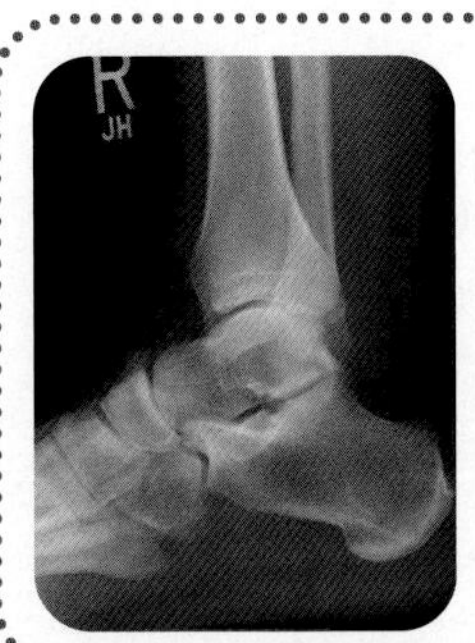

A 35-year-old man injures his right ankle when he trips at a curb. He complains of moderate pain, swelling, and tenderness along the outside of the ankle.

Clinical Presentation

Accessory ossification centers are nontraumatic occurrences; the **mechanism of injury** is failure to fuse during development. They are incidental findings seen on routine radiographs. Although accessory ossification centers may appear in one of several different locations in the hindfoot and midfoot (even the forefoot), they usually occur alongside the inferior lateral border of the cuboid, the proximal tuberosity of the fifth metacarpal, or the posterior talus (Fig. 24.1). Usually, they are asymptomatic. The absence of pain, swelling, and tenderness along with their characteristic sesamoid appearance should prevent the examiner from confusing them with an acute fracture. Accessory ossification centers rarely require surgical removal.

CLINICAL POINTS

- Discovery of accessory ossification is incidental.
- No treatment is necessary.

Radiographic Evaluation

Accessory ossification centers are visible on radiographs taken for other purposes. Unlike acute fractures, they are not associated with soft swelling and tenderness and usually do not fit into larger bones like pieces of a puzzle. Common ossicles include the os peroneum (peroneal ossicle), which lies inferior laterally to the cuboid (Fig. 24.2) and the os vesalianum (vesalian ossicle), which is proximal inferior border of the tuberosity of the fifth metatarsal (Fig. 24.3). The os trigonum (trigone ossicle) lies posterior to the talus (Fig. 24.4). The peroneal ossicle and the vesalian ossicle may be identified on the lateral or the oblique view. The trigone ossicle is best appreciated on the lateral view.

PATIENT ASSESSMENT

1. Asymptomatic
2. Seldom require surgery

Treatment

No treatment is generally necessary. Surgical removal for symptomatic cases is rare.

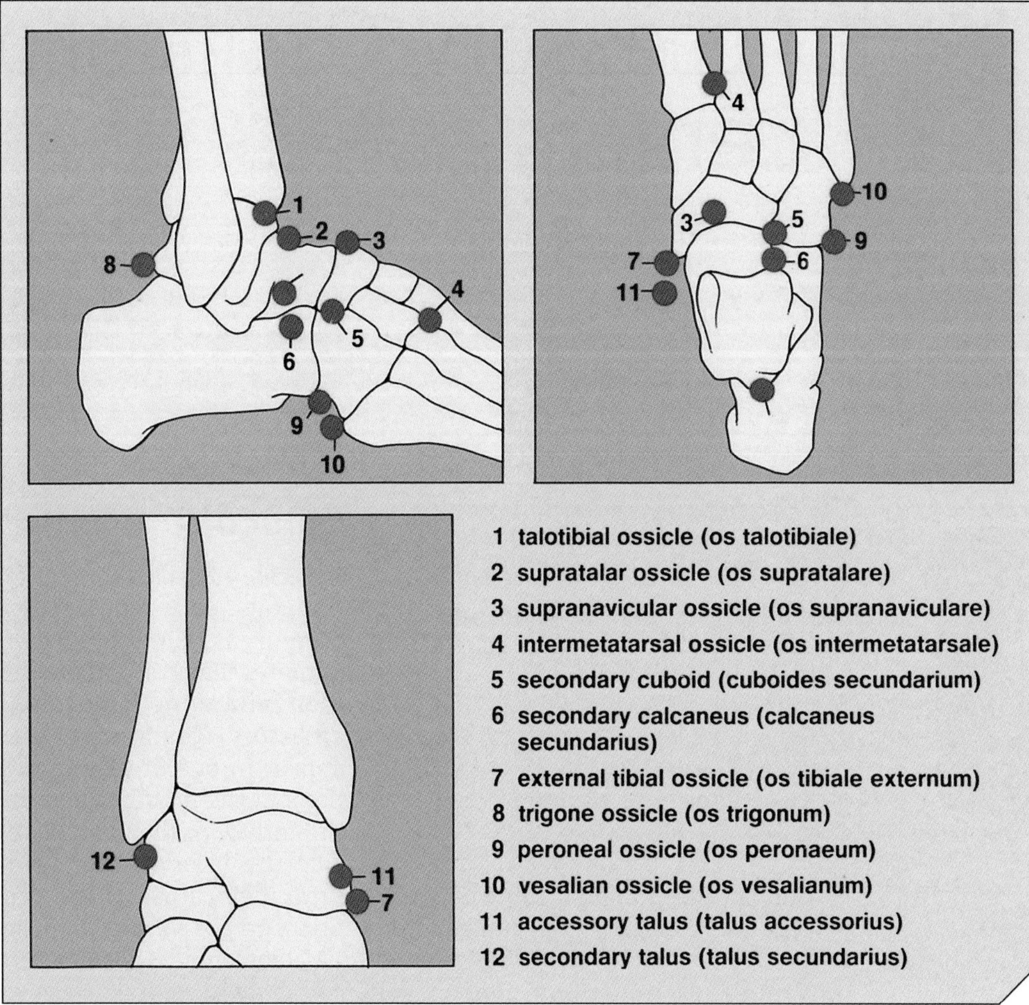

Figure 24.1 Accessory ossification centers. (From Greenspan A. *Orthopedic Imaging: A Practical Approach*. 4th ed. Philadelphia, PA: Lippincott Williams & Wilkins; 2004:309.)

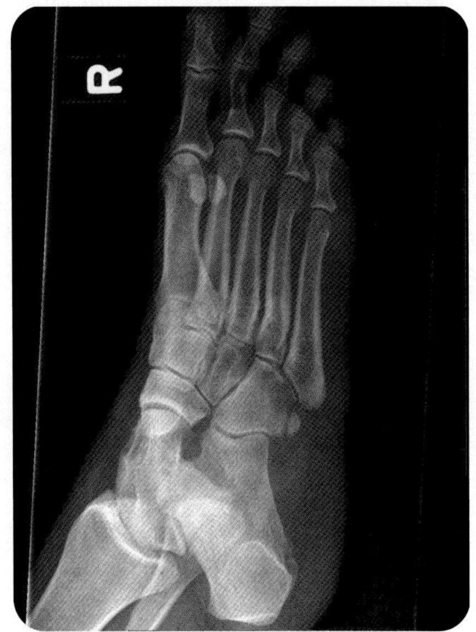

Figure 24.2 Os peroneum (peroneal ossicle), which lies inferior laterally to the cuboid.

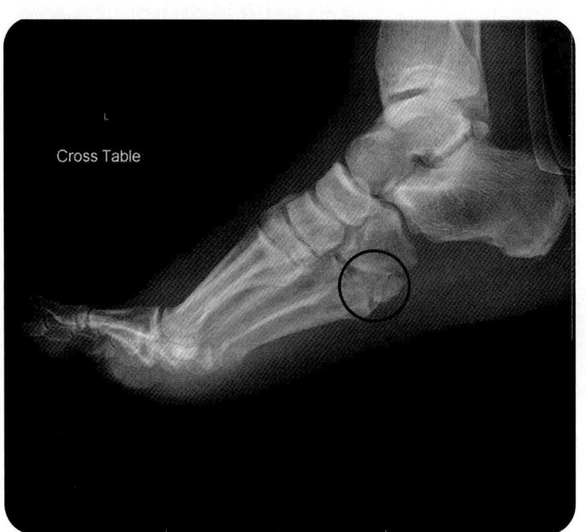

Figure 24.3 Os vesalianum (vesalian ossicle).

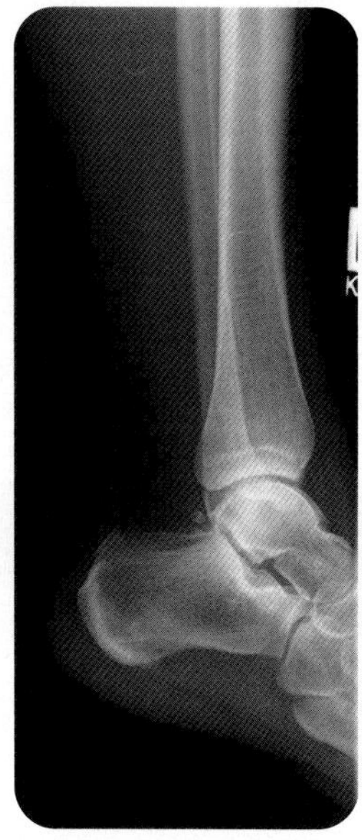

Figure 24.4 Os trigonum (trigone ossicle).

Suggested Readings

Ahn JM, El-Khoury GY. Radiologic evaluation of chronic foot pain. *Am Fam Physician*. 2007;76:975–983.

Greenspan A. *Orthopedic Imaging: A Practical Approach*. 4th ed. Philadelphia, PA: Lippincott Williams & Wilkins; 2004.

Judd DB, Kim DA. Foot fractures frequently misdiagnosed as ankle sprains. *Am Fam Physician*. 2002;66: 785–794.

Magee DJ. *Orthopedic Physical Assessment*. 4th ed. Philadelphia, PA: WB Saunders; 2002:829.

McKinnis LN. *Fundamentals of Orthopedic Radiology*. Philadelphia, PA: FA Davis; 1997:320–321.

Mellado JM, Ramos A, Salvado E, et al. Accessory ossicles and sesamoid bones of the ankle and foot: imaging findings, clinical significant and differential diagnosis. *Eur Radiol*. 2003;13(4):164–177.

Miller TT. Painful accessory bones of the foot. *Semin Musculoskelet Radiol*. 2002;6(2):153–161.

SECTION 5

Foot

Functional Anatomy

The foot may be divided into three regions: the forefoot, the midfoot, and the hindfoot. The forefoot includes the phalanges and the metatarsals. The first, or great, toe has two phalanges, whereas the second through fifth toes contain three phalanges each (proximal, middle, and distal). The interphalangeal joints are hinge joints (with one degree of freedom), which allow for limited flexion (downward movement toward the floor) and extension (sometimes referred to as dorsiflexion). The first metatarsal bone has two oval sesamoid bones (the medial and the lateral sesamoid) within the tendon of the flexor hallucis brevis tendon. Weight bearing means standing and walking. These sesamoids help shield the tendon while weight bearing and allow for greater dorsiflexion (upward movement in a cranial direction) of the great toe. Approximately 15% to 25% of patients have a bipartite sesamoid (i.e., an incomplete bony fusion of the sesamoid, resulting in two small bony fragments). The condition is frequently bilateral and does not require any treatment.

The metatarsals are column-shaped structures and consist of a distal head, a shaft, and a proximal base. Like the phalanges, the articulating metatarsals are numbered one through five, starting with the medial metatarsal that articulates with the great toe. Range of motion at the metatarsophalangeal joints is across two planes. It consists of limited flexion and extension, approximately 30 degrees in each direction. In addition, there is limited adduction (inward movement of the forefoot) and abduction (outward movement of the forefoot). Injuries to the metatarsals are sometimes classified as rays; these are based on the major contact points of the foot when striking the ground. The first ray contains the first metatarsal, the second ray the second through fourth metatarsals, and the third ray the fifth metatarsal.

The midfoot contains the first, second, and third cuneiforms; the cuboid; and the navicular (Fig. 1). The cuneiforms consist of three wedge-shaped bones that makeup the medial portion of the midfoot. The first cuneiform (sometimes called the medial cuneiform) articulates distally with the base of the first metatarsal. The second cuneiform (sometimes called the intermediate or middle cuneiform) articulates distally with the base of the second metacarpal, and it forms a wedge between the first and the third cuneiforms. The third cuneiform (sometimes called the lateral cuneiform) articulates with the base of the third metatarsal, and it forms a wedge between the second cuneiform and its lateral neighbor, the cuboid. All three cuneiforms articulate proximally with the navicular. The cuboid is located laterally to the navicular and third cuneiform. It provides structural support to the bases of the fourth and the fifth metatarsals.

The articulation between the tarsal structures (the three cuneiforms and the bases of the metatarsals) receives structural reinforcement from the tarsometatarsal (Lisfranc) ligament. The Lisfranc ligament connects the forefoot with the midfoot. The proximal midfoot is connected to the hindfoot at the talonavicular joint (sometimes called Chopart's joint) by the transverse tarsal ligament. In addition, the cuboid articulates with the calcaneus at the calcaneocuboid joint.

The hindfoot contains the talus and the calcaneus. The talus has a rounded head, a neck, and a body. The head of the talus articulates with the distal tibia to form the talocrural joint—a hinge joint. The talocrural joint is primarily responsible for ankle plantar flexion (depression of the toes) and dorsiflexion (elevation of the toes). The body of the talus articulates with the calcaneus to form the subtalar joint.

As a whole, the foot (excluding the toes) has two movements: supination and pronation. The gait cycle (walking) consists of a stance phase and a swing-through phase. The stance phase accounts for approximately 60% of

Frontal View

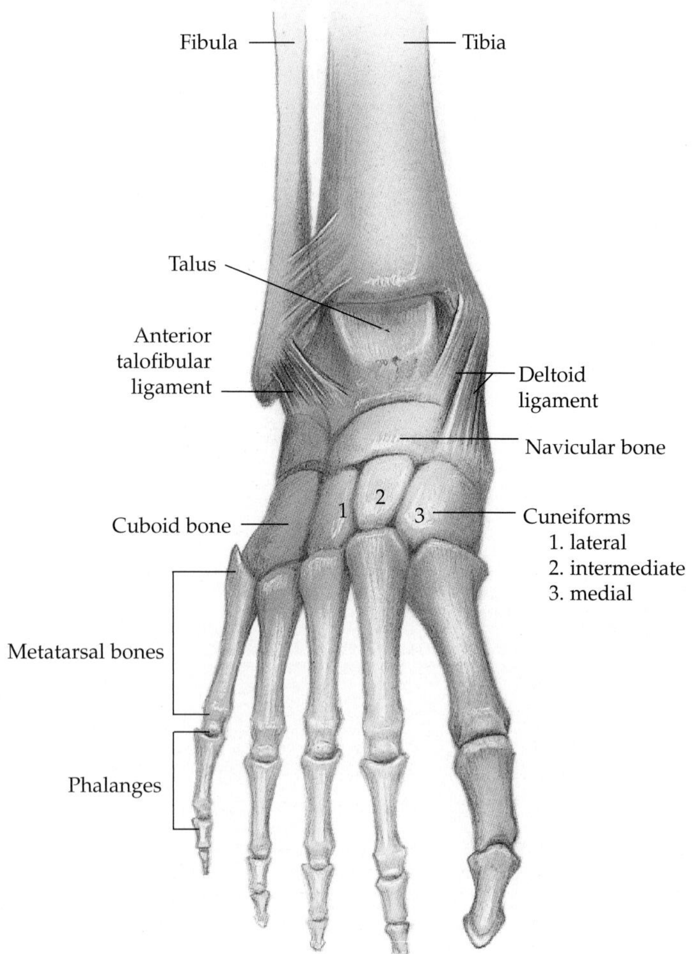

Figure 1 Frontal view of foot and ankle skeletal anatomy with deltoid and anterior talofibular ligaments. Asset provided by Anatomical Chart Co.

the gait cycle, and the swing-through phase accounts for the other 40%. The stance phase is subdivided into three phases: heel strike, midstance, and push-off ("toe-off"). Heel strike occurs when the foot first hits the ground when walking or jogging. During heel strike, the foot begins to pronate. Pronation is a complex triplanar motion in which the foot and ankle dorsiflexes and rolls outward. It accounts for approximately 25% of the stance phase. During the early part of midstance, the foot begins to supinate. Supination is a complex triplanar motion during which the foot and ankle flexes and rolls inward. This primes the foot as a lever for the push-off phase; it is primed for the next heel strike.

CHAPTER 25

Fifth Metatarsal Fractures

George M. Bridgeforth and George Holmes

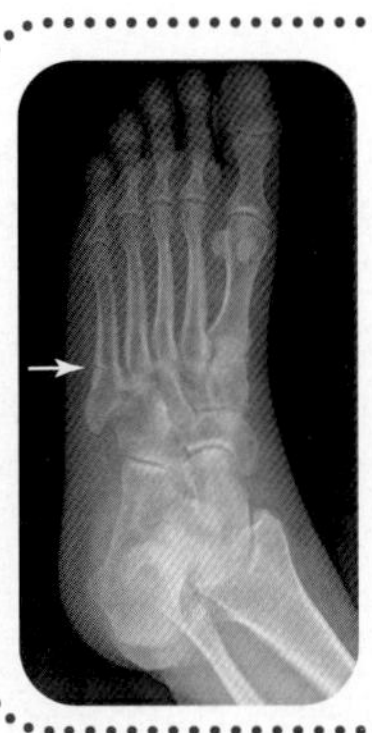

A 55-year-old woman slipped and fell on her icy driveway yesterday. She presents with pain over the base of the left fifth metatarsal.

Clinical Presentation

Fractures of the foot are common and often involve the fifth metatarsal, the bone that runs from the middle of the foot to the base of the small toe (Fig. 25.1). There are basically three types of fifth metatarsal injuries.

- Avulsion fractures: These fractures have a mechanism of injury that is similar to an ankle sprain.* Patients may complain of tripping or missing a curb or the rung of ladder. Avulsion fractures are transverse fractures that generally involve the tuberosity of the metatarsal base—the site of attachment of the avulsed peroneus brevis tendon.
- Jones fractures: True Jones fractures, more rare than avulsion fractures, occur at the proximal diaphysis (shaft). These result from laterally directed force on the forefoot with the ankle in plantar flexion (see "Radiographic Evaluation" for more information); they are caused by inversion of the foot. The resulting injury is more serious (Fig. 25.2).
- Stress fractures: Stress fractures of the metatarsals may occur distally at the metatarsal neck in runners. However, some stress fractures may appear more proximally, especially in dancers; axial loads with torsion result in more proximal fractures. These result from the placement of abnormal stress on a normal bone.

CLINICAL POINTS

- Patients complain of pain and swelling.
- Weight-bearing is limited.
- Tenderness at the base of the fifth metatarsal may be present.

PATIENT ASSESSMENT

1. Swelling and point tenderness with an inability to bear weight along the lateral border of the foot
2. Sometimes caused by placement of abnormal stress
3. Easily missed in many cases, because the examiner focuses on the ankle injury. The examiner should always check for point tenderness of the metatarsal tenderness with any ankle injury.

Patients with a fifth metatarsal styloid fracture or a Jones fracture (proximal diaphysis) exhibit marked tenderness at the proximal fifth metatarsal, and bruising may be present. In the case of fifth metatarsal styloid fracture, the pain and soreness is at the tuberosity of the fifth metatarsal base. There is pain-limited weight-bearing along the lateral aspect of the foot.

When examining a patient for a fracture of the fifth metatarsal, the examiner should

- specifically palpate for a fifth metatarsal fracture. An associated metatarsal fracture is easily missed because the examiner focuses on the pain and swelling caused by the ankle injury.

*Avulsion fractures to the base (or proximal shaft) of the fifth metatarsal are caused by the lateral band of the planar ligament as an inverted ankle strikes the ground.

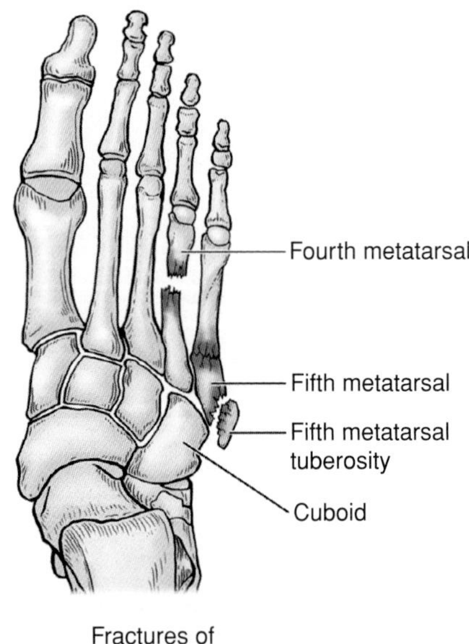

Figure 25.1 Anatomical diagram demonstrating a displaced transverse of the fourth metatarsal shaft. Note the avulsion fracture of the fifth metatarsal tuberosity. Jones fractures are uncommon but are characterized by transverse fractures of the proximal shaft (diaphysis) of the fifth metatarsal. (From Moore KL, Agur A. *Essential Clinical Anatomy*. 2nd ed. Philadelphia, PA: Lippincott Williams & Wilkins; 2002.)

- observe the Ottawa rules. Look for pain, swelling, or tenderness of the lateral malleolus or both malleoli. It is important to check for navicular and fibular head tenderness as well.
- always check and record the neurovascular status

Radiographic Evaluation

Radiographs to order include anteroposterior (AP), lateral, and oblique views. If there is associated metatarsal tenderness of the base or proximal shaft and the area is not well visualized on standard ankle radiographs, then AP, lateral, and oblique foot radiographs should be obtained as well. It is always necessary to check all foot radiographs (and lateral ankle radiographs) for a fifth metatarsal fracture (Fig. 25.3). An avulsion fracture usually is located at or proximal to the metatarsal–cuboid joint (Fig. 25.4). True Jones fractures must be distinguished from avulsion fractures at the base of the fifth metatarsal. Also, true Jones fractures are rare and occur near (about 1 inch distal to) the metaphyseal–diaphyseal junction (i.e., right at the proximal fifth metatarsal shaft) (Fig. 25.5). This region must be visualized on all ankle radiographs. Generally, Jones fractures are at or distal to a transverse line drawn from the metatarsal–cuboid joint. The zonal classification is helpful in this case. Fractures at the tuberosity of the fifth metatarsal are avulsion fractures (zone 1). Fractures at the proximal diaphysis (shaft) are Jones fractures (zone 2). Fractures of the mid or distal shaft are stress fractures (zone 3) (Fig. 25.6).

It is important to note that in stress fractures, the fracture line may not appear (if at all) until 2 to 3 weeks after the initial injury. However, soft tissue swelling may be evident on the initial radiographs. Callus formation, which is characterized by a subtle periosteal thickening, may take 4 to 6 weeks. If a stress fracture is suspected, repeat images may be necessary. Although bone scans are highly sensitive for detecting early stress fractures, they are highly nonspecific as well. Bone scans are highly sensitive but provide poor anatomical detail, and magnetic resonance imaging scans provide more specific anatomical detail.

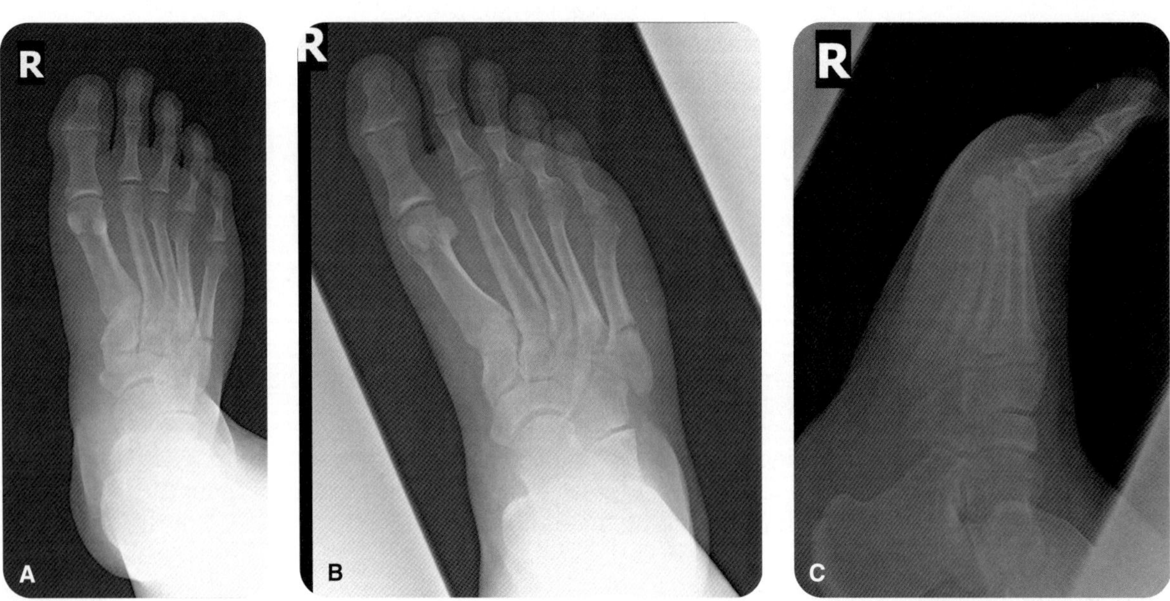

Figure 25.2 (A–C) Three views of the right foot, all showing an incomplete transverse fracture in the base of the fifth metatarsal bone. The fracture line does not extend to the tarsometatarsal joint. (Courtesy of Richard Kim, MD.)

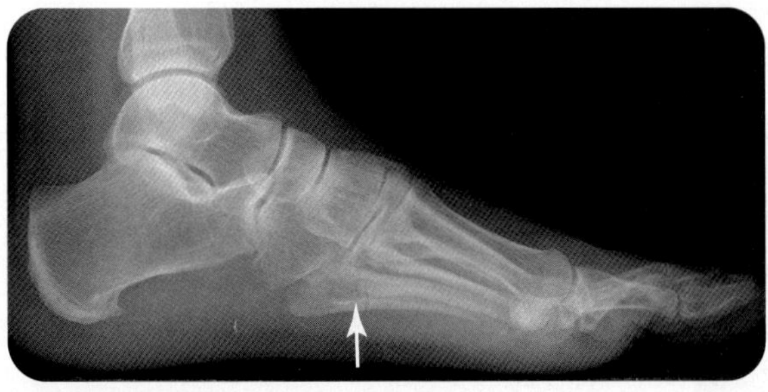

Figure 25.3 Lateral radiograph of the foot demonstrates an acute fracture of the fifth metatarsal.

Treatment

AVULSION FRACTURES

Patients with nondisplaced avulsion fractures may be treated with crutches and an orthopedic shoe. Patients may engage in limited weight-bearing. Some patients may require a short walking cast for 2 to 3 weeks or a hard-soled orthopedic shoe for approximately 6 to 8 weeks. For severe injuries, additional assistive devices (canes, crutches) may be required. If the examiner is not sure whether or not the fracture is a true Jones fracture, it is advisable to keep patients on non–weight-bearing status until they have been evaluated by an orthopedic specialist.

NOT TO BE MISSED

- Foot contusion
- Styloid fracture
- Accessory ossification centers (usually asymptomatic)
- Bone tumors (rare)

JONES FRACTURES

Unfortunately, true Jones fractures may be complicated by delayed healing. Because of the history of nonunion, a Jones fracture should be followed up by an orthopedic specialist; some fractures may require pinning. Pending the orthopedic referral, patients may be placed on crutches, a posterior mold, and maintained on non–weight-bearing status (on the affected leg). Many acute Jones fractures may be treated with a non–weight-bearing cast for 6 to 8 weeks. Treatment failures and chronic nonhealing fractures are candidates for surgery.

STRESS FRACTURES

Most patients with stress fractures may be placed in an orthopedic shoe or a short leg walking cast for 6 to 12 weeks. Non–weight-bearing status is necessary. Fifth metatarsal stress fractures are more prone to malunion, and surgery is rarely indicated unless the patient has chronic pain with radiographic evidence of nonunion.

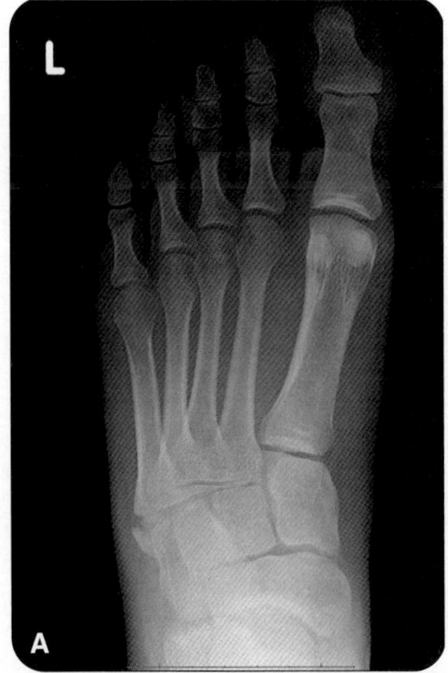

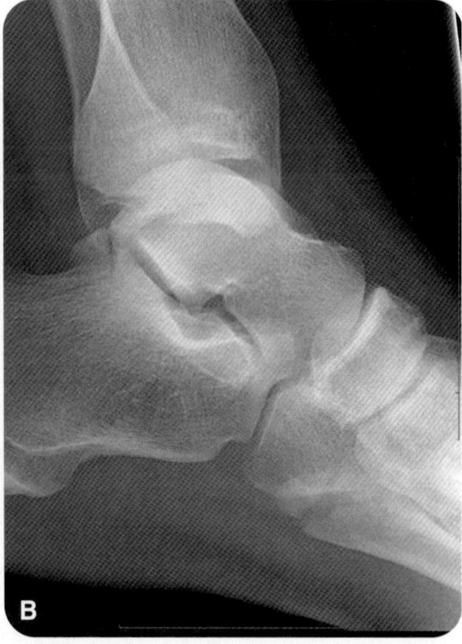

Figure 25.4 **(A)** Anterior–posterior and **(B)** lateral radiographs of the left foot demonstrating an avulsion fracture of the base of the fifth metatarsal in a 22-year-old man who jumped a fence and twisted his ankle.

WHEN TO REFER

- Most patients with avulsion fractures require referral if the primary care physician is not experienced with fracture management.
- Immediate referral is necessary for:
  - patients with Jones fractures and stress fractures
  - patients with cold cyanotic limbs with diminished or absent pulses

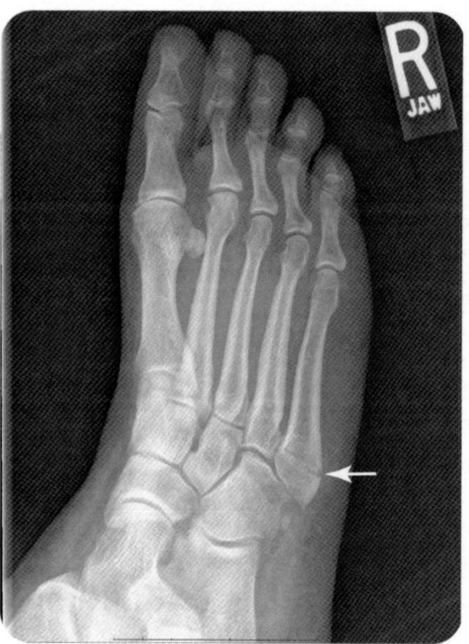

Figure 25.5 Oblique radiograph of the right foot, demonstrating a Jones fracture.

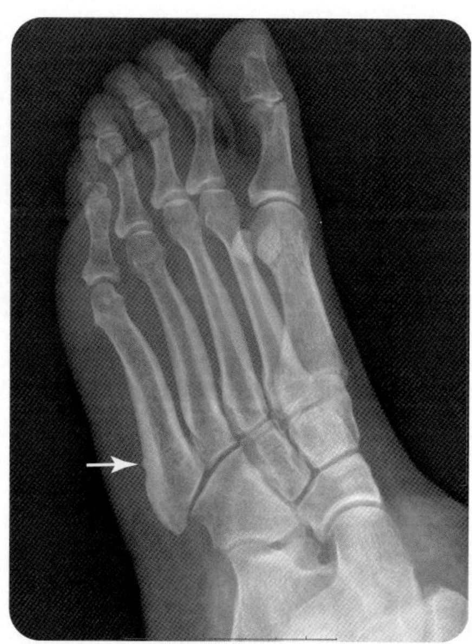

Figure 25.6 Oblique radiograph demonstrating a zone 3 Jones fracture.

Suggested Readings

Den Hartog BD. Fracture of the proximal fifth metatarsal. *J Bone Joint Surg*. 2009;17:458–464.

Eiff MP, Hatch RL, Calmbach WL. *Fracture Management for Primary Care*. Philadelphia, PA: Saunders; 2003: 348–350.

Greenspan A. *Orthopedic Imaging: A Practical Approach*. 4th ed. Philadelphia, PA: Lippincott Williams and Wilkins; 2004:336–342.

Harris JH, Harris WH, Novelline RA. *The Radiology of Emergency Medicine*. 3rd ed. Baltimore, MD: Lippincott Williams & Wilkins; 1993:1030–1032.

Hatch RL, Alsobrook JA, Clugston JR. Diagnosis and management of metatarsal fractures. *Am Fam Physician*. 2007;76:817–826.

Kavanaugh JH, Brower TD, Mann RV. The Jones fracture revisited. *J Bone Joint Surg*. 1978;60:776–782.

McKinnis L. *Fundamentals of Orthopedic Radiology*. Philadelphia, PA: FA Davis; 1997:317.

Rosen P, Doris PE, Barkin RM, Markovchick VJ. *Diagnostic Radiology in Emergency Medicine*. St Louis, MO: Mosby; 1992:209.

Rosenberg GA, Sferra JJ. Treatment strategies for acute fractures and nonunions of the proximal fifth metatarsal. *J Bone Joint Surg*. 2000;8:332–338.

Strayer SM, Reece SG, Petrizzi MJ. Fractures of the proximal fifth metatarsal. *Am Fam Physician*. 1999;59:2516-2522.

Theodorou DJ, Theodorous SJ, Kakitsubata Y, et al. Fractures of proximal portion of fifth metatarsal bone: anatomic and imaging evidence of pathogenesis of avulsion of the plantar aponeurosis and the short peroneal muscle tendon. *Radiology*. 2003;226:857–865.

Torg JS, Balduini FC, Zelko RR, et al. Fractures of the base of the fifth metatarsal distal to the tuberosity: classification and guidelines for non-surgical and surgical management. *J Bone Joint Surg*. 1984;66:209–214.

Other Metatarsal Fractures

George M. Bridgeforth and George Holmes

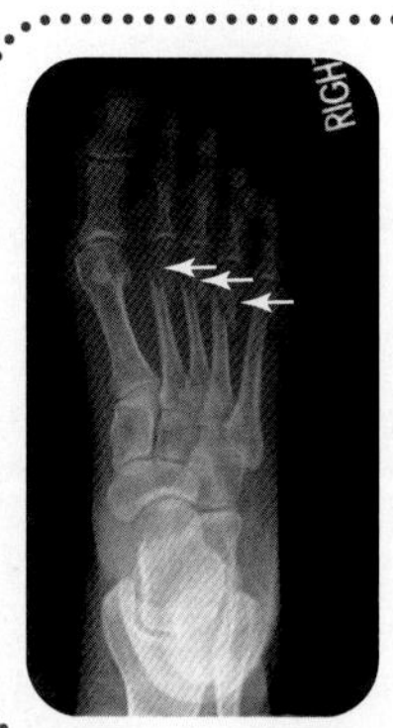

A 26-year-old woman presents after falling 4 weeks earlier. She complains of moderate-to-severe pain, swelling, and tenderness of her foot, with pain on movement and difficulty putting weight on it.

Clinical Presentation

Metatarsal injuries are common, because there is minimal soft tissue to protect the top of the foot. These injuries usually involve direct trauma (impact) but may result from an axial load with torsion. Injuries to the first, second, third, and fourth metatarsals are considered in this chapter, and fractures of the fifth metatarsal fractures are discussed in Chapter 25. Patients with acute metatarsal fractures have moderate-to-marked pain, swelling, and tenderness at the midfoot, which are always important clues that direct the examiner to the fracture site. In addition, patients commonly have pain-limited dorsiflexion and plantar flexion with limited weight bearing.

CLINICAL POINTS

- Metatarsal fractures are often caused by trauma.
- People with diabetes have a greater risk of infection as a result of a metatarsal injury.
- Stress fractures may manifest as point tenderness, especially over the second or third metatarsal or the fifth metatarsal shaft.

The clinician should perform a careful neurovascular examination to check the neurovascular status of the foot for evidence of sensory loss, marked swelling, coldness, pallor, and impaired pulses. It is important to document the results. It is necessary to inspect the foot, including each phalanx, carefully for coldness and cyanosis, and palpate the posterior tibial pulse at the posterior medial malleolus just behind the distal tibia. The dorsalis pedis pulse lies medially to the extensor hallucis tendon as it runs along the first metatarsal shaft.

In addition, the clinician should inspect the foot carefully for open wounds. Even with small open wounds without fractures, patients with diabetes are at increased risk for developing a serious cellulitis of the foot (Fig. 26.1). These patients require close follow-up to watch for signs of infection, especially with penetrating wounds, and serious consideration for possible antibiotic therapy with close follow-up. It is also necessary to closely monitor people with diabetes and closed foot injuries for infection (Fig. 26.2).

Patients with multiple metatarsal fractures may have an associated Lisfranc ligament injury. The Lisfranc ligament is at the midfoot and anchors the tarsal bones to the proximal metatarsals. It is important to note that patients with moderate swelling and tenderness over the midfoot may have associated damage to the Lisfranc ligament with or without accompanying metatarsal fractures. In addition, these patients exhibit an antalgic gait (i.e., a pronounced limp). Moreover, they may have trouble wearing regular shoes because of pronounced

PATIENT ASSESSMENT

1. Pain, swelling (bruising), and point tenderness at the fracture site
2. Limited weight bearing

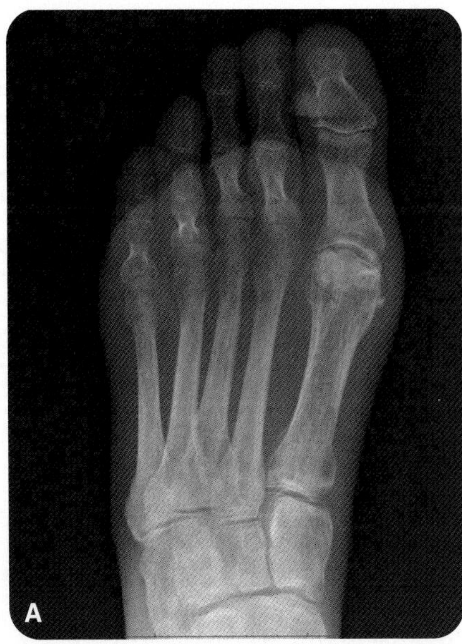

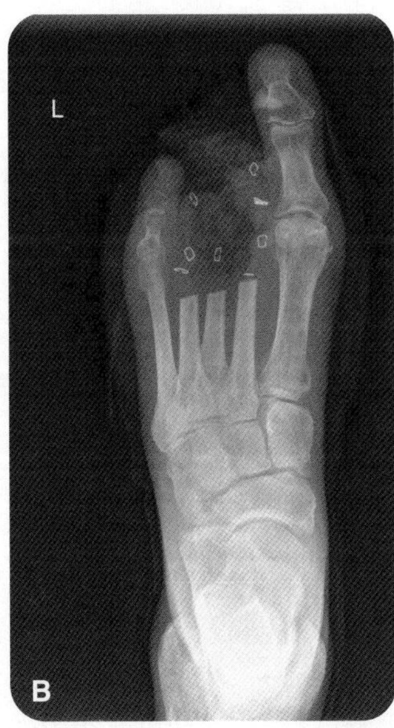

Figure 26.1 (A) Notice the lucent areas over the middle metatarsal–phalangeal joints compatible with subcutaneous gas from gas-forming bacteria in left foot cellulitis in this 83-year-old diabetic male. **(B)** Follow-up radiograph demonstrates midtarsal amputation of the second, third, and fourth digits in the same patient.

pain at the dorsal midfoot. Lisfranc injuries may be easily missed, and a high index of suspicion is required (see Chapter 27). The examiner should suspect an associated Lisfranc injury if there is marked tenderness over the Lisfranc (tarsometatarsal) joint (Fig. 26.3).*

*In addition, patients with Lisfranc injuries exhibit pain-limited weight bearing. Underlying fracture may or may not be apparent on radiographs.

NOT TO BE MISSED

- Lisfranc injury
- Foot contusion
- Associated talar fracture
- Osteomyelitis (especially in diabetic patients)

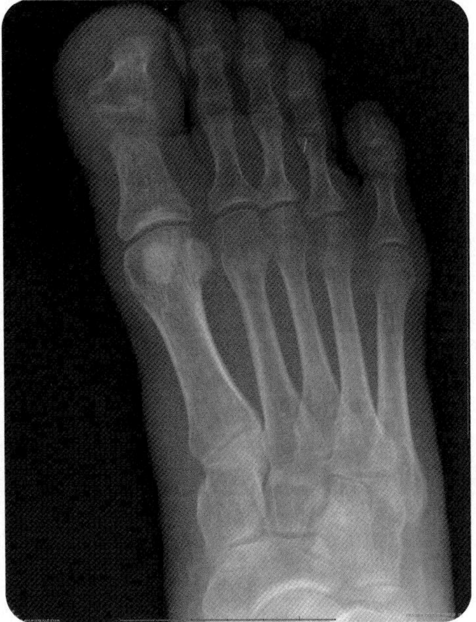

Figure 26.2 Anteroposterior radiograph of the foot demonstrates soft tissue swelling of the first digit with juxta-articular bone resorption compatible with osteomyelitis of the first interphalangeal joint.

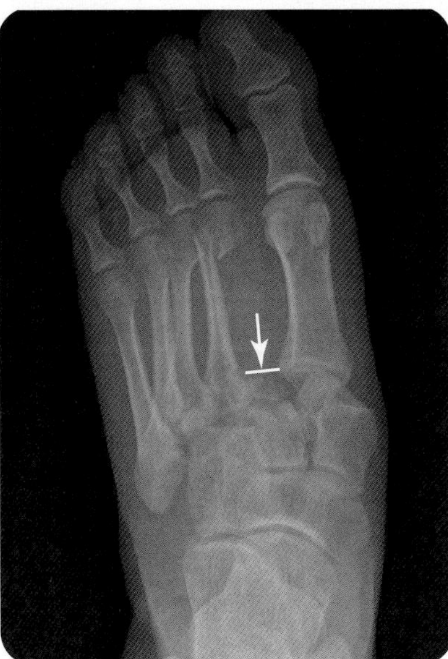

Figure 26.3 Lisfranc fracture, with acute fractures of the second and third metatarsals with widening of the Lisfranc interval (*arrow*).

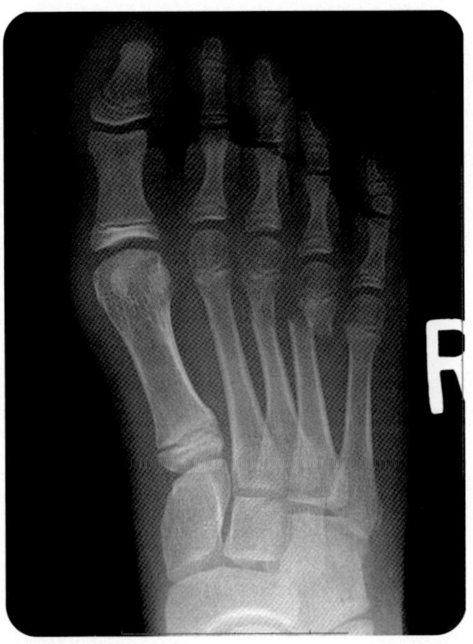

Figure 26.4 Anteroposterior radiograph, demonstrating acute fractures of the distal third and fourth metatarsals.

Radiographic Evaluation

Anteroposterior (AP), oblique, and lateral views should be obtained. Many metatarsal fractures are best appreciated on the AP view (Fig. 26.4). However, the examiner cannot rely on the AP view along to determine the degree of displacement. The lateral view should be used to check for evidence of displacement, although metatarsal displacement in a dorsal (top of the foot) or plantar (bottom of the foot) direction may be obscured by bony overlap on the lateral view. The degree of angulation of bony separation for these planes may be difficult to determine by the AP view alone. In these situations, comparison with the oblique view can be extremely helpful. If there is evidence of displacement, an immediate orthopedic referral is indicated. Weight-bearing views are usually taken by specialists to determine if there is any metatarsal displacement.

A metacarpal stress fracture may present with nonspecific swelling around the shaft or callus formation (a slight bulge in the midshaft). A thin translucent fracture line may not be apparent, especially during the first several weeks of injury.

Treatment

First metatarsal fractures should be kept non–weight bearing for a minimum of 4 to 6 weeks.

Generally, patients with nondisplaced metatarsal fractures of the second through the fourth metatarsals are generally treated with a walking cast or an orthopedic shoe. Many of those with displaced fractures of the second through the fourth metatarsals are treated with a closed reduction followed by casting for approximately 6 weeks. However, affected patients should remain on non–weight-bearing status. Displaced fractures of the metatarsal neck are more difficult to treat and may require an open reduction and internal fixation. The decision about whether or not to operate is made on a case-by-case basis. Unlike nondisplaced fractures of the second through the fourth metatarsals, some practitioners keep patients with nondisplaced first metatarsal fractures on non–weight-bearing status. It is recommended that these fractures should be discussed with orthopedics. Oblique and spiral fractures are generally unstable. Metatarsal neck fractures and transverse fractures may be unstable despite without any evidence of displacement on standard (AP and lateral) radiographs.

Fractures of the first metatarsal may require surgery, but fractures of the second, third, and fourth metatarsals usually do not require surgery unless displacement of the bone is significant.

Patients without metatarsal fractures who exhibit limited weight bearing with marked pain, soreness, and tenderness over the Lisfranc (tarsometatarsal joint) should be placed in a posterior mold and kept on non–weight-bearing status. A magnetic resonance imaging scan should be obtained for a possible Lisfranc injury.

WHEN TO REFER

- Patients with open, displaced, or unstable fractures, as well as possible Lisfranc injuries warrant immediate referral. Those with neurovascular compromise should also require immediate referral.
- Referral is necessary for:
  - patients with fractures with displaced bone fragments greater than 3 to 4 mm or with intra-articular fractures (fracture lines that extend to the joint spaces).
  - patients with angulations (in a dorsal or plantar direction) of greater than 10 degrees warrant referral (Eiff et al.)

Suggested Readings

Eiff MP, Hatch RL, Calmbach WL. *Fracture Management for Primary Care.* Philadelphia, PA: Saunders; 2003:348–350.

Greenspan A. *Orthopedic Imaging: A Practical Approach.* 4th ed. Philadelphia, PA: Lippincott Williams & Wilkins; 2004:336–342.

Harris JH, Harris WH, Novelline RA. *The Radiology of Emergency Medicine.* 3rd ed. Baltimore, MD: Williams & Wilkins; 1030–1032.

McKinnis L. *Fundamentals of Orthopedic Radiology.* Philadelphia, PA: FA Davis; 1997:317.

Rosen P, Doris PE, Barkin RM, Markovchick VJ. *Diagnostic Radiology in Emergency Medicine.* Saint Louis, MO: Mosby Year Book; 1992:209.

Torg JS, Balduini FC, Zelko RR, et al. Fractures of the base of the fifth metatarsal distal to the tuberosity. Classification and guidelines for non-surgical and surgical management. *J Bone Joint Surg JBJS.* 1984;66:209–214.

CHAPTER 27

Lisfranc Injuries

George M. Bridgeforth and George Holmes

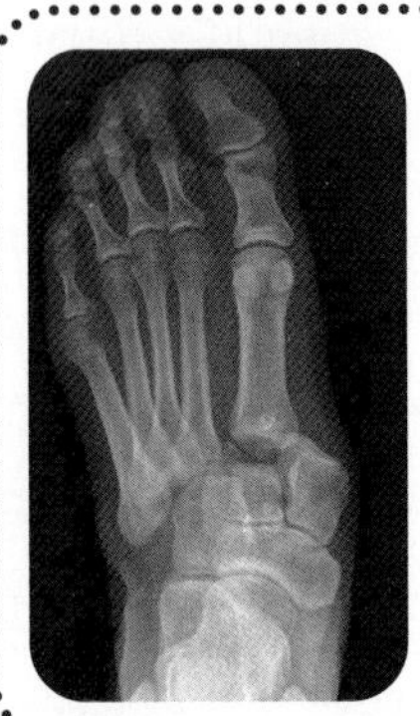

A 33-year-old woman fell down the stairs. She presents with a gross deformity of the left foot.

Clinical Presentation

A Lisfranc injury is damage to the joints in the midfoot—the Lisfranc joint, or tarsometatarsal articulation of the foot. The most common mechanism of injury is torsion/impaction against the plantar flexed foot (i.e., foot is pointed downward). Common examples would include being involved in a motor vehicle accident or forklift accident, when the foot gets caught under a brake. Another example would be having the foot caught on the rung of a ladder or falling down the stairs (with the foot in a plantar flexed position). However, Lisfranc injures may be also be caused by axial loads (heavy items) that land directly on the dorsal foot.

Lisfranc injuries are rare but are associated with a high risk of chronic secondary disability. They are easily missed during the initial evaluation, and the best way to detect these injuries is to have a high index of suspicion. Normal radiographs do not rule out an associated Lisfranc injury. Valuable clinic clues include marked pain, swelling, and tenderness over the midfoot, especially over the tarsometatarsal joint; some inability to bear weight; and limited range of motion. The presence of these signs and symptoms and a lack of any improvement may point to a Lisfranc injury.

CLINICAL POINTS

- Lisfranc injuries vary in severity from sprains to fractures/dislocations.
- These injuries are difficult to diagnose.
- The neurovascular status of all patients should be checked carefully.

Radiolographic Evaluation

Anteroposterior (AP), lateral, and oblique views of the foot should be obtained. Radiographs are helpful but are not always diagnostic. If a Lisfranc injury is suspected but radiographs show only soft tissue swelling, a computed tomography scan or a magnetic resonance imaging scan may be necessary (Fig. 27.1).

Basically, there are two types of Lisfranc injuries: homolateral and divergent.

PATIENT ASSESSMENT

1. Marked pain, swelling, and tenderness over the midfoot
2. Pain-limited weight bearing and range of motion

HOMOLATERAL LISFRANC INJURY

With a homolateral Lisfranc injury (Fig. 27.2), all of the metatarsal fractures are pointing in the same direction. There is marked lateral displacement of the forefoot at the Lisfranc (tarsometatarsal) joint on the AP view. On the lateral view, there is a pronounced step-off between the cuboid–cuneiforms and the proximal metatarsals (at the Lisfranc joint). Although Lisfranc injuries are one

NOT TO BE MISSED

- Foot fracture
- Foot contusion
- Osteomyelitis (especially in patients with diabetes)

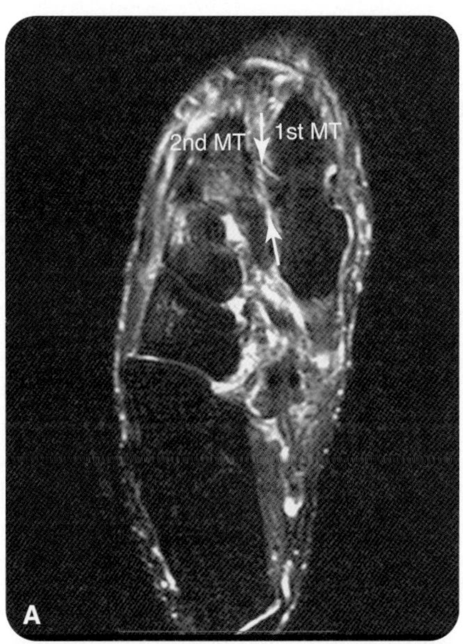

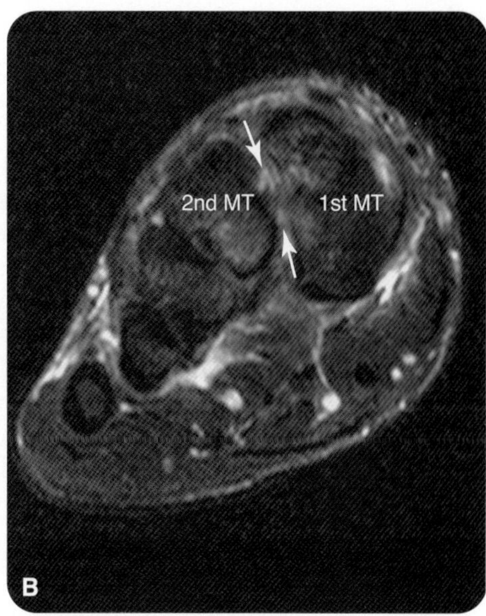

Figure 27.1 Lisfranc ligament injury. Selected **(A)** oblique and **(B)** coronal T2-weighted, fat-saturated images from magnetic resonance imaging scan of the right foot after a twisting injury in a 43-year-old man. Abnormal increased fluid signal is demonstrated in the Lisfranc ligament (*arrows*).

of the most common injuries of the foot, they are frequently missed. Large fracture dislocations are easy to identify.

DIVERGENT LISFRANC INJURY

With a divergent Lisfranc fracture/dislocation, the first metatarsal is displaced medially; the remaining metatarsals are displaced laterally in the opposite direction. Lisfranc injures are unstable injures, and the fractures are associated with tears in the tarsometatarsal ligament (Fig. 27.3).

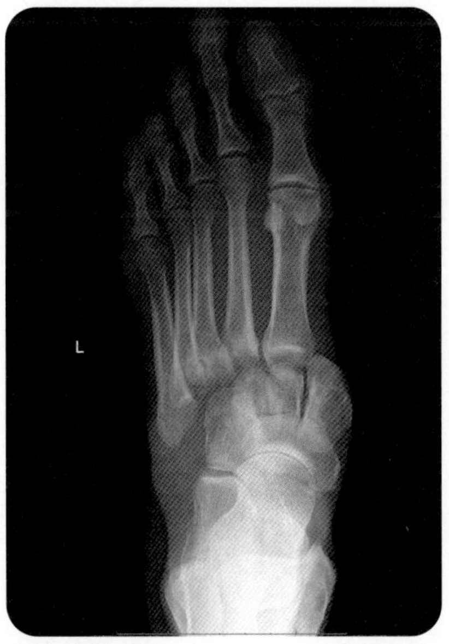

Figure 27.2 Anteroposterior radiograph, demonstrating homolateral Lisfranc fracture/dislocation.

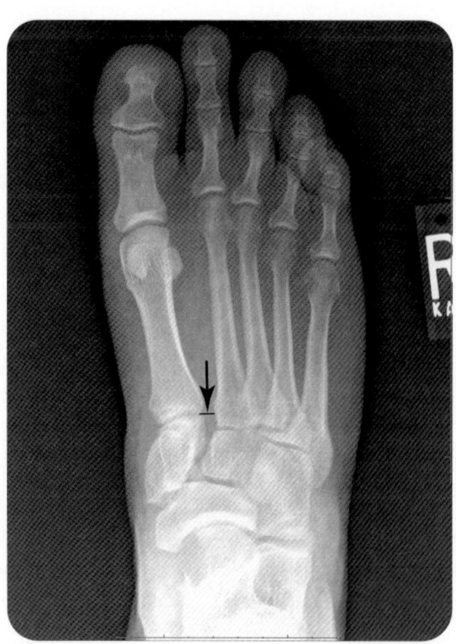

Figure 27.3 Anteroposterior radiograph, demonstrating widening of the Lisfranc interval in a divergent Lisfranc fracture/dislocation.

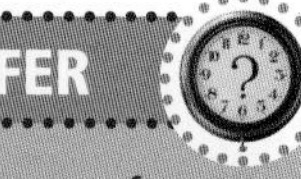

WHEN TO REFER

- Patients with open fractures, fracture dislocations, and neurovascular compromise require immediate referral.

OTHER RADIOGRAPHIC CLUES

A disruption of the Lisfranc ligament may be present if there is an increase in the space between the base of the first and the second metatarsal greater than 1 mm on the AP view. If a subtle separation between the first and the second metatarsal base is not readily apparent on the standard AP view, then a weight-bearing view may be helpful. (Subtle findings may not be apparent on weight-bearing views.) Sometimes, a tiny avulsion fracture (a fleck fracture) can be identified between the bases of the first and the second metatarsals on the AP view. The examiner should specifically look for a fleck fracture; clinicians commonly miss these. Moreover, they should suspect a Lisfranc injury if there is a fracture at the base of the second metatarsal. The American College of Emergency Physicians notes that a Lisfranc injury may occur if there is an isolated fracture of the cuboid or the cuneiforms. In addition, dorsal displacement of the second cuneiform on the lateral view indicates a possible Lisfranc injury.

Treatment

If a Lisfranc injury is suspected, the patient should be placed on non–weight-bearing status on the affected leg. The patient should be placed in a posterior mold and on crutches. The patient should be referred to orthopedics.

Suggested Readings

Aronow MS. Treatment of the Missed Lisfranc Injury. *Foot Ankle Clin*. 2006;11(1):127–142.

Burroughs KE, Reimer CD, Fields KB. Lisfranc injury of the foot: a commonly missed diagnosis. *Am Fam Physician*. 1998;58(1):118–127.

Englanoff G, Anglin D, Hutson HR. Lisfranc fracture-dislocation: a frequently missed diagnosis in the emergency department. *Ann Emerg Med*. 1995;26:229–233.

Foster SC, Foster RR. Lisfranc's Tarsometatarsal Fracture-Dislocation. *Radiology*. 1976;120:79–83.

Goossens M, DeStoop N. Lisfranc's fracture-dislocations: etiology radiology, and results of treatment. A review of 20 cases. *Clin Orthop Relat Res*. 1983;176:154–162.

Haapamaki V, Kiuru M, Koskinen S. Lisfranc fracture-dislocation in patients with multiple trauma: diagnosis with multidetector computer tomography. *Foot Ankle Int*. 2004;25(9):614–619.

Myerson MS, Cerrato RA. Current management of tarsometatarsal injuries in the athlete. *JBJS*. 2008;90: 2522–2533.

Raikin SM, Elias I, Dheer S, et al. Prediction of midfoot instability in the subtle Lisfranc injury. *JBJS*. 2009; 91:892–899.

Thompson MC, Normino MA. Injury to the tarsometatarsal joint complex. *J Am Acad Ortho Surg*. 2003;11: 260–267.

Thuan VL, Coetzee JC. Treatment of primarily ligamentous Lisfranc joint injuries; primary arthrodesis compared with open reduction and internal fixation. *JBJS*. 2006;88:514–520.

CHAPTER 28

Phalangeal Fractures

George M. Bridgeforth and George Holmes

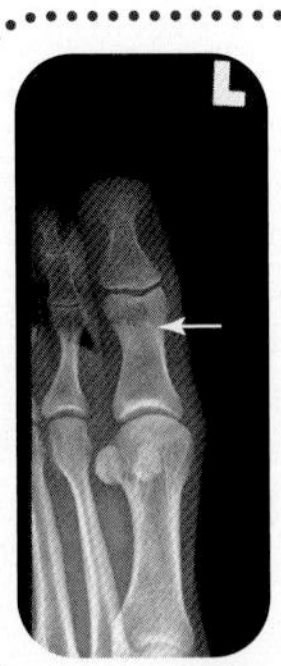

A 41-year-old woman presents with severe toe pain several hours after a horse stepped on her toe.

CLINICAL POINTS

- Evidence of infection (swelling, warmth, erythema, and purulent drainage), especially in patients with diabetes, may be seen.
- Throbbing pain may be a common complaint.
- Delayed capillary refill indicates impaired blood flow and necessitates a "stat" referral.

PATIENT ASSESSMENT

1. Pain, swelling, and tenderness of the affected phalanx/phalanges
2. Poor range of motion
3. Antalgic gait (limp) with a poor push-off

Clinical Presentation

Fractures of the phalanges (toes) are rather common and are often diagnosed and treated by primary care physicians. They are characterized by pain, swelling, and tenderness of the fractured phalanx. Patients commonly complain that they are not able to wear a regular shoe. When walking, they characteristically exhibit a poor push-off, with limited weight bearing of the forefoot. The mechanism of injury in toe fractures is direct trauma (e.g., from stubbed toes or falling objects).

The clinician should perform a careful physical examination. Assessment and documentation of deformity of the injured digit is essential. (The phalanges [toes] are numbered one through five, starting with the big toe.) To distinguish contusions from fractures, it is necessary to view the radiographs. In addition, the examiner should inspect the skin for open wounds or significant injury that may lead to necrosis. It is also necessary to inspect the nails for subungual hematomas and other nail injuries such as paronychia, an infection that subsequently develops along the nail edge. Patients with painful subungual hematomas who do not have associated phalangeal fractures may undergo a trephination in which a small hole is placed in the nail with a sterile heated needle or electrical cautery. The pressure under the nail caused by the hematoma is relieved. Pain and soreness between the third and the fourth phalanges may be secondary to a Morton's neuroma. This is a painful irritation of the plantar digital nerve. It is more common in females and may be caused by high heels or tightly fitting shoes. It does not appear on radiographs and it is marked characterized by tenderness of the web space. Lastly, the examiner should check the pulses and inspect for coldness, cyanosis, and discoloration. The neurovascular examination should always be well documented.

Patients with diabetes who have foot contusions or fractures are more likely to develop serious infections and should be monitored carefully. Severe infections in these patients may lead to an associated osteomyelitis (i.e., an infection of the bone), and close follow-up is critical. They present initially with minor foot (phalangeal fractures) or contusions; without careful monitoring, they can decompensate within a 3- to 4-week period.

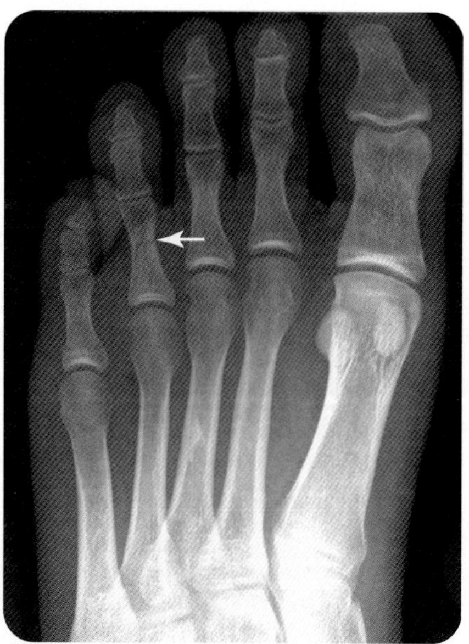

Figure 28.1 Anteroposterior radiograph demonstrates a comminuted fracture of the fourth proximal phalanx.

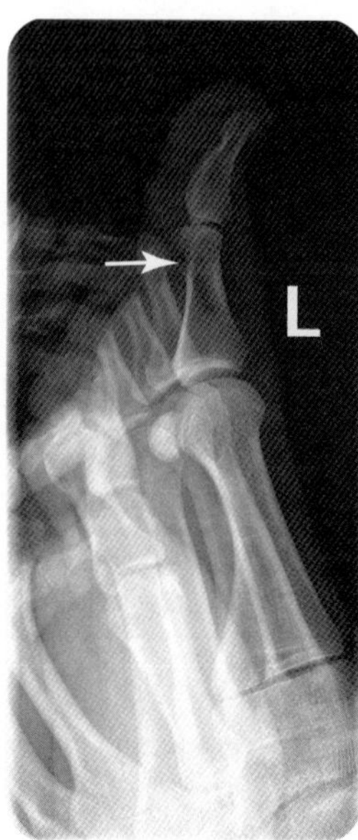

Figure 28.2 Lateral radiograph of the first digit of the left foot of the patient in the introductory case, demonstrating an acute fracture of the first proximal phalange.

Radiographic Evaluation

Anteroposterior (AP) (Fig. 28.1), lateral (Fig. 28.2), and oblique views should be obtained.

NONDISPLACED PHALANGEAL FRACTURES

From a clinical as well as radiographic standpoint, areas of soft tissue swelling and tenderness direct the examiner to the fracture site. Generally, nondisplaced fractures appear as thin translucent lines that break the cortex. They are best appreciated on the AP view. The lateral view contains significant overlap and is sometimes difficult to interpret (Fig. 28.3).

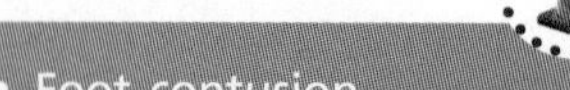

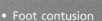

NOT TO BE MISSED

- Foot contusion
- Open fractures/dislocations
- Subungual hematoma
- Paronychia
- Osteomyelitis (patients with diabetes)
- Gout (great toe)
- Hallux valgus (bunions of the great toe)
- Hallux rigidus (turf toe)
- Hammer toes/claw toes
- Morton's neuroma

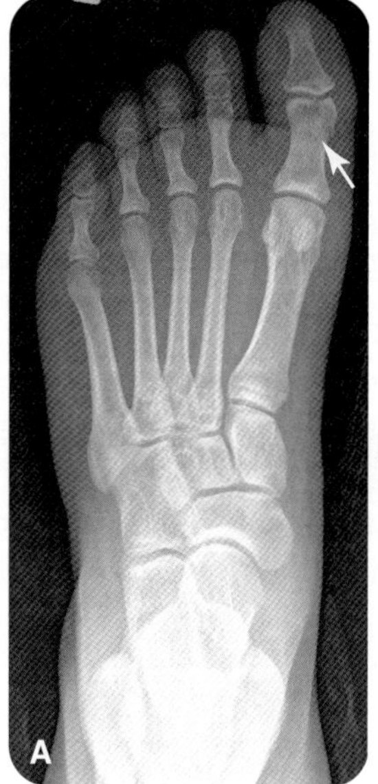

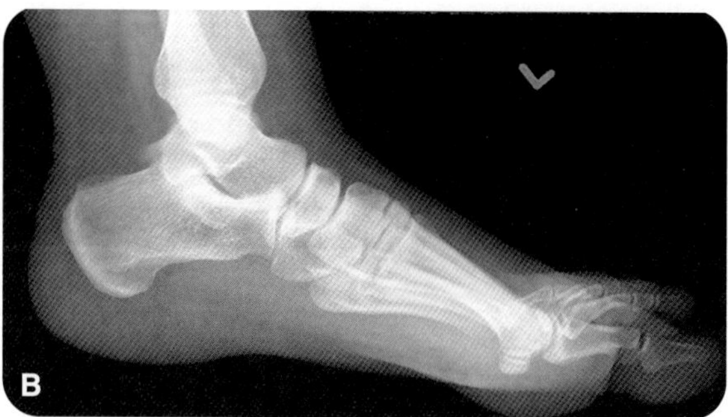

Figure 28.3 Anteroposterior (A) and lateral (B) radiographs demonstrates an acute fracture of the first proximal phalanx.

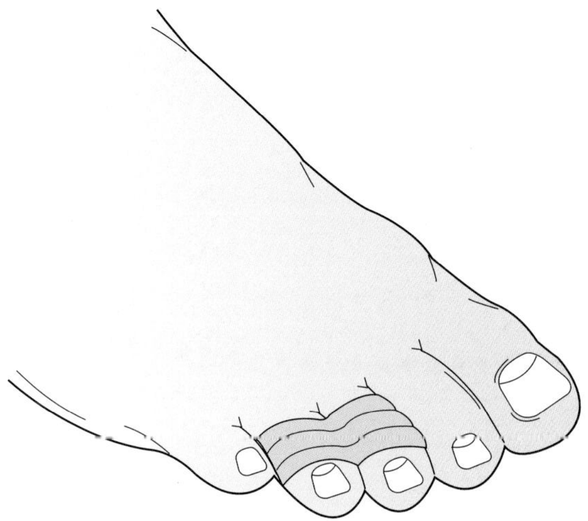

Figure 28.4 Buddy taping. It is helpful to place a small piece of cotton or adaptic between the taped phalanges to help prevent maceration. The distal portion of the phalanges should remain uncovered so that the area between the phalanges can be inspected for signs of maceration or infection.

Osteomyelitis causes destruction of the cortex and bony erosion. Harris notes that this process may take 3 weeks before radiologic changes are apparent. Acute changes consist of soft tissue swelling with moderate tenderness. Advanced changes may consist of widespread destruction and inflammation extending across the joint space, although they are often "hidden" under open wounds, especially in patients with diabetes.

TUFT FRACTURES

Tuft fractures are comminuted (more than two bone fragments) fractures of the distal phalanx of the foot (or hand). They may occur as skin infections, usually from open wounds that form tracks into bones, especially in elderly, diabetic, and immunocompromised patients.

Treatment

Most phalangeal fractures can be treated conservatively. Nondisplaced fractures should be treated with buddy taping for at least 3 weeks (Fig. 28.4). Splinting may be necessary for up to 6 weeks if healing is slow or pain continues. Gauze padding should be placed between the taped phalanges to prevent skin maceration. Generally, therapy also involves an orthopedic shoe with a rigid sole and weight bearing as tolerated. Moreover, it is recommended that it is helpful to keep the nail beds exposed to check for any "rotational deformities." Gait training is rarely necessary but may be considered for refractory cases that do not improve with conservative therapy.

WHEN TO REFER

- Immediate referral is necessary for patients with:
  - Open fractures or neurovascular compromise
  - Osteomyelitis (usually those with diabetes)
  - Fracture/dislocation of the phalanx (fracture of the first metatarsal but are not routinely for the great toe)
- If patients do not improve in 4 to 6 weeks, it may be necessary to consider an orthopedic referral.

Suggested Readings

Eiff MP, Hatch RL, Calmbach WL. *Fracture Management for Primary Care.* 2nd ed. Philadelphia, PA: Saunders; 1998:40–42.

Harris JH, Harris WH, Novelline RA. *The Radiology of Emergency Medicine.* 3rd ed. Baltimore, MD: Williams & Wilkins; 1993:460–468.

Henry MH. Fractures of the proximal phalanx and metacarpals in the hand: preferred methods of stabilization. *J Am Acad Orthop Surg.* 2008;16:586–595.

Kozin SH, Thoder JJ, Liberman G. Operative treatment of metacarpal and phalangeal shaft fractures. *J Am Acad Orthop Surg.* 2000;8:111–121.

Leggit JC, Medko CJ. Acute finger injuries: Part II. Fractures, dislocations and thumb injuries. *Am Fam Physician.* 2006;73(5):827–834.

McKinnis LN. *Fundamentals of Orthopedic Radiology.* Philadelphia, PA: FA Davis; 1997:410–411.

Rosen P, Doris PE, Barkin RM, Barkin SZ, Markovchick SZ. *Diagnostic Radiology in Emergency Medicine.* Saint Louis, MO: Mosby Year Book; 1992:178–181.

Wang QC, Johnson BA. Fingertip injuries. *Am Fam Physician.* 2001;63:1961–1969.

Calcaneal Fractures

George M. Bridgeforth and George Holmes

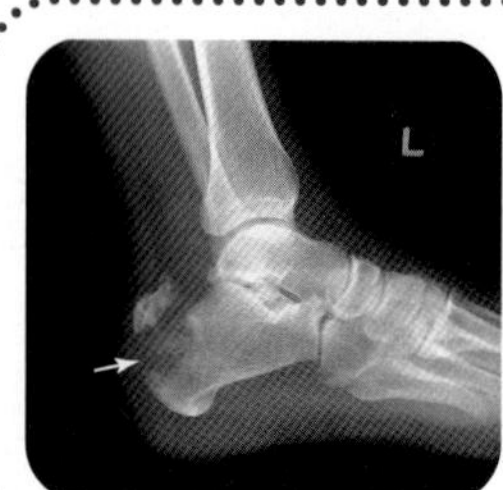

A 47-year-old man fell off a ladder and landed on his feet. He complains of marked pain, swelling, and tenderness in his left foot.

Clinical Presentation

Calcaneal fractures account for approximately 2% of all fractures seen in adults. These fractures most often occur in young men. The calcaneus has three subtalar articular facets—the anterior, middle, and posterior facets—that support the talus. The fourth articular facet articulates with the cuboid of the midfoot. Approximately 33% of all calcaneal fractures are extra-articular and include all fractures that do not involve the posterior facet. Approximately 67% of calcaneal fractures are intra-articular fractures, which are calcaneal fractures that involve all four articular facets.

Most calcaneal fractures are caused by direct trauma—direct impact resulting from falls from heights or high-impact motor vehicle collisions (Fig. 29.1). When evaluating calcaneal fractures, it is important to remember the 10% rule:

- 10% of calcaneal fractures are bilateral (Fig. 29.2).
- 10% (approximately) are associated with burst fractures of the thoracolumbar region. It is essential to examine both feet and the spinal column carefully for pain and tenderness, bruising, and swelling.
- 10% (approximately) of affected individuals may have a compartment syndrome (marked swelling of the extremity, resulting in neurovascular compromise). When conducting a neurovascular examination, it is important to always check for swelling, coldness, and pallor of the ankle and the foot. The posterior tibial arterial pulses may be detected along the posterior medial malleolus. The dorsal pedis arterial pulses lie just medially to the extensor hallucis tendon at the midfoot. It is necessary to ensure that capillary refill is 2 seconds or less. Patients at risk for developing compartment syndrome should be referred and kept under observation.

CLINICAL POINTS

- Most calcaneal fractures are unilateral.
- 10% rule:
  - 10% of the injuries are bilateral.
  - 10% may be associated with burst fractures of the spine.
  - 10% may be associated with a compartment syndrome.
- These fractures are sometimes associated with compression fractures of the spinal vertebrae.

Patients may complain of pain, bruising, and swelling as well as an inability to bear weight on the injured foot. They frequently have an impaired heel strike during weight bearing. The examiner should check the contralateral heel to exclude the presence of bilateral injury. Also, it is necessary to inspect and palpate other areas at high risk for fracture, such as the bony part of the ankle, as well as the metatarsals. Patients with marked comminuted calcaneal fractures may exhibit a heel deformity, but this finding is absent with nondisplaced fractures.

It is also important to document the integrity of the Achilles tendon. Patients with an intact Achilles tendon have a normal Thompson's test. A normal test is

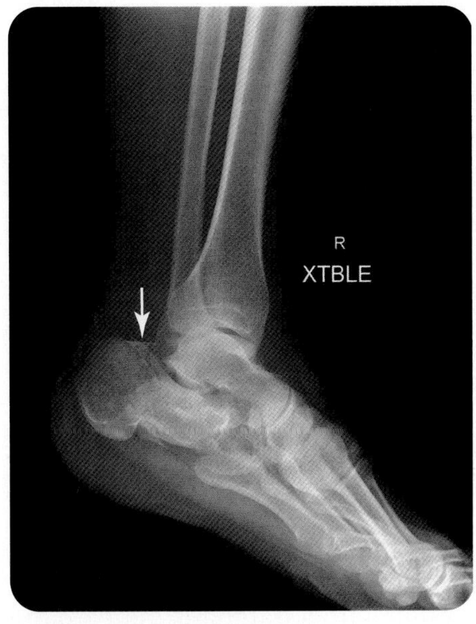

Figure 29.1 Lateral radiograph of the right calcaneus in a 47-year-old man involved in a motor vehicle collision, demonstrating an acute fracture from an axial load on the calcaneus.

characterized by plantar flexion (downward toward the floor) of the foot when the calf is squeezed by the examiner.

As previously stated, calcaneal fractures may be accompanied by compression fractures of the spinal vertebrae. The axial load from falls may cause a burst fracture in the lower thoracic/upper lumbar spine. Although uncommon, lower burst fractures involving L5 have been reported in the literature. Therefore, patients who are seen in acute settings following major falls should have an assumed spinal cord injury until proven otherwise. Patients with burst fractures commonly exhibit marked focal tenderness over the fracture site. Neurological findings with acute burst fractures of the lower thoracic/upper lumbar region are variable. The findings may range from no functional neurological deficits to acute paraplegia at T10 (the umbilicus) with neurological damage (lower motor neuron injury), impairing bowel and bladder function. See Chapter 5 for more information about burst fractures.

Radiographic Evaluation

Anteroposterior (AP), lateral, oblique, and calcaneal views should be ordered. For acute occult fractures, computed tomography (CT) scans are necessary. For ruptures of the plantar fascia, magnetic resonance imaging (MRI) scans should be obtained (Fig. 29.3).

PATIENT ASSESSMENT

1. Pain and tenderness of the heel
2. Inability to bear weight (on the heel)
3. Deformity of the heel or plantar arch

Boehler's angle helps identify a calcaneal fracture. One line is drawn from the posterior tubercle to the apex of the calcaneus. Another line is drawn from the anterior tubercle to the apex of the calcaneus. The angle formed in front of the two intersecting lines is the Boehler's angle. An angle of less than 25 degrees should prompt suspicion for an underlying calcaneal fracture.

With strong axial loads (usually the weight of the body from falls), there is a fracture of the calcaneus, which is usually characterized by a flattening of the calcaneus. With this type of injury, there is a reduced Boehler's angle, which is very strong evidence of an associated calcaneal fracture. However, this finding may not be readily apparent on the initial radiographs. It is important to note that a normal Boehler's angle (Fig. 29.4) does not rule out a small nondisplaced calcaneal fracture, such as a stress fracture. In this instance, a CT scan may be very helpful; it is a very useful test for detecting acute fractures. However, an MRI is useful for detecting surrounding soft tissue injuries as well.

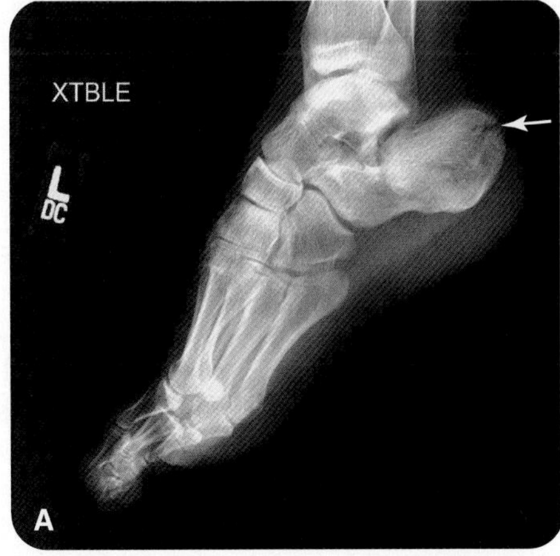

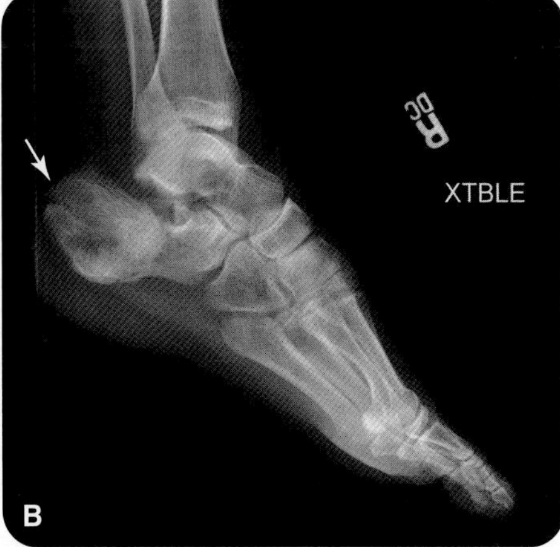

Figure 29.2 Lateral radiographs of the (A) left foot and (B) right foot, demonstrating bilateral comminuted calcaneus fractures.

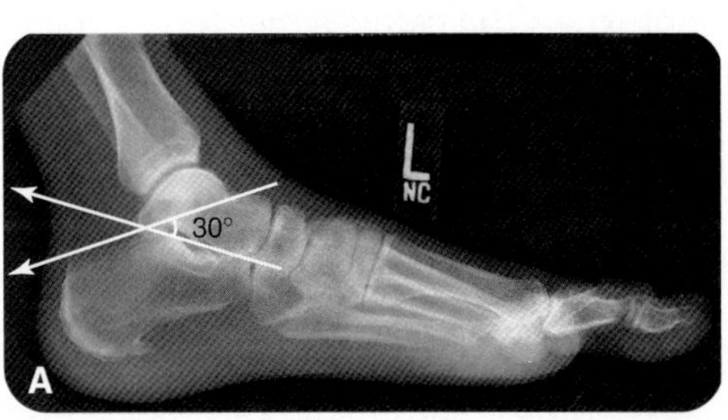

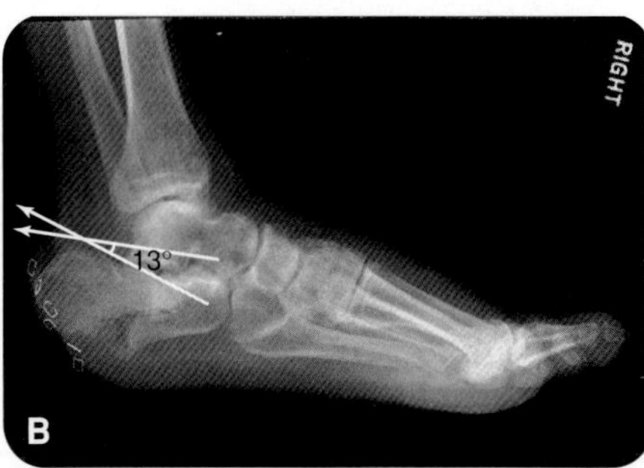

Figure 29.3 Normal and abnormal Boehler's angles. Lateral radiographs of the bilateral feet in a 70-year-old man with diabetes demonstrating **(A)** a normal left foot and **(B)** a right calcaneal fracture with osteomyelitis.

STRESS FRACTURES

Small stress fractures may occur with traumatic injuries to the heel, especially with sports injuries. Patients with stress fractures of the heel have marked heel pain but a normal Boehler's angle. In any patient with a traumatic injury to the heel, calcaneal views may be very useful. Calcaneal views may be very helpful in detecting small nondisplaced fractures of the heel. However, small stress fractures may not appear on the initial radiographs. Greenspan notes that stress fractures may appear as small sclerotic bands 14 days after the injury.

Although patients may not recall that they injured their foot 2 weeks ago while jogging, they may report that they have pronounced unexplained heel pain with weight bearing. Therefore, patients with resolved pronounced heel pain with limited weight bearing should have an MRI scan for a suspected stress fracture. Some practitioners prefer bone scans for the detection of stress fractures. However, bone scans are very sensitive but nonspecific.

PLANTAR FASCIITIS

Traumatic injuries may cause a plantar fasciitis. Generally, this is a strain placed on the plantar fascia from prolonged exercise, walking, and standing. However, along with heel contusions, this condition may occur with axial load injuries as well. Individuals with this condition have negative radiographs but present with persistent point tenderness along the anterior border of the calcaneus. In addition, there is marked tenderness with weight bearing; the pain generally occurs at the anterior heel where the plantar aponeurosis inserts into the calcaneus. When this area is palpated, patients commonly withdraw their foot in pain.

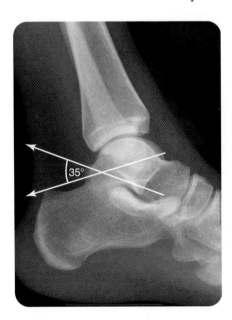

Figure 29.4 Lateral view of the left calcaneus in a 21-year-old man who was shot in the left lower extremity. This demonstrates a normal Boehler's angle.

Treatment

Treatment of calcaneal stress fractures generally consists of analgesic medication, proper orthotics (not heel pads), and stretching. Most cases resolve within a period of about 6 months. Patients should be non–weight-bearing for 6, possibly 8, weeks, followed by gradual increasing weight bearing, determined by the patient's postinjury pain. With respect to long-term management, orthotics or additional cushioning in the shoe may be necessary. For patients in physical therapy, they undergo a regimen of active and passive stretching that emphasizes dorsiflexion (elevation of the foot with the ankle fixed). These exercises are designed to stretch the tight plantar fascia and the heel cord (Achilles tendon). Multiple steroid injections should be avoided because they may cause the plantar fascia to rupture.

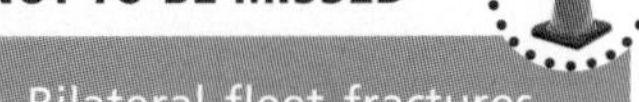

WHEN TO REFER

- Patients with open fractures, neurovascular impairment, or large or displaced fractures should be seen immediately.
- Patients with nondisplaced calcaneal fractures should be referred promptly.

NOT TO BE MISSED

- Bilateral fleet fractures
- Thoraco-lumbar burot fractures
- Open fractures
- Neurovascular compromise

In plantar fasciitis, treatment generally consists of analgesic medication, proper orthotics (not heel pads), stretching, and possibly steroid injections. For patients who are placed in physical therapy, a regimen of active and passive stretching emphasizes dorsiflexion (elevation of the foot with the ankle fixed). These exercises are designed to stretch the tight plantar fascia and the heel cord (Achilles tendon). Most cases resolve within a few weeks with conservative therapy.

Suggested Readings

Ahn JM, El-Khoury GY. Radiologic evaluation of chronic foot pain. *Am Fam Physician*. 2007;76:975–983.

Aldrige T. Diagnosing heel pain in adults. *Am Fam Physician*. 2004;70:332–338.

Ballas MT, Tytko J, Mannarino F. Commonly missed orthopedic problems. *Am Fam Physician*. 1998;57:267–277.

Barret SL, O'Malley RO. Plantar fasciitis and other causes of heel pain. *Am Fam Physician*. 1999;59:2200–2209.

Buckely R, Tough S, McCormackl R, et al. Operative compared with nonoperative treatment of displaced intra-articular calcaneal fractures. *JBJS*. 2002;84:1733–1744.

Daftary A, Haims AH, Baumgaertner MR. Fractures of the calcaneus: a review with emphasis on CT. *Radiographics*. 2005;25:1215–1226.

Geerling J, Kendoff D, Citak M, et al. Intraoperative 3D imaging in calcaneal fracture care—clinical implications and decision making. *J Trauma*. 2009;66(3):768–773.

Greenspan A. Orthopedic imaging: a practical approach. 4th ed. Philadelphia, PA: Lippincott, Williams & Wilkins; 2004:332.

Judd DB, Kim DH. Foot fractures frequently misdiagnosed as ankle sprains. *Am Fam Physicians*. 2002; 66:785–794.

Mazzone MF, McCue T. Common conditions of the Achilles tendon. *Am Fam Physician*. 2002;65:1805–1810.

Niceklbur S, Dixon TB, Probe RA. Calcaneus fractures. eMedicine Orthopedic Surgery. http://emedicine.medscape.com/. Accessed July 15, 2009.

Potter MQ, Nunely JA. Long-term functional outcomes after operative treatment for intra-articular fractures of the calcaneus. *JBJS*. 2009;9198:1854–1860.

Shearman CM, El-Khoury GY. Pitfalls in the radiologic evaluation of extremity trauma: Part ll. The lower extremity. *Am Fam Physician*. 1998;57(6):1314–1322.

Swanson SA, Clare MP, Sanders RW. Management of intra-articular fractures of the calcaneus. *Foot Ankle Clin*. 2008;13(4):659–678.

SECTION 6

Shoulder

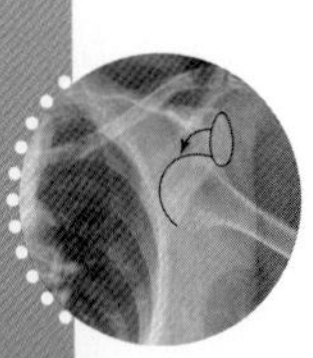

Functional Anatomy

The shoulder has three major joints: the glenohumeral, acromioclavicular, and sternoclavicular. The glenohumeral joint is a ball-and-socket joint that is formed by the articulation between the head of the humerus and the lateral scapula. It is capable of flexion (anterior elevation of the arm), abduction (outward elevation of the arm), flexion (posterior elevation of the arm), internal rotation (rotating the fist toward the body with the elbow flexed at 90 degrees), external rotation (rotating the fist away from the body with the elbow flexed at 90 degrees), and circumduction (rotation of the arm in a clockwise or counterclockwise direction). In addition to the head, the (proximal) humerus comprises the anatomical neck, surgical neck, and shaft (diaphysis). The head, a rounded structure, contains the greater and lesser tuberosities.

The greater tuberosity, which is more prominent and is lateral to the lesser tuberosity (and slightly higher), allows for the insertion of the tendons from three of the four rotator cuff muscles: the supraspinatus, infraspinatus, and teres minor. The supraspinatus muscle initiates shoulder abduction, and the infraspinatus and teres minor insert laterally (from the outside) to promote external rotation. The fourth rotator cuff muscle, the subscapularis, originates along the inside of the shoulder blade (in the subscapular fossa) and traverses medially in front of the head of the humerus to the lesser trochanter. It rotates the shoulder internally. During shoulder abduction, the infraspinatus and the teres minor externally rotate the greater tubercle and pull the head of the humerus inferiorly into the glenoid socket. The rotator cuff muscles counteract the upward and lateral pull of the deltoid to stabilize the humeral head during shoulder rotation. The greater and lesser trochanters are separated by the bicipital (intertubercular) groove, which anchors the tendon from the long head of the biceps (the short head inserts into the coracoid process of the shoulder). This (long head tendon) tendon inserts into the superior labrum. The biceps is the major flexor and supinator (palm facing upward) of the elbow and forearm.

The anatomical neck of the humerus, which connects the head and the shaft, has a medial (inward) angulation of 130 to 150 degrees. There is a slight angulation posteriorly (~30 degrees) as well in the sagittal (anterior–posterior) plane. This medial posterior angulation allows for better articulation of the humerus with the glenoid fossa. Just above the anatomical neck (but below the tuberosities) is the surgical neck, a more frequent site of fractures. The head of the humerus articulates with a shallow concave structure called the "glenoid fossa." The glenoid labrum forms a wedge-shaped cartilaginous cushion around the rim of the articulating humerus. This cushion, which is several millimeters thick, deepens the concavity of the glenoid fossa and allows for better contact and joint stability.

The acromioclavicular joint connects the acromion, a bony process that represents the most superior extension from the scapula, with the distal clavicle. This diarthrodial joint contains a synovial lining and is encased by a joint capsule. The acromioclavicular ligament, which supports the acromioclavicular joint, helps prevent posterior dislocations of the clavicle. The sternoclavicular joint connects the medial end of the clavicle to the sternum.

The clavicle acts like a strut that prevents compression between the arm and the sternum. Moreover, it provides protection for the subclavian neurovascular bundles. The conical middle third is its weakest part and is the most common area of clavicle fractures. The costoclavicular ligament receives additional support from the medial first rib and the sternal capsule. This supporting ligament helps anchor the medial clavicle from dislocating not only during shoulder movements but also when the arms are carrying heavy loads.

Located medially and inferiorly to the acromion is the coracoid process of the scapula. This knob-shaped extension of the scapula lies beneath the clavicle. The coracoclavicular ligament attaches the coracoid process to the outer third of the overlying clavicle (Fig. 1). This ligament may be subdivided into the medial trapezoid and the conoid, its lateral counterpart (the ligaments are named for their shapes), which help prevent superior displacement of the clavicle. The acromioclavicular ligament connects the coracoid process to the acromion.

During shoulder abduction (outward movement of the arm in a superior direction), the scapula glides across the thoracic cavity in a 2 to 1 ratio. In other words, for every two degrees of abduction of the humerus at the

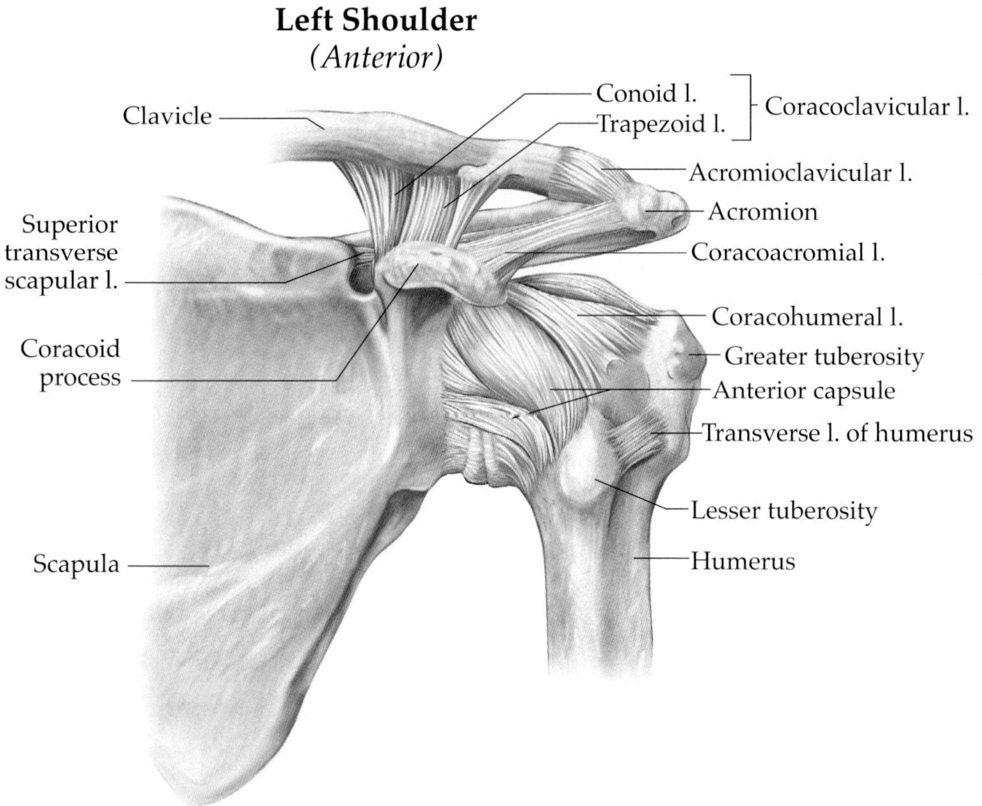

Figure 1 Left shoulder ligaments, anterior labeled. Asset provided by Anatomical Chart Co.

glenohumeral joint, there is a one-degree abduction of the tip of the scapula across the thorax. However, the scapular thoracic glide is not a true joint. Rather, winging of the scapula is prevented by its surrounding muscular attachments.

Regarding shoulder movement, it is important to note the complex relationship between the static stabilizers and the dynamic stabilizers. The static stabilizers hold the shoulder in place at rest. The major static stabilizers are the glenoid labrum, the ligaments (joining various shoulder structures), and the joint capsule. The dynamic stabilizers include the major surrounding muscle groups: the rotator cuff, deltoid, pectoralis muscles, rhomboids, and latissimus dorsi. These muscles work in concert with the static stabilizers to help maintain shoulder stability when the shoulder is in motion.

CHAPTER 30

Shoulder Dislocations

George M. Bridgeforth, Shane J. Nho, Rachel M. Frank, and Brian J. Cole

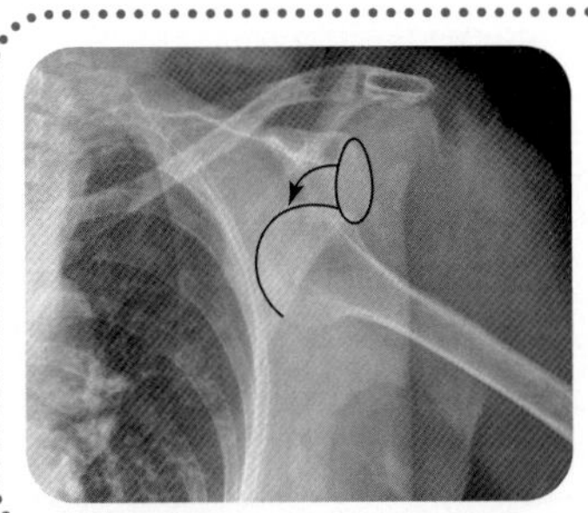

An 83-year-old woman who fell from a treadmill now complains of pain and soreness in both shoulders.

CLINICAL POINTS

- Most shoulder displacements occur in an anterior–inferior direction.
- Posterior dislocations are uncommon, and inferior dislocations (luxatio erecta) are rare.
- Gross dislocations may be associated with rotator cuff tears.

Clinical Presentation

A shoulder dislocation occurs at the glenohumeral joint when the humerus separates from the scapula (Fig. 30.1). The shoulder's great range of motion makes it especially susceptible to dislocation, and it is the most commonly dislocated joint. Shoulder dislocations have a bimodal incidence; they occur more frequently in younger men and older women. The cause of most of these dislocations is generally a direct force applied to the arm; this force could result from a fall or a collision with another person or object.

Approximately 95% of all shoulder dislocations are anteroinferior. Posterior dislocations are uncommon, and pure inferior dislocations are rare. Most anteroinferior dislocations are characterized by displacement of the humeral head. Signs and symptoms include:

- Difficulty with arm movement together with impaired range of motion
- Marked pain
- Numbness of the arm
- Palpable gap in the subdeltoid region

Tears of the rotator cuff contribute to shoulder instability and may occur in shoulder dislocation. Patients with rotator cuff tears, with or without an associated dislocation, have impaired range of motion with a positive drop arm test—an inability to sustain abduction (in which the arm is raised laterally) against resistance. The ability to abduct the arm to 90 to 120 degrees with limited resistance may indicate a partial tear or strain of a rotator cuff. The presence of limited extension (i.e., in which the arm is placed behind the shoulder) and weak external rotation (in which the forearm is rotated away from the body against resistance) commonly signifies complete tears of the rotator cuff. Supraspinatus tendinopathy also results unimpaired abduction and marked pain with resistance.

It is always important to rule out cervical disc disease, because a C5 radiculopathy can mimic or be associated with a shoulder injury. Patients with a C5 radiculopathy have a positive Spurling's test (cervical pain with axial compression), pain-limited cervical pain, and sensory loss along the lateral deltoid. In advanced cases, deltoid function may be pain limited and mimic a shoulder injury. Patients with C6 radiculopathies have numbness of the thumb

Dislocation of the Humerus

The shoulder joint is the most frequently dislocated joint in the body. It can become dislocated when a strong force pulls the shoulder outward (abduction) or when extreme rotation of the joint causes the head of the humerus to pop out of the shoulder socket.

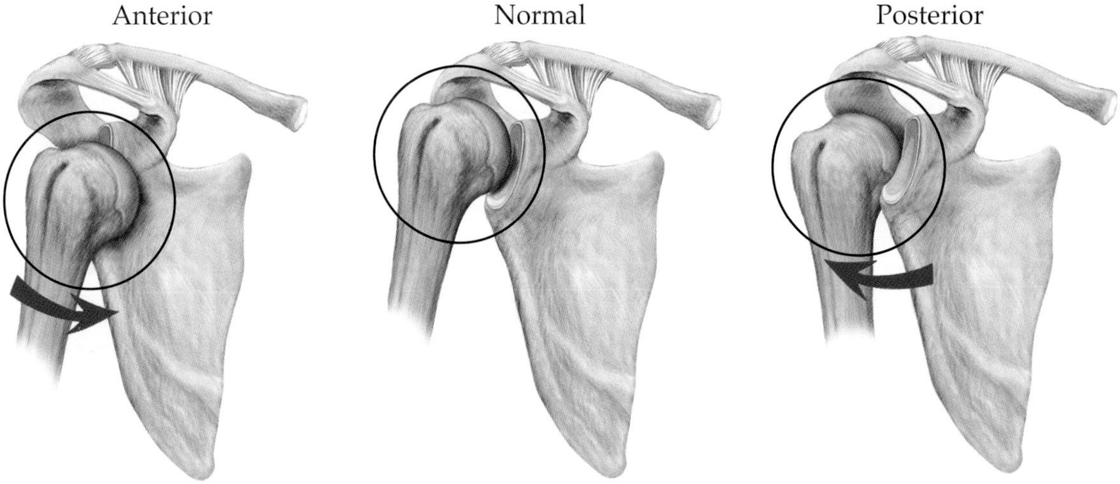

Figure 30.1 Anatomy and injuries of the shoulder. Instability. Dislocation of the humerus. Asset provided by Anatomical Chart Co.

and forefinger (Hoppenfeld's "six shooter"). C7 radiculopathies present with numbness to the middle finger, and C8 radiculopathies are characterized by cervical pain and numbness that radiates to the little finger. More advanced cases (C8 radiculopathy) demonstrate triceps weakness (elbow extension) with an impaired triceps reflex.

Posterior dislocations account for less than 5% of all shoulder dislocations. Unlike anterior–inferior dislocations, they can be missed on the clinical examination. It is strongly recommended that clinicians obtain a "Y" view (see section, "Radiographic Evaluation").

PATIENT ASSESSMENT

1. Marked pain and tenderness
2. Inability to abduct the affected arm (i.e., raise the arm away from the body)
3. The arm is adducted at the shoulder and flexed at the elbow

Radiographic Evaluation

An anteroposterior (AP) view, AP view with internal rotation, and "Y" (transscapular) view (used in acute trauma to determine whether there is an anterior or posterior dislocation of the humerus; Fig. 30.2) should be ordered. An axillary view is optional (some physicians prefer an axillary view to a "Y" view to rule out a shoulder dislocation).

Normally, the humeral head fits into the glenoid fossa like a golf ball on a tee. The golf ball analogy is very important. In a normal radiograph, a plumb line (a downward vertical line dropped at a 90 degree angle from a point on a horizontal plane) that goes directly below the coracoid process should lie medial to the humeral head. The head of the displaced humerus lies directly inferior to the coracoid process as the dislocated humeral head crosses the scapula. Note the anterior and inferior displacement of the humeral head. It lies medial to the glenoid rim and below the glenoid fossa as well.

The overwhelming majority of anterior dislocations are identified on the standard AP and AP view with internal rotation. If the head of the humerus lies inside and inferior to the glenoid fossa, the examiner should immediately suspect a shoulder dislocation. However, some shoulder dislocations, especially

NOT TO BE MISSED

- Shoulder fractures
- Shoulder contusions
- Associated chronic shoulder instability
- Associated Bankart fractures, Hill–Sachs fractures, and superior labrum anterior posterior (SLAP) lesions
- Rotator cuff strains/tears
- C5 radiculopathy
- Subacromial bursitis
- Upper biceps tendonitis
- Acromioclavicular joint strains
- Clavicular fractures
- Pneumothoraces
- Upper lobe pneumonia
- Pancoast tumors

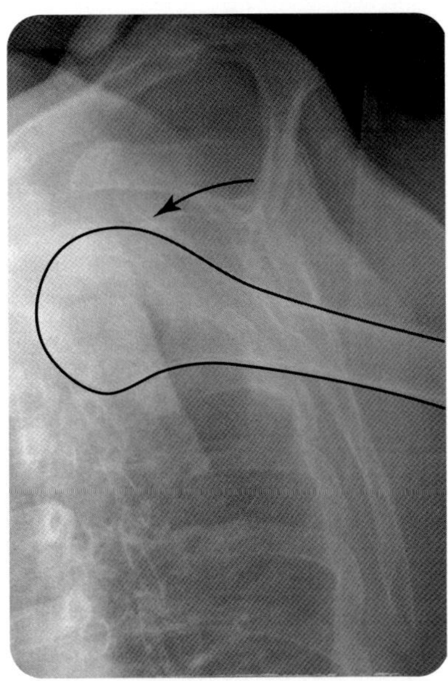

Figure 30.2 Scapular "Y" view of the left shoulder, demonstrating anterior shoulder dislocation from the patient in the introductory case. Note that on the anteroposterior view shown at the beginning of the chapter, the shoulder is inferiorly displaced and that the scapular "Y" view confirms and anterior dislocation.

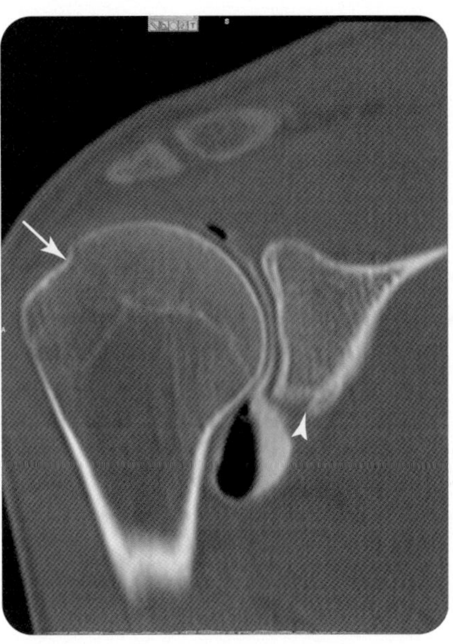

Figure 30.3 Selected coronal image from a right shoulder computed tomography arthrogram with iodinated contrast and air contrast demonstrating Hill–Sachs lesion (*arrow*) and Bankart fracture (*arrowhead*). This 23-year-old man dislocated his right shoulder 6 weeks earlier when he fell off the back of a moving truck.

posterior dislocations, are best identified on the "Y" view. In this projection, the anterior arm of the "Y" is formed by the coracoid process, and the posterior arm of the "Y" is formed by the acromion. Normally, the long axis of the humerus should bisect the "Y" (Fig. 30.2). The long axis of the humerus clearly lies in front of the "Y". Therefore, the "Y" view provides additional evidence of an anterior dislocation. On the other hand, with a posterior dislocation, the long axis of the humerus would lie behind the "Y".

HILL–SACHS FRACTURES

Acute anterior dislocations may result in an impaction of the humerus head against the glenoid rim. The force of the impact may cause a fracture along the posterolateral head of the humerus. This type of injury is called a Hill–Sachs fracture (Fig. 30.3). Hill–Sachs deformities appear in 20% to 38% of anterior shoulder dislocations and are more common with chronic recurrent dislocations. A flattening along the posterior lateral segment of the humerus identifies an old Hill–Sachs fracture. Another sign of a Hill–Sachs fracture is a poorly defined sclerotic margin along the posterior lateral head (Harris).

Hill–Sachs fractures may have a variety of appearances, which vary from minimal cortical flattening to a notch (hatchet) defect of the humeral head. However, the classic hatchet deformity is uncommon and occurs in approximately 15% of cases. These defects of the humeral head may be associated with a sclerotic density along the posterior lateral humeral heads; these radiological findings are important clues to a prior Hill–Sachs fracture. In addition, the presence of an old Hill–Sachs fracture is important radiological evidence of chronic instability secondary to recurrent dislocations.

The AP view is best for appreciating Hill–Sachs fractures. An axillary view may reveal a hatchet-shaped deformity in the posterior lateral portion of the humeral head.

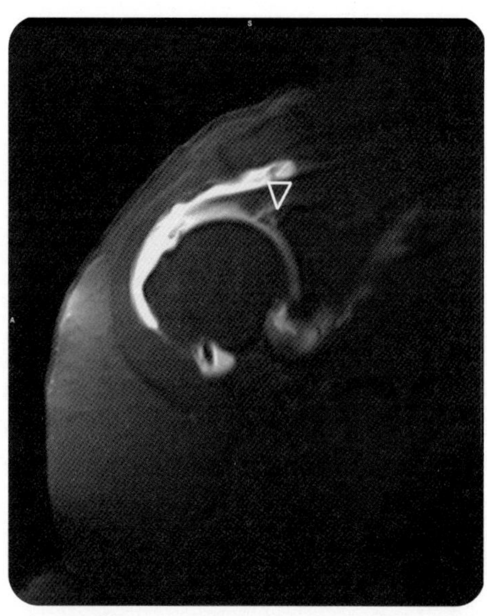

Figure 30.4 A selected coronal magnetic resonance imaging scan from a gadolinium-injected left shoulder arthrogram, demonstrating contrast extending between a torn superior labrum (*arrow*). Additionally, contrast is demonstrated in the subacromion space from a full thickness tear of the supraspinatus tendon.

BANKART FRACTURES

In addition, the impact of the humeral head may cause a fracture of the anterior–inferior glenoid rim. This type of fracture is called a Bankart fracture (see Fig. 30.3). From a clinical standpoint, Bankart fractures should be suspected in any patient with an anterior dislocation who has palpable pain and tenderness along the inferior glenoid labrum, which forms a fibrocartilaginous rim around the glenoid fossa. However, it is important to note that if the impact is limited to the cartilaginous labrum, the injury to the inferior rim of the glenoid may not be identified on routine radiographs. Following a reduction, consideration should be given to obtaining a computed tomography scan to rule out an occult Bankart fracture. A magnetic resonance imaging (MRI) scan or an MRI arthrogram may be necessary (Fig. 30.4).

SLAP LESIONS

These injures may occur in individuals who engage in overhead sports and work activities. The injury damages the superior glenoid labrum near the insertion of the long head of the biceps, which is an important stabilizer of the shoulder joint. Detachment of the long head of the biceps may result in superior instability of the shoulder. In addition, patients may complain of shoulder popping from the detached labral–biceps tendon complex. Moreover, the popping may be accentuated with overhead activities. Associated complaints may include shoulder pain with elevation and external rotation. If a SLAP lesion is suspected, an MRI arthrogram should be obtained.

Treatment

The treatment options for shoulder instability caused by shoulder dislocation have evolved over the years, and patients must be evaluated on a case-by-case basis. Treatment decisions are based on patient factors (sport-specific injury, timing of athlete's dislocation relative to the sport season, work-related injury, single traumatic dislocation versus a chronic, recurrent dislocation). In addition, some patients present without frank instability yet have pain due to excessive laxity that might be considered pathologic.

In general, treatment for shoulder dislocation can be divided into nonoperative and operative courses. The first step in the management of nearly any shoulder dislocation should be attempted closed reduction. This can be done at the site of injury, or preferably, in the emergency department. It is critical to obtain an axillary lateral view of the shoulder to confirm the direction of dislocation, as they can occur anterior, posterior, or inferior. A number of reduction maneuvers have been described; however, appropriate pain control and muscle relaxation is critical for a successful reduction. In many instances, a simple 10-mL injection of 1% lidocaine into the glenohumeral joint and placing the patient in the prone position with the affected arm hanging freely facilitate reduction and can avoid the need for a traumatic traction–induced reduction. Following reduction, nonoperative treatment involves immobilization of the glenohumeral joint with a sling as well as rehabilitation of the joint with an experienced physical therapist. Nonsteroidal anti-inflammatory drugs tif tolerated as well as ice therapy may also be used to relieve pain and reduce swelling. Early return to play for in-season athletes has been documented following this type of nonoperative treatment; however, it should be noted that athletes may need to undergo stabilization surgery if they continue to experience recurrent dislocations. See Figure 30.5 for postreduction radiographs.

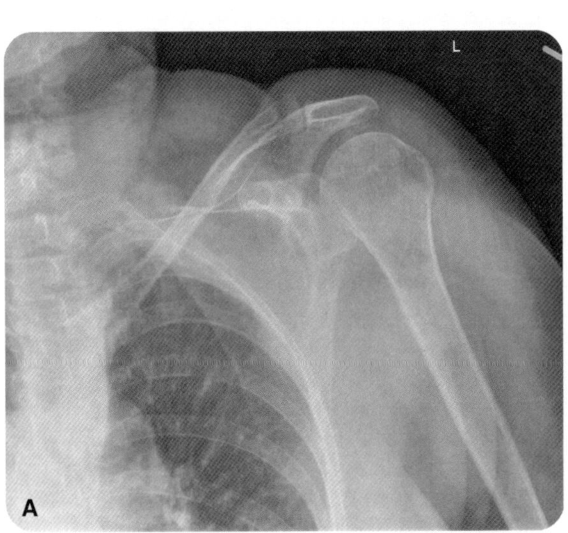

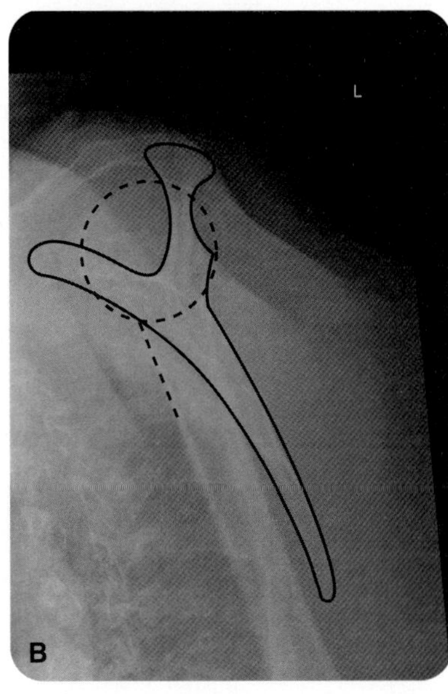

Figure 30.5 (A and B) Postreduction radiographs of the left shoulder in a more normal alignment.

Operative intervention is generally reserved for cases of recurrent dislocation, and factors such as age, type of sport or work, activity level, number of dislocations, and type of motions that cause instability may help guide the decision for operative intervention. Operative treatment for shoulder dislocation injuries usually involves minimally invasive arthroscopic surgery, during which the surgeon addresses any pathology associated with the glenohumeral joint. Specific attention is paid to the anteroinferior glenoid labrum and capsule (Bankart lesion), and repair of the Bankart lesion with or without capsular plication may be performed to reduce any capsular redundancy. The surgeon also examines the entire shoulder joint to assess for any concomitant pathology, including anteroinferior glenoid bone loss, Hill–Sachs lesions, additional labral tears, rotator cuff tears, or biceps pathology, and he or she makes treatment decisions depending on the operative findings. Return to sports generally occurs within 4 to 6 months, but this period can be somewhat longer when the dominant arm of a throwing athlete is involved.

WHEN TO REFER

- Immediate referral is necessary for patients with significant dislocations for reduction.
- Patients with chronic instability may be surgical candidates

Suggested Readings

Burbank KM, Stevenson JH, Czarneck GR, Dorfman J. Chronic shoulder pain; Part l. evaluation and diagnosis. *Am Fam Physician*. 2008;77(4):453–460.

Buss DD, Lynch GP, Meyer CP, Huber SM, Freehill MQ. Nonoperative management for in-season athletes with anterior shoulder instability. *Am J Sports Med*. 2004;32(6):1430–1433.

Hendry GW. Necessity of radiographs in the emergency department management of shoulder dislocations. *Ann Emerg Med*. 2000;36:108–113.

Hoppenfeld S. Physical examination of the spine and extremities. Norwalk, CT: Appleton-Century-Crofts; 1976:121.

Hovelius L, Olofsson A, Sandstrom B, et al. Nonoperative treatment of primary anterior shoulder dislocation in patients forty years of age and younger. A prospective twenty-five-year follow-up. *J Bone Joint Surg Am*. 2008;90(5):945–952.

Millett PJ, Clavert P, Warner JJ. Open operative treatment for anterior shoulder instability: when and why? *JBJS*. 2005;87:419–432.

O'Connor DR, Schwarze D, Fragomen AT, Perdomo M. Painless reduction of acute anterior shoulder dislocation without anesthesia. *Orthopedics*. 2006;29(6):528–532.

Perron AD, Ingerski MS, Brady WJ, Erling BF. Acute complications associated with shoulder dislocations at an academic emergency department. *J Emerg Med*. 2003;24(2):141–145.

Quillen DM., Wuchner M, Hatch RL. Acute shoulder injuries. *Am Fam Physician*. 2004;70:1947–1954.

Robinson CM, Adertinto J. *Posterior shoulder dislocations and fracture–dislocations. JBJS*. 2005;87:639–650.

Woodward TW, Best TM. The painful shoulder: Part 1. Clinical evaluation. *Am Fam Physician*. 2000;61:3079–3088.

Woodward TW, Best TM. The painful shoulder: Part ll. Acute and chronic disorders. *Am Fam Physician*. 2000;61:3291–3300.

CHAPTER 31

Clavicle Fractures

George M. Bridgeforth, Shane J. Nho, Rachel M. Frank, and Brian J. Cole

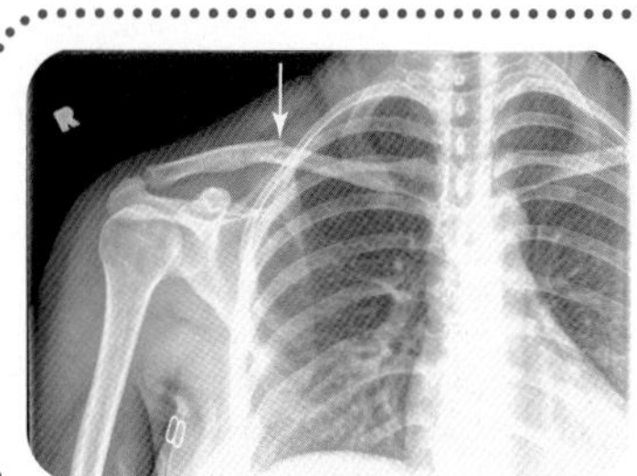

A 25-year-old woman who fell on her right arm complains of marked pain and soreness around her right collarbone.

Clinical Presentation

The clavicle is the only bony connection between the upper arm—shoulder and the thorax. It is the most frequently broken bone in the human body. The clavicle is divided into thirds. Fractures of the middle third are the most common, accounting for 80% of cases. Many of these fractures are caused by direct blows or falls, including falls onto an outstretched hand. Fractures of the lateral third account for 15% of cases. Generally, these types of fractures are caused by a direct impact injury at the top of the shoulder (Fig. 31.1). Fractures of the medial third account for 5% of cases and are usually caused by direct chest trauma. Patients with clavicle fractures complain of marked pain, particularly with movement; swelling and bruising; and tenderness.

The clinician should evaluate clavicle fractures, especially those involving the medial and middle thirds, for any associated thoracic and cervical injuries. It is essential to treat any associated cervical injury as an unstable acute spinal cord injury until it is proven otherwise. Stabilization of the patient on a spine board and in a hard cervical collar is necessary until a cervical injury is excluded by radiographs and a computed tomography scan. Thorough examination of the patient's neurovascular status (associated compartment syndrome, cold cyanotic limb with decreased or absent pulses), with careful documentation, is necessary.

CLINICAL POINTS

- Most clavicle fractures affect the middle third of the bone.
- Fractures affecting the medial third of the bone may be associated with more serious thoracic injuries.
- Most of these fractures heal without serious sequelae; however, complications can occur.

It is important to examine the acromioclavicular (AC) joint and the upper humerus for any evidence of associated swelling and ecchymosis. Lateral clavicular fractures may be associated with AC joint separations or upper humeral fractures. It is necessary to palpate the humeral head and neck (Fig. 31.2). In the AC joint, there may be a nondisplaced fracture, a grade 1 joint separation, or a step-off deformity with possible fracture displacement. In addition, the clinician should inspect the shoulder girdle for any acute dislocations. In addition, the clinician be on the alert for several associated conditions.

It is necessary to strongly consider a thorough chest examination with rib films if there is accompanying chest wall trauma. Radiographs show an effacement of the vascular tree. Sometimes with smaller pneumothoraces (<10%), the effacement may hide in the apical portions of the lungs. This is easy to miss (Fig. 31.3).

The examiner should also check for any focal chest wall tenderness associated with absent breath sounds (and hyperresonance to percussion), which is suspicious for an associated pneumothorax. Patients with an effusion have shortness of breath, dullness at the bases (if they are able to sit up), and absent

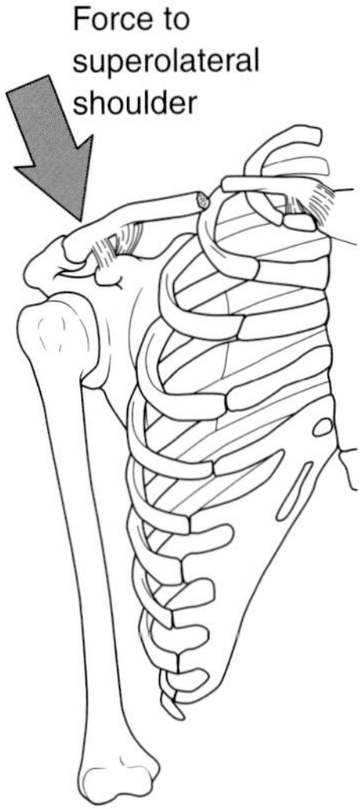

Figure 31.1 The most common mechanism of clavicle fracture is a fall on the superolateral shoulder. Since the sternoclavicular ligaments are extremely strong, the force exits the clavicle in the midshaft. (From Bucholz RW and Heckman JD. *Rockwood & Green's Fractures in Adults.* 5th ed. Philadelphia, PA: Lippincott, Williams & Wilkins, 2001.)

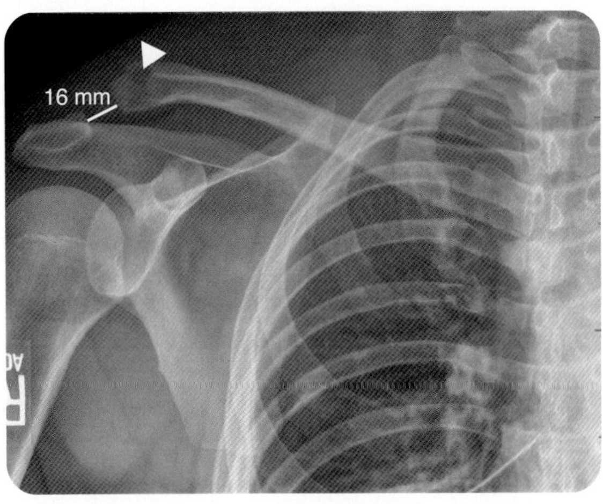

Figure 31.2 An anteroposterior radiograph of the right shoulder in a 30-year-old patient who was involved in a motorcycle collision, demonstrating an acute fracture through the distal third clavicle (*arrow*) and widening of the acromioclavicular joint by 16 mm.

breath sounds. Radiographs show blunting of the affected diaphragm(s). The normally sharp costophrenic angle is effaced with an effusion. A pneumothorax may occur with or without an associated chondral (rib) or clavicular fracture. A tension pneumothorax is rare, but it is characterized by an acute pneumothorax that is associated with tracheal deviation. The ruptured lung operates like a one-way valve. It allows air to accumulate in the pleural space (between the pleural lining and the collapsed lung) during inspiration. As the pressure in the pleural cavity increases, it can cause deviation of the trachea and move the cardiac structures to the opposite side. Decompression with chest tube placement must be performed immediately.

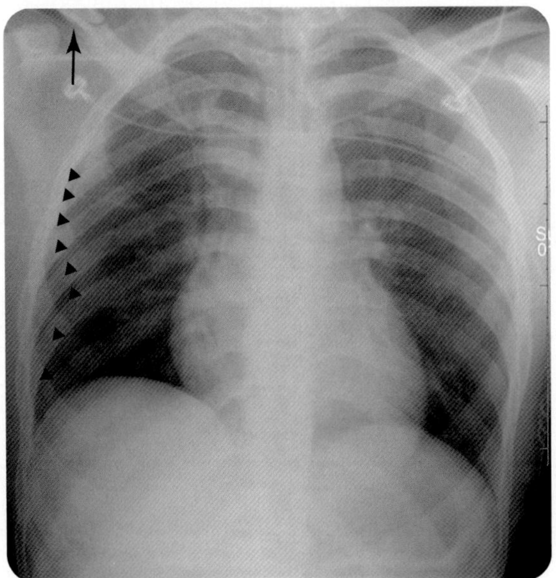

Figure 31.3 A portable chest radiograph in a trauma patient, demonstrating an acute right clavicle fracture (*arrow*) associated with a moderate-sized right pneumothorax (*arrowheads*). A computed tomography scan of the chest demonstrated nondisplaced fractures of the right ribs.

PATIENT ASSESSMENT

1. Pain, swelling, and tenderness at the fracture site (usually at the middle of the clavicle)
2. Possible clinical and radiological evidence of displacement
3. Limited range of motion

Although cardiac tamponade is a rare complication, the clinician should suspect it in any patient who presents with jugular venous distention, diminished heart sounds, and hypotension. An emergency pericardiocentesis is a lifesaving procedure. Aortic injuries (transections) may cause a widening of the mediastinum on a posteroanterior (PA) or anteroposterior (AP) radiograph. Many of the radiographs taken in the emergency setting on unstable patients are portable AP projections that normally may show slight enlargement of the cardiac structures.

Radiographic Evaluation

The clinician should obtain standard radiographs of the shoulder and AP views of the clavicle in external and internal rotation. Clavicle fractures are usually evident on standard views. In addition, he or she may order optional radiographs, including

- "Y" view: recommended for suspected acute shoulder trauma. It substitutes for the lateral view and is very useful for detecting anterior (95% of cases) and posterior (<5% of cases) shoulder dislocations.
- Angled frontal view: not commonly used by primary care physicians. This projection is angled 15 degrees above the clavicle and is used to identify fractures of the middle third of the clavicle.

Displaced fractures of the middle third of the clavicle are usually characterized by a cephalic ("upward") displacement of the proximal fragment. The distal fragment is pulled inferiorly by the unopposed pectoralis major and the weight of the arm. The pectoralis major attaches to the coracoid process.

The Neer classification is used to evaluate fractures of the distal third of the clavicle.

- Type I: nondisplaced fracture of the distal clavicle. The coracoacromial ligament and the coracoclavicular ligaments are attached. The coracoclavicular ligament is made up of the conoid ligament and the trapezoid ligament; both these ligaments prevent displacement of the clavicle (Fig. 31.4).
- Type II fracture: displaced fracture. The medially placed conoid ligament is torn, and there is an associated cephalic (upward) displacement of the proximal fractured segment. However, the distal segment (which includes an intact AC joint) remains anchored by the intact trapezoid ligament and intact coracoacromial ligament (Fig. 31.5).
- Type III: displaced fracture that extends to the AC joint. However, the supporting coracoacromial and coracoclavicular ligaments remain attached. In patients with serious impact injuries to the upper thoracic region, chest radiographs and rib films (of the affected area) should be obtained as well (Fig. 31.6).

NOT TO BE MISSED

- Associated shoulder fractures
- Shoulder contusions
- AC joints strains/separations
- Rotator cuff strains/tears
- Subacromial bursitis
- Associated cardiac and pulmonary injuries
- Associated cervical injuries, including C5 radiculopathies
- Brachial plexus injuries (uncommon)

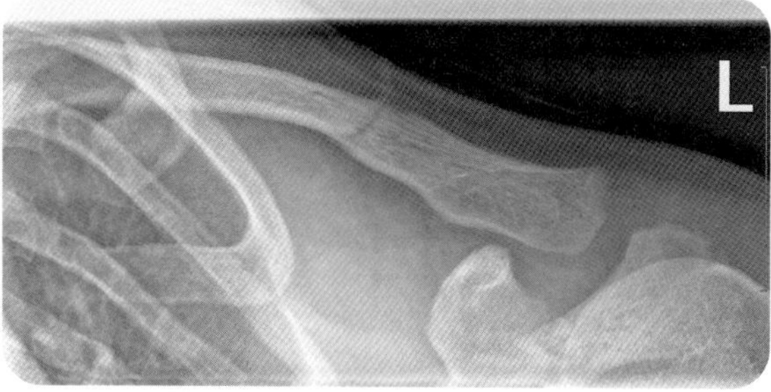

Figure 31.4 Neer type I. Anteroposterior radiograph of the left clavicle, demonstrating an acute nondisplaced fracture of the distal third left clavicle.

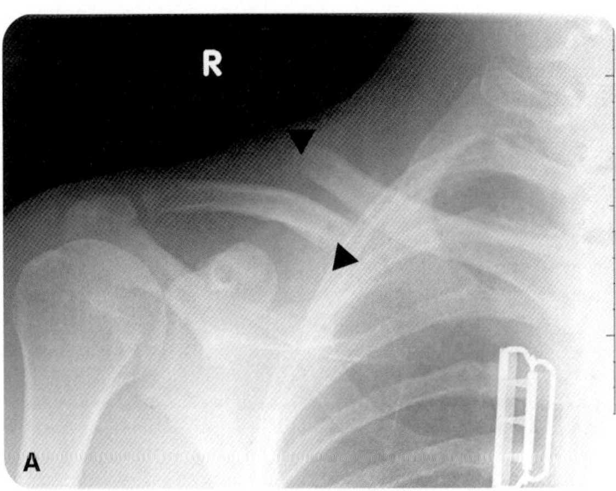

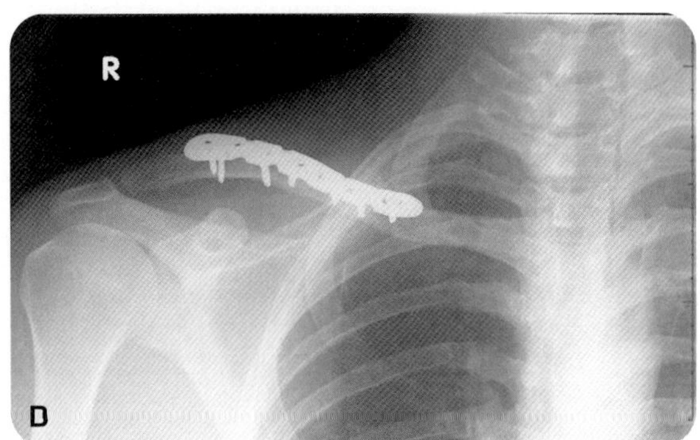

Figure 31.5 Neer type II. **(A)** Anteroposterior radiograph of the right clavicle, demonstrating an acute fracture of the middle of the clavicle with cephalad displacement of the proximal fracture fragment that overrides the distal fragment (*arrows*). However, the right acromioclavicular joint is intact. **(B)** A follow-up radiograph, demonstrating a clavicle fixation plate and screws from open reduction and internal fixation in the same patient.

Treatment

The course of treatment typically depends on the type of fracture, because some fractures have a much better chance of healing without surgery than others. Most minor nondisplaced fractures are treated conservatively. The large majority of fractures of the middle third of the clavicle can usually be treated with immobilization, either with a sling or with a figure-of-eight bandage. There has, however, been no determination that immobilization for pain relief only using anything other than a sling is necessary. However, nonsteroidal anti-inflammatory drugs (NSAIDs) and ice applications may be used to relieve pain and reduce swelling. Patients who cannot tolerate NSAIDs may be treated with other analgesics. However, the long term use of narcotics should be discouraged. Fractures of the proximal third of the clavicle can also be treated nonoperatively with a sling, especially if the fracture is nondisplaced. It should be noted that neonatal and pediatric clavicle fractures typically respond to conservative treatment within a few weeks.

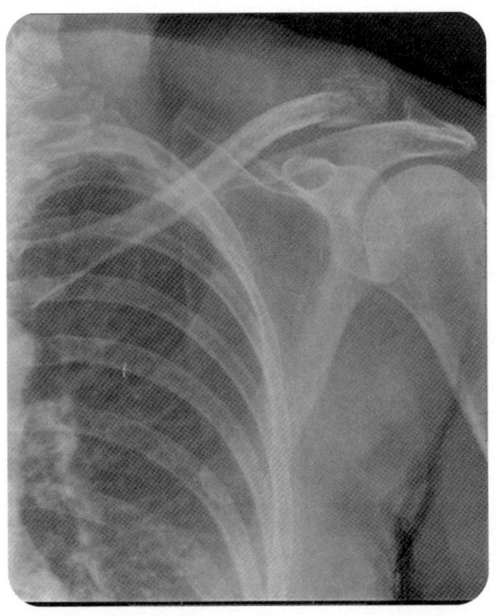

Figure 31.6 Neer type III. Anteroposterior radiograph of the left shoulder, demonstrating a comminuted fracture of the distal left clavicle with extension to the acromioclavicular joint without significant displacement of the joint.

However, recent studies have suggested improved clinical outcomes with open reduction internal fixation (ORIF) of clavicle fractures. Operative treatment indications had traditionally been reserved for cases of open fractures, tenting of the skin, neurovascular injury, floating shoulder, and polytrauma. In addition, despite the propensity to heal, many fractures unite in a significantly shortened position (i.e., more than 2 cm of shortening), which can lead to significant biomechanical abnormalities about the shoulder and scapula with associated pain and dysfunction. Thus, a decision to use ORIF may still be made for clavicle fractures that have a propensity to heal in an overlapping position. The current recommendations for displaced clavicle fractures with greater than 2 cm of shortening is operative management with ORIF; recent studies have reported improved functional outcomes and lower rates of malunion and nonunion with operative management. Treatment of fractures of the distal third depends on the specific nature of the fracture. Distal type I and type III (articular facing) fractures may need only nonoperative treatment with a sling and immobilization. Distal type II fractures, which are inherently unstable, typically require surgery.

Surgical options involve use of a intramedullary cannulated threaded screw or open reduction of the fracture followed by plate fixation with a compression or locking plate. Anatomically precontoured

WHEN TO REFER

- Immediate referral is warranted for:
  - Patients with open fractures, displaced fractures, and complicated fractures
  - Cases involving serious chest injuries or neurovascular impairment

clavicle plates are available, and surgical use has have been successful. During surgery, the surgeon must pay special attention to important nerves (brachial plexus) and vessels (subclavian artery). In the postoperative setting, NSAIDs and ice may also be useful.

Suggested Readings

Altamimi SA, McKee MD. Nonoperative treatment compared with plate fixation of displaced midshaft clavicular fractures. Surgical technique. *J Bone Joint Surg Am.* 2008;90(Suppl 2 Pt 1):1–8.

Grassi FA, Tajana MS, D'Angelo F. Management of midclavicular fractures: comparison between nonoperative treatment and open intramedullary fixation in 80 patients. *J Trauma.* 2001;50(6):1096–1100.

Jeray KJ. Acute midshaft clavicular fracture. *J Am Acad Orthop Surg.* 2007;15(4):239–248.

Khan LA, Bradnock TJ, Scott C, Robinson CM. Fractures of the clavicle. *J Bone Joint Surg Am.* 2009;91(2):447–460.

Low AK, Duckworth DG, Bokor DJ. Operative outcome of displaced medial-end clavicle fractures in adults. *J Shoulder Elbow Surg.* 2008;17(5):751–754.

Pecci M, Kreher JB. Clavicle fractures. *Am Fam Physician.* 2008;77(1):65–70.

Postacchini F, Gumina S, DeSantis P, Albo F. Epidemiology of clavicle fractures. *J Shoulder Elbow Surg.* 2002;11(5):452–456.

Pujalte G, Housner JA. Management of clavicle fractures. *Curr Sports Med Rep.* 2008;7(5):275–280.

Robinson CM. Fractures of the clavicle in the adult: epidemiology and classification. *J Bone Joint Surg JBJS (Br).* 1998;80-B:476–484.

CHAPTER 

Acromioclavicular Joint Injury

George M. Bridgeforth, Shane J. Nho, Rachel M. Frank, and Brian J. Cole

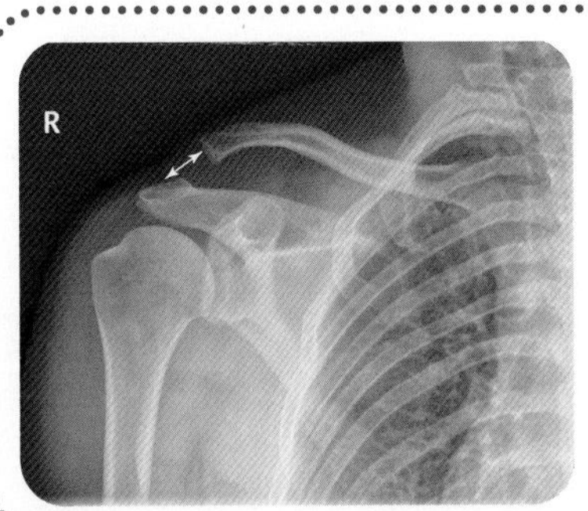

A 38-year-old man who fell on outstretched hand complains of right shoulder pain, and he has trouble moving his shoulder.

CLINICAL POINTS

- A fall on an outstretched hand may injure the AC joint.
- Associated fractures of the wrist, collarbone, scapula, and humerus may be present.
- Patients commonly hold the affected arm adducted at the shoulder, flexed at the elbow, and pronated at the wrist.

Clinical Presentation

Acromioclavicular (AC) joint injuries are relatively common. They are commonly caused by a downward force applied to the AC joint. In the workplace, they can be caused by following objects and falling onto the outstretched hand. In sports, such as hockey or football, they can be caused by hard checks or tackles. AC injuries occur most often in males in the second decade of life.

Patients with AC joint injuries often have pain and limited range of motion above the shoulder level (90 degrees), with abduction (raising the forearm outward laterally toward the head) being affected more severely than flexion (raising the forearm in front of the body toward the head). Injuries can be classified as follows (Table 32.1):

- Grade 1: point tenderness at the AC joint but no pronounced dislocation
- Grade 2: moderate pain and soreness with a mild step off
- Grade 3: moderate–to-severe pain and soreness but with a more prominent step-off
- Grade 4: severe pain; marked but unusual deformity in which the clavicle is pushed behind the AC joint
- Grade 5: severe pain; end of clavicle punctures muscle above the AC joint, causing a significant bump
- Grade 6: very pronounced and rare cosmetic deformity in which the clavicle is pushed downward

During the patient assessment, it is necessary to perform a thorough evaluation of the patient. The clinician should

- Rule out a fracture to the clavicle, humerus, or scapula.
- Rule out head or cervical trauma. Patients with C5 radiculopathies may complain of pain or numbness that radiates from the cervical region to the lateral shoulder. To help diagnose acute cervical radiculopathy, the examiner should perform a Spurling's test by placing downward (axial) force on the head while rotating the head and tilting it laterally. Patient complaint of radicular symptoms is a positive test. **Note that patients with unstable cervical injuries are not candidates for a Spurling's test.**
- Always check the lower extremities for upper motor neuron signs (spasticity, hyperreflexia, upgoing plantar responses [positive Babinski test]) for all

Table 32.1 Acromioclavicular (AC) Joint Injuries

DEGREE	GRADE	DESCRIPTION	RADIOGRAPHIC APPEARANCE	COMMENTS
Mild	1	Partial tear	Unremarkable	Localized tenderness at AC joint
Moderate	2	Capsule and AC ligament are ruptured	Widening of AC joint with 25%–50% elevation of clavicle	Tenderness with palpable step defect at AC joint
Severe	3	Capsule AC and coracoclavicular (CC) ligaments are disrupted	Complete dislocation of AC joint with AC joint and CC widening Marked displacement	Dropped shoulder Distal end of clavicle is prominent and palpable
Severe	4	Complete disruption	Posterior displacement of the clavicle	
Severe	5	Complete disruption	More than 300% superior displacement of clavicle	
Severe	6	Complete disruption	Subcoracoid displacement of the clavicle	

cervical injuries. The presence of bilateral upper motor neuron signs in a patient with cervical trauma is indicative of spinal cord damage at the cervical region (e.g., severe central cervical stenosis).

- Suspect an accompanying pneumothorax in any patient with direct shoulder trauma who complains of shortness of breath. It is necessary to perform a cardiovascular examination to rule out a pneumothorax, especially with high-impact injuries. Be wary of associated chest trauma. With any bruising of the chest wall and shortness of breath, obtain two-view chest radiographs and rib films of the affected area.
- Rule out rotator cuff tears, which may result in pain-limited abduction, such as AC joint injuries. However, rotator cuff tears are usually accompanied by weak external rotation (outward rotation of the forearm away from the body when the elbow is flexed at 90 degrees). Both conditions may lead to pain-limited extension (i.e., when the hand is placed on the lower back), but with an AC injury, the pain is usually localized to the AC joint.

PATIENT ASSESSMENT

1. Pain and tenderness
2. Limited range of motion
3. Possible associated fracture of the collarbone, scapula, or humerus

Radiographic Evaluation

Standard radiographic views are two anteroposterior (AP) views (one with the arm in internal rotation). The two AP views are helpful in identifying fracture of the humeral head and neck. A "Y" (transscapular) view may be necessary if a shoulder dislocation is suspected. It should be noted that some clinicians prefer an axillary view to rule out a shoulder dislocation. An enhanced view (digital radiograph) is optional (Fig. 32.1).

The standard AP view shows a slight elevation of the clavicle without a pronounced increase in the AC space. This increase is associated with a 25% to 50% elevation of the clavicle. A 25% to 50% elevation of the clavicle is diagnostic of a grade 2 AC joint dislocation (see Table 32.1). An elevated clavicular tip is suspicious for an AC joint dislocation (Fig. 32.2).

Another way to determine whether there is increased AC separation is to take a stress view of the AC joint with the patient holding a 5- to 7-lb weight (Fig. 32.3). However, most grade 1, 2, and 3 injuries are treated conservatively, and some clinicians have begun to question the useful of stress views.

NOT TO BE MISSED

- Shoulder fractures or contusions
- Shoulder dislocations: acute or chronic
- Rotator cuff strains or tears
- Clavicle fractures
- C5 radiculopathy
- Subacromial bursitis
- SLAP lesions
- Upper biceps tendonitis
- Pneumothorax
- Upper lobe pneumonia
- Pancoast tumor (rare)

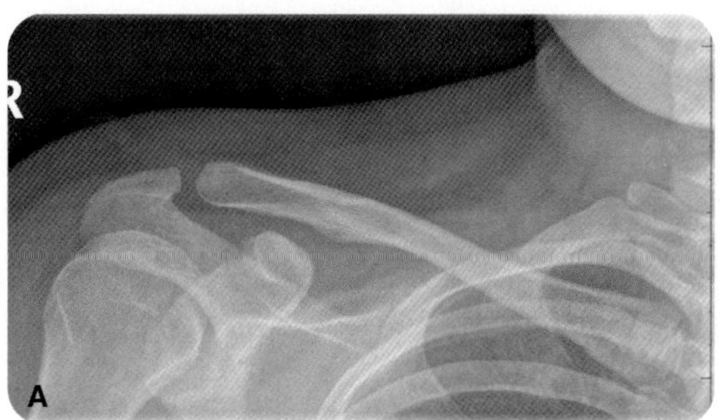

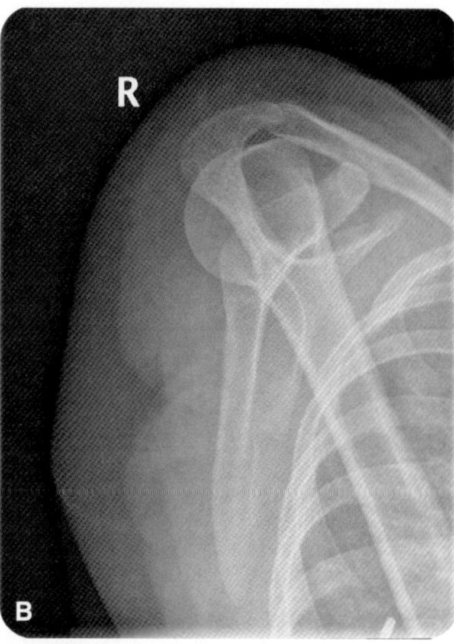

Figure 32.1 Normal **(A)** anteroposterior and **(B)** Y-views of the right clavicle.

Treatment

Treatment of AC dislocations, also known as separations, may be conservative or surgical, depending on the situation. Conservative treatment, involving a combination of ice, use of sling of brace, nonsteroidal anti-inflammatory (NSAIDs), and rehabilitation with an experienced physical therapist, is generally adequate for grade 1 and 2 AC joint injuries. Patients who cannot tolerate NSAIDs may be treated with other analgesics medications. However, the long term use of narcotics should be discouraged. Similar therapy is also effective for most grade 3 injuries, although this is more controversial. Refractory cases may require steroid injections. Operative intervention for patients with grade 3 separations remains controversial and is limited to overhead athletes or laborers. Patients can expect to return to activity after 2 (grade 1) to 12 weeks (grade 3), after painless range of motion has been achieved.

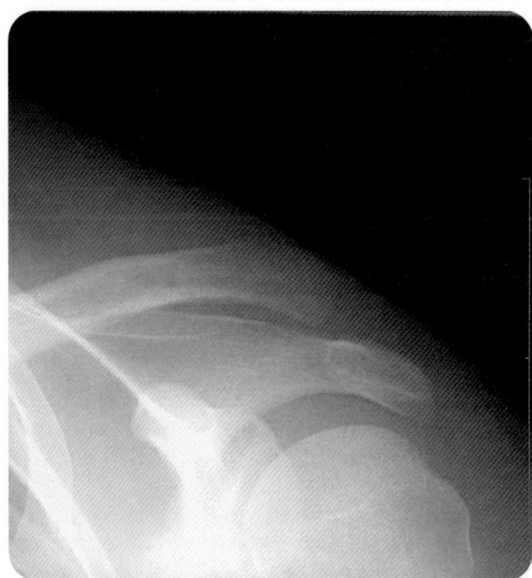

Figure 32.2 Grade 2 acromioclavicular (AC) joint separation. This anteroposterior radiograph of the left shoulder in a 27-year-old man complaining of left shoulder pain after a football injury demonstrates elevation of the clavicle in relation to the acromion, consistent with an AC joint separation.

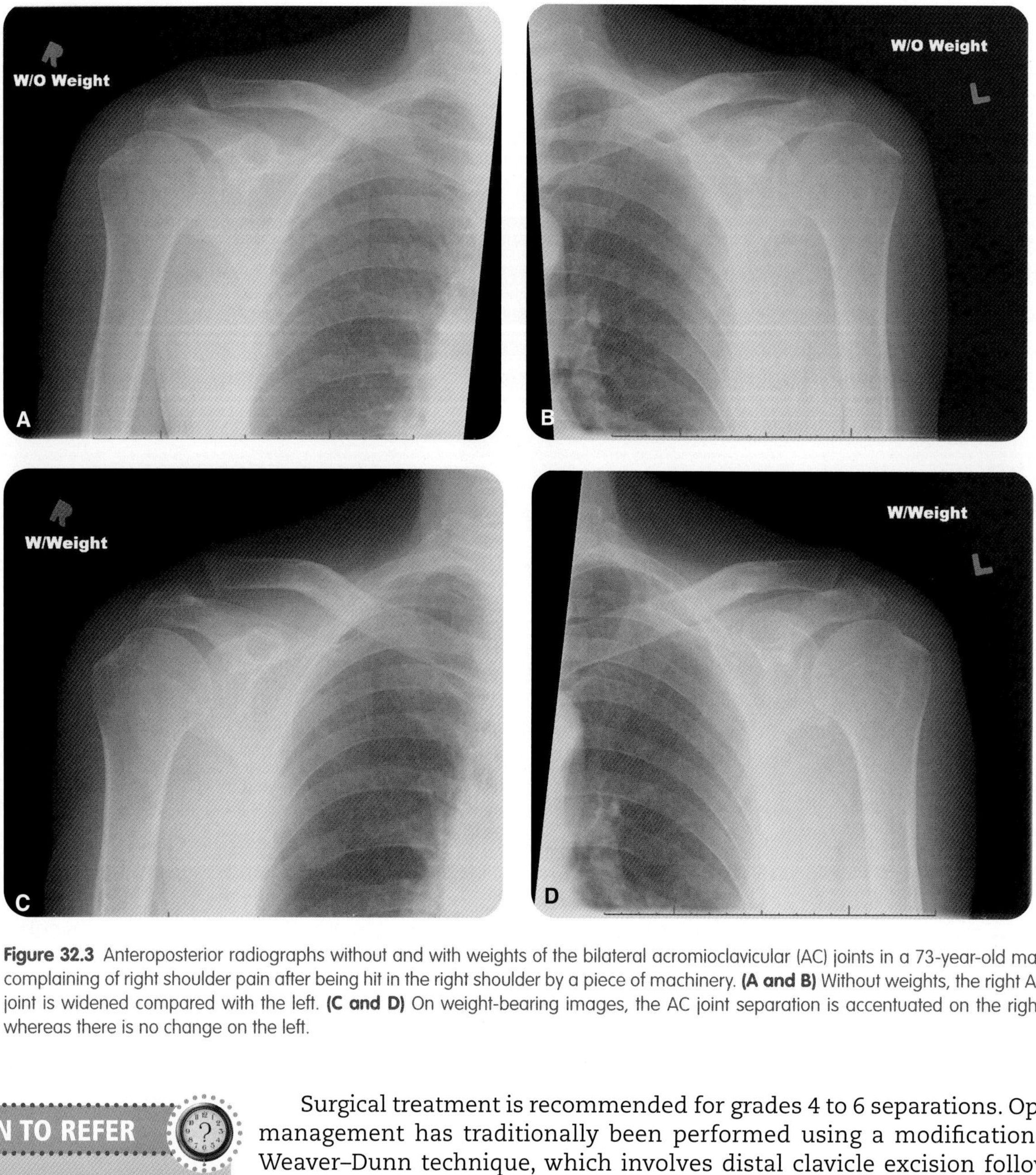

Figure 32.3 Anteroposterior radiographs without and with weights of the bilateral acromioclavicular (AC) joints in a 73-year-old man complaining of right shoulder pain after being hit in the right shoulder by a piece of machinery. **(A and B)** Without weights, the right AC joint is widened compared with the left. **(C and D)** On weight-bearing images, the AC joint separation is accentuated on the right, whereas there is no change on the left.

- Immediate referral is warranted for:
  - Cases with pronounced deformities (grades 4–6), especially if there is a risk of chest wall trauma
  - Associated neurovascular impairment
  - Associated serious cervical or chest injuries
- Referral is up to the discretion of the primary care physician for patients with grade 1 to 3 injuries.

Surgical treatment is recommended for grades 4 to 6 separations. Operative management has traditionally been performed using a modification of the Weaver–Dunn technique, which involves distal clavicle excision followed by stabilization of the AC joint with the coracoacromial ligament. A recent technique described by Mazzocca and colleagues involves allograft reconstruction of the coracoclavicular ligaments with interference screw fixation. Postoperatively, patients are immobilized in a sling to help eliminate gravity and minimize the downward pull of the scapula and shoulder girdle for at least 6 weeks; this protects the soft tissues while healing occurs. After 6 weeks, the patient may begin active assistive range of motion exercises with physical therapy. At approximately 3 months, a strengthening program may be initiated.

Suggested Readings

Aval SM, Durand P, Shankwiler JA. Neurovascular injuries to the athlete's shoulder: Part II. *J Am Acad Orthop Surg*. 2007;15(5):281–289.

Bishop JY, Kaeding C. Treatment of the acute traumatic acromioclavicular separation. *Sports Med Arthrosc*. 2006;14(4):237–245.

Egol KA, Connor PM, Karunakar MA, Sims SH, Bosse MJ, Kellam JF. The floating shoulder: clinical and functional results. *J Bone Joint Surg Am*. 2001;83-A(8):1188–1194.

Fraser-Moodie JA, Shortt NL, Robinson CM. Injuries to the acromioclavicular joint. *J Bone Joint Surg Br.* 2008;90(6):697–707.

Lemos MJ. The evaluation and treatment of the injured acromioclavicular joint in athletes. *Am J Sports Med.* 1998;26(1):137–144.

Mazzocca AD, Arciero RA, Bicos J. Evaluation and treatment of acromioclavicular joint injuries. *Am J Sports Med.* 2007;35(2):316–329.

Mazzocca AD, Santangelo SA, Johnson ST, Rios CG, Dumonski ML, Arciero RA. A biomechanical evaluation of an anatomical coracoclavicular ligament reconstruction. *Am J Sports Med.* 2006;34(2):236–246.

Nuber GW, Bowen MK. Acromioclavicular joint injuries and distal clavicle fractures. *J Am Acad Orthop Surg.* 1997;5(1):11–18.

Quillen DM, Wuchner M, Hatch RL. Acute shoulder injuries. *Am Fam Physician.* 2004;70:1947–1954.

Simovitch R, Sanders B, Ozbaydar M, et al. Acromioclavicular joint injuries: diagnosis and management. *J Am Acad Orthop Surg.* 2009;17(4):207–219.

Wolf AB, Sethi P, Sutton KM, et al. Partial-thickness rotator cuff tear. *J Am Acad Orthop Surg.* 2006;14:715–725.

Woodward TW, Best TM. The painful shoulder: Part l. Clinical evaluation. *Am Fam Physician.* 2000;61: 3079–3088.

Woodward TW, Best TM. The painful shoulder: Part ll. Acute and chronic disorders. *Am Fam Physician.* 2000,61.3291–3300.

SECTION 7

Elbow and Arm

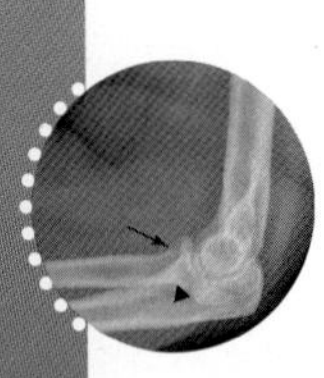

Chapter 33 **Radial Head Fractures (Elbow)**

George M. Bridgeforth, David S. Wellman, and Charles Carroll IV

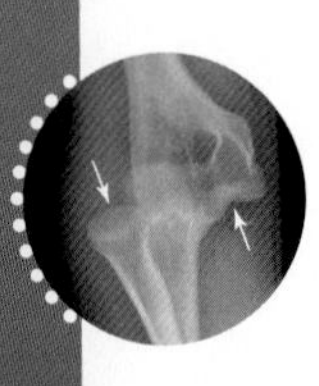

Chapter 34 **Elbow Dislocations**

George M. Bridgeforth, David S. Wellman, and Charles Carroll IV

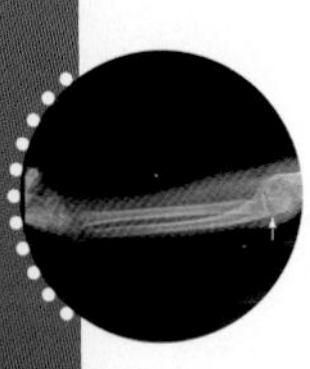

Chapter 35 **Olecranon Fractures**

George M. Bridgeforth, David S. Wellman, and Charles Carroll IV

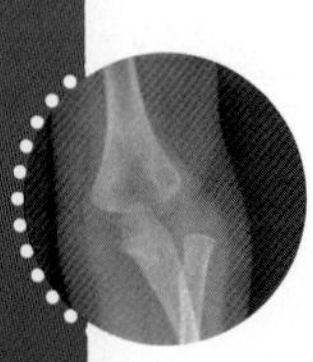

Chapter 36 **Forearm Fractures**

Joan Williams, George M. Bridgeforth, and Charles Carroll IV

Functional Anatomy

The elbow has three major articulations: the ulnohumeral joint, the radiohumeral (radiocapitellar) joint, and the radioulnar joint. A fibrous capsule encases all of these joints. The ulnohumeral joint allows for flexion and extension. Rotation of the radius around the ulna allows for supination (palm facing upward) and pronation (palm facing downward).

The (distal) humerus consists of an obliquely slanted trochlea (pulley's wheel) and its lateral counterpart, the knob-shaped capitulum (Fig. 1). The

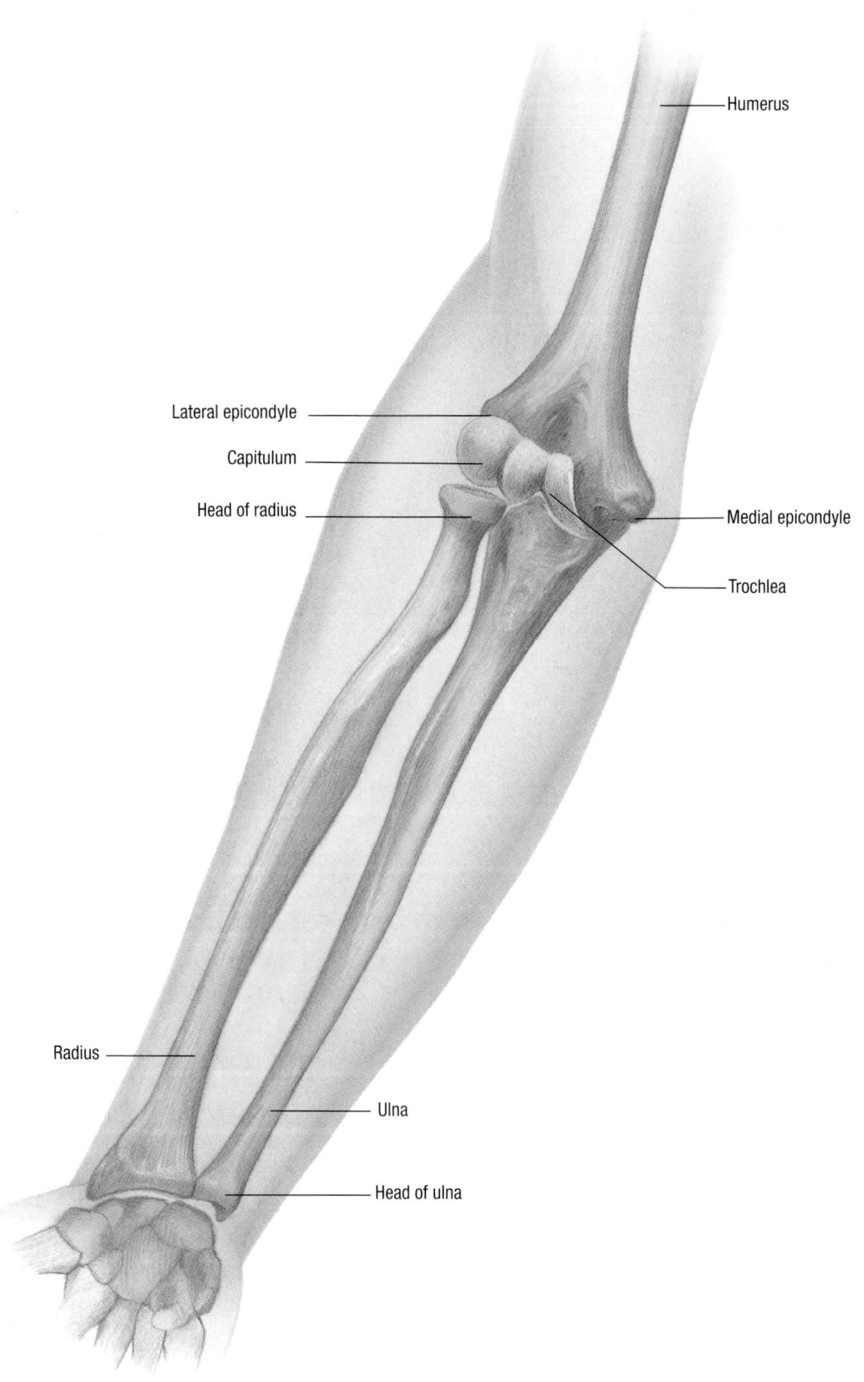

Figure 1 Elbow and forearm bones. Asset provided by Anatomical Chart Co.

trochlea articulates with the olecranon process of the ulna (see later), and the capitulum articulates with the head of the radius. The proximal radius has a rounded edge, which is shaped like the bottom of a baseball bat. It articulates with the lateral surface of the distal humerus (capitelum).

The medial edge of the trochlea is larger than its lateral counterpart. This anatomical feature, along with the ulnar collateral ligament, provides greater support and stability against medial dislocation from valgus forces (i.e., forces from a lateral to a medial direction). The smaller lateral edge of the trochlea allows for greater rotation of the radius during supination and pronation. During flexion, the radial head rotates around a groove between the capitulum and the trochlea (i.e., the capitulotrochlear groove). Flexion is stabilized as the head of the radius enters the radial fossa, a concave cavity proximal to the capitulum.

The proximal ulna has a hook-like projection that wraps underneath the trochlea to form a hinge joint. The proximal portion of the ulna's articular surface is called the olecranon, and it articulates with the olecranon fossa on the posterior aspect of the humerus in extension. It provides added mechanical stability during extension. The distal portion of the articular surface has an anterior prominence called the coronoid, which articulates with the coronoid fossa of the anterior distal humerus during flexion.

The major ligaments of the elbow are the medial collateral ligament, the annular ligament, and the lateral collateral ligament. The medial collateral ligament is composed of three bundles; it is a very strong ligament that assists with valgus stability (i.e., preventing inward dislocations of the elbow from outside forces that are directed inward). The fibers of the lateral collateral ligament blend in with the circular annular ligament. The lateral collateral ligament helps prevent varus strain (lateral dislocation of the elbow from medial forces moving in an outward direction). The annular ligament wraps around the proximal radius and ulna, thus providing stabilization of the proximal radius as it rotates around the ulna during supination and pronation.

CHAPTER

Radial Head Fractures (Elbow)

George M. Bridgeforth, David S. Wellman, and Charles Carroll IV

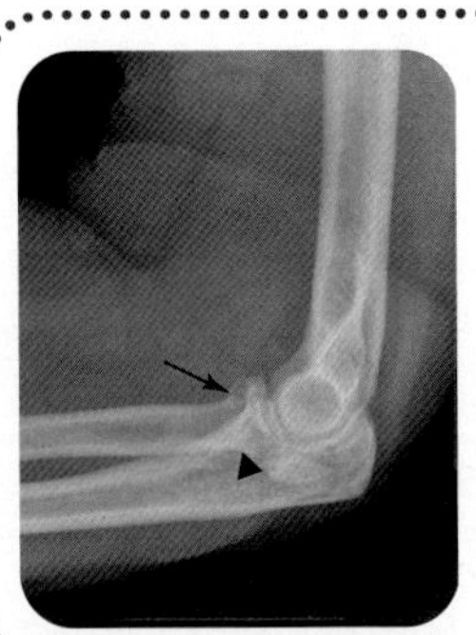

A 60-year-old woman fell on her outstretched wrist and hand when she tripped on a sidewalk. She presents with pain and tenderness in her elbow.

CLINICAL POINTS

- Fractures and dislocations of the radial head are usually caused by trauma.
- Pain is prominent with passive flexion/extension of the digits.
- Wrist pain may occur.
- Compartment syndrome is uncommon.

Clinical Presentation

Elbow fractures account for 6% to 7% of all fractures. Radial head fractures are the most common type of elbow fracture in adults; they account for approximately 30% of all elbow fractures. Olecranon fractures account for an additional 10% to 20%. Distal humeral fractures are uncommon (2% of all elbow fractures), capitellar fractures are even more uncommon (0.5%), and trochlear fractures are rare. Fractures of the radial head and neck generally result from a hard fall on the arm, with the hand outstretched. The wrist is usually in an extended position.

In a patient presenting with elbow pain, the examiner must maintain a high index of suspicion and carefully palpate the radial head as there may be a paucity of clinical findings. Often, patients display only a loss of terminal extension. The examiner must keep in mind other conditions on the differential diagnosis: compartment syndrome, medial epicondylitis, and biceps rupture.

While neurological findings are more frequently associated with ulnar neuropathies from a medial epicondylitis, a high index of suspicion must be kept for compartment syndrome. Compartment syndromes are characterized by marked swelling of the forearm, coldness, pallor, numbness, and diminished pulses. Pain is the first clinical sign.

Patients with a medial epicondylitis of the elbow have pain and soreness over the medial epicondyle with resisted wrist flexion. When it is present, an associated ulnar entrapment is characterized by numbness and sensory loss along the ulnar border of the forearm. Associated findings with ulnar entrapment include a sensory loss of the ulnar border of the ring finger and the little finger. Patients may also exhibit interosseous muscle weakness of the hand, characterized by an inability to hold a small piece of paper between the fingers when it is removed by an examiner.

Patients with acute biceps tears complain of feeling a “pop” in the upper arm while lifting. Extreme tears present with a bulging knot in the arm. Moderate tears present with pain soreness and tenderness with pronounced swelling and bruising over the medial biceps. The ecchymosis and swelling may extend into the antecubital fossa and medial upper forearm. Range of motion, including supination, is limited. With complete tears of the biceps tendon, the biceps tendon cannot be palpated when the elbow is flexed with the hand supinated (palm facing upward) (Fig. 33.1).

PATIENT ASSESSMENT

1. Tenderness of the radial head with palpation
2. Soreness and swelling around the elbow
3. Impaired range of motion
4. Possible open fractures

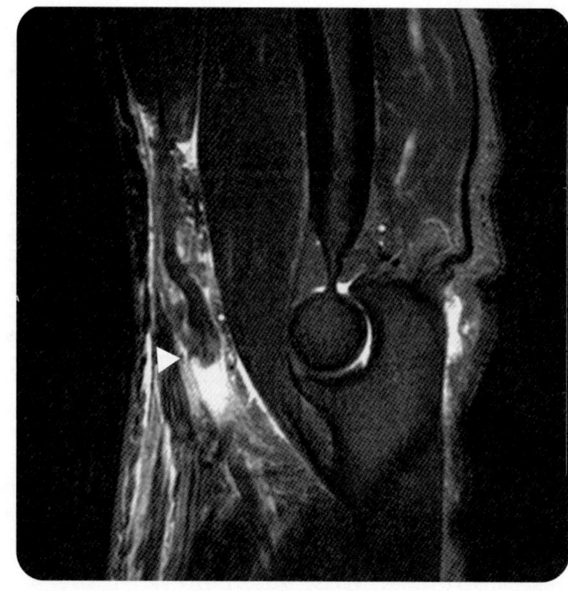

Figure 33.1 A sagittal image of the left elbow, demonstrating a complete tear of the biceps tendon (*arrow*) from its radial insertion with approximately 4 cm of retraction.

During the physical examination, the clinician should:

- palpate the radial head for tenderness (radial head fracture).
- palpate the olecranon and distal humerus for tenderness (associated fractures).
- assess range of motion in supination, pronation, flexion, and extension. Fracture fragments may restrict motion. The contralateral extremity is useful for comparison.
- check for elbow dislocations (articulation between ulna and humerus).
- assess for concomitant distal radius (wrist) fracture, scaphoid fracture, carpal injury, hand fracture, and shoulder injury.
- assess for soft tissue injuries by palpating around the medial and lateral collateral ligaments and checking varus/valgus stability.
- check for neurovascular compromise (cold, cyanotic limb, absent, or diminished pulses).

NOT TO BE MISSED

- Elbow contusions
- Elbow dislocations
- Coronoid fractures
- Olecranon bursitis/fractures
- Medial or lateral epicondylitis
- Torn collateral ligaments
- Septic joint
- Septic bursitis
- Forearm and biceps strains; biceps tears
- Gout
- Rheumatoid arthritis

Radiographic Evaluation

Plain radiographs should be obtained. A complete elbow series consists of anteroposterior (AP), lateral (Fig. 33.2), and oblique views of the elbow with the beam centered on the radiocapitellar joint. In more severe trauma settings, the radial head fracture can be isolated or exist in conjunction with other elbow injuries, with possible associated fractures, dislocations, subluxations, and ligament injuries. A computed tomography (CT) scan may be ordered to evaluate these injuries further and to assist with preoperative planning. Magnetic resonance imaging (MRI) scans are helpful in defining soft tissue injury components.

The AP and lateral plain views should be evaluated first for evidence of a radial head fracture. Radial head fractures are described using the Mason classification, which was expanded by Johnston and Morrey to form the system most commonly used today (Table 33.1). Occasionally, when fracture lines are difficult to see, the x-radiograph may only demonstrate a positive fat pad sign. The anterior fat pad forms a small dark (radiolucent) oblique triangle that extends from the distal humerus to the proximal radius (Fig. 33.3). Enlargement of this radiolucency represents displacement of the soft tissue by the hemarthrosis. A second fat pad sign may be present posteriorly at the distal

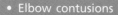

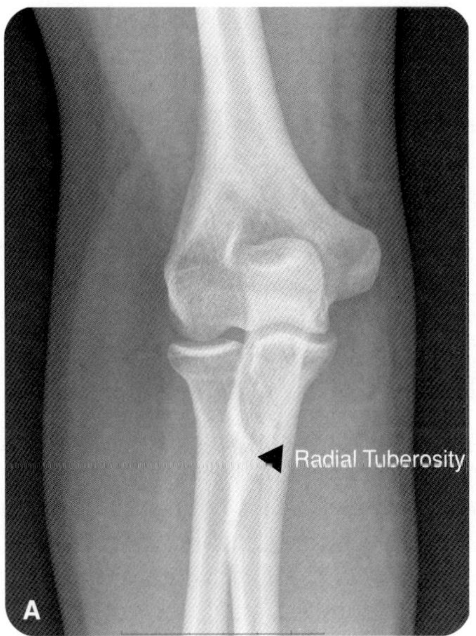

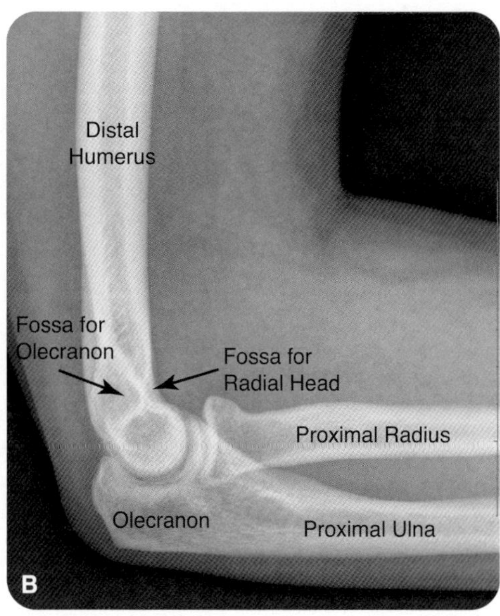

Figure 33.2 Anteroposterior **(A)** and lateral **(B)** views of a normal right elbow.

humerus. Small nondisplaced radial head fractures are notorious for not appearing on initial radiographs, so it is important to always examine the fat pads carefully. A positive fat pad sign may occur with use of warfarin (Coumadin) as well as with such disorders as rheumatoid arthritis, neoplasms, and gout. The examiner can rule out these alternate diagnoses based on a comprehensive history and physical examination, including a detailed description of the mechanism of injury. When there is a positive fat pad sign in the setting of trauma, the examiner should assume that there is a radial head fracture until proven otherwise. Normally, the anterior fat pad forms a thin dark oblique line along the distal humerus (lateral view). It looks like a thin sail. When there is a hemarthrosis, the fat pad enlarges and looks like a sail billowing in the wind. Posterior fat pad sign are less common but only be seen with severe injuries. A capitellar view x-ray with the beam focused on the radiocapitellar joint offers an additional study to assist the physician. If a fracture is still not visible, a CT or MRI may assist with the diagnosis.

After higher energy trauma, the radial head fracture may be quite complex (Fig. 33.4). In the setting of a more complex radial head fracture, the treating physician must assume that there is an associated injury until proven otherwise. CT and MRI should be considered early in the workup process to evaluate for these injuries. Associated injuries occurring with radial head fractures include

- Ruptured medial collateral ligament from valgus loading
- Capitellum fracture

Table 33.1 Modified Mason Classification of Radial Head and Neck Fractures

TYPE	DESCRIPTION
I	Nondisplaced or minimally displaced fractures with depression, angulation, and impaction
II	Displaced fractures (at least 2 mm) involving more than 30% of articular surface
III	Comminuted and displaced fractures involving entire radial head
IV	Radial head or neck fracture with dislocation

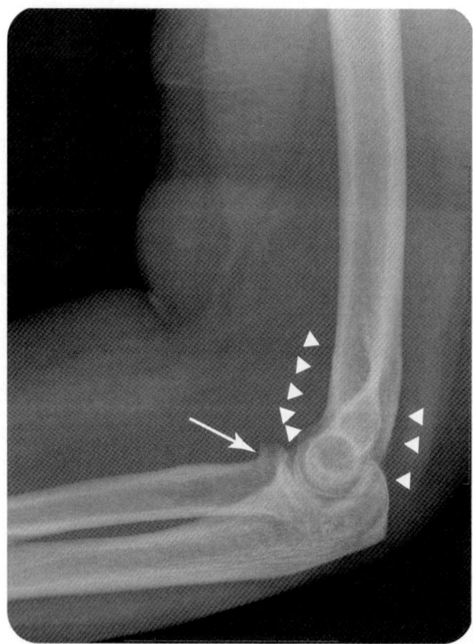

Figure 33.3 Lateral radiograph of the left elbow in a 28-year-old woman who fell while roller skating, demonstrating an acute, nondisplaced fracture of the radial head (*arrow*). A joint effusion is also present, as outlined by bowing the anterior and posterior fat pads (*arrowheads*).

- Elbow dislocation/subluxation
- Dislocation with coronoid fracture and radial head fracture (terrible triad injury)
- Olecranon fracture dislocations
- Essex-Lopresti injury: radial head fracture with associated wrist instability

Treatment

Treatment is based on the severity of the fracture. The Mason classification is useful.

- Type I fractures: conservative treatment is generally adequate. The key in physical examination nondisplaced or minimally displaced fractures is to document range of motion in flexion, extension, pronation, and supination. If no mechanical block to motion is present, it is acceptable to initiate conservative treatment. Use a sling followed by physical therapy within several days. As pain subsides, patients may discard the sling.
- Type II fractures: this currently represents an area of controversy in orthopaedics. Although clinical studies describing successful conservative treatment do exist, most patients with these types of injuries do well with surgery. Primary care physicians who encounter displaced radial head fractures (type II) should refer these patients to an orthopaedic surgeon for operative decision making.
- Types III and IV fractures: these are typically associated with higher energy trauma mechanisms and usually have associated injuries, often including dislocations and subluxations even if the joints appear anatomic in the initial workup phase. Even small fractures of the coronoid process can represent global instability of the elbow joint. Instability is common in the higher energy elbow injuries; these patients require placement of a well-padded posterior mold splint to hold the elbow in a reduced position prior to referral.

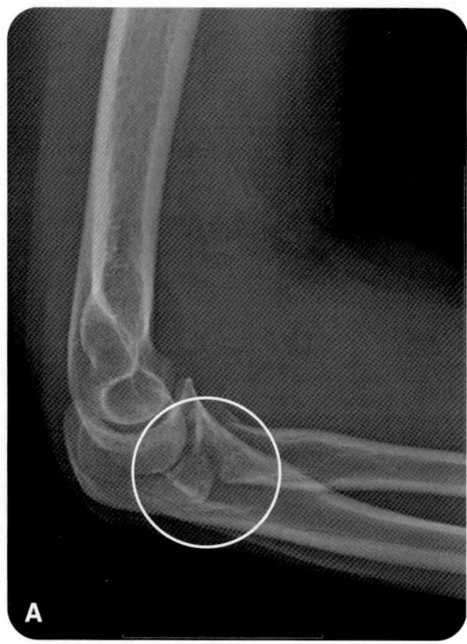

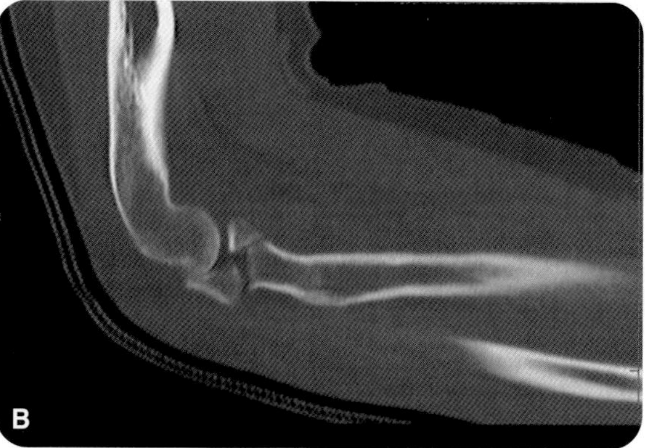

Figure 33.4 **(A)** A lateral radiograph of the right elbow, demonstrating an acute, comminuted fracture of the radial head with intraarticular extension. **(B)** A sagittal computed tomographic scan in the same patient, redemonstrating the findings in the plain radiographs.

WHEN TO REFER

- Open fractures, fractures with neurovascular impairment (or compartment syndromes), displaced fractures (includes radial head fractures 2 mm or greater), associated elbow injuries, or locked joints (representing interposed bone fragments) require immediate referral. Compartment syndromes warrant evaluation and possible fasciotomy to prevent ischemia and potential loss of the extremity.
- Uncomplicated nondisplaced radial head fractures with full range of motion may be referred at the discretion of the primary care physician, especially if the physician is not experienced in fracture management.

Any patient with a suspected complex radial head fracture pattern requires an orthopaedic referral. Surgery is often necessary. Operative treatments for radial head fractures include pins, plate/screw constructs, bioabsorbable screws, and radial head replacements. Excision of the radial head can even be considered. More complex and comminuted patterns of injury typically require radial head replacement.

Suggested Readings

Akesson T, Herbertsson P, Josefsson PO, et al. Primary nonoperative treatment of moderately displaced two-part fractures of the radial head. *J Bone Joint Surg Am*. 2006;88(9):1909–1914.

Bernstein J, Adler JM, Blank JE, Dalsey RM. Evaluation of the Neer system of classification of proximal humeral fractures with computerized tomographic scans and plain radiographs. *J Bone Joint Surg JBJS*. 1996;78:1371–1375.

Goswant G. The fat pad sign. *Radiology*. 2002;222:419–420.

Greenspan A, Norman A, Rosen H. Radial head-capitellum view in elbow trauma: clinical application and radiographic-anatomic correlation. *AJR*. 1984;143(2):355–359.

Johnston GW. A follow-up of one hundred cases of fracture of the head of the radius with a review of the literature. *Ulster Med J* 1962;31:51–56.

Kijowski R, Tuite M, Sanford M. Magnetic resonance imaging of the elbow. Part I: Normal anatomy, imaging technique, and osseous abnormalities. *Skeletal Radiol*. 2004;33(12):685–697.

Kijowski R, Tuite M, Sanford M. Magnetic resonance imaging of the elbow. Part II. Abnormalities of the ligaments, tendons and nerves. *Skeletal Radiol*. 2005;34(1):1–18.

Mason ML. Some observations on fractures of the head of the radius with a review of one hundred cases. *Br J Surg*. 1954;42(172):123–132.

McGinley JC, Roach N, Hopgood BX, Kozin SH. Nondisplaced elbow fractures. A commonly occurring and difficult diagnosis. *Am J Emerg Med* 2006;24(5):560–566.

Morrey BF. *Radial Head Fractures. The Elbow and Its Disorders*. Philadelphia, PA: WB Saunders; 1985:355–381.

Morrey BF. Current concepts in the treatment of fractures of the radial head, the olecranon, and the coronoid. *JBJS*. 1995;77:316–327.

Murphy BJ. MR imaging of the elbow. *Radiology*. 1992;184:525–529.

Murphy WA, Siegel MJ. Elbow fat pads with new signs and extended differential diagnosis. *Radiology*. 1977;124:659–665.

O'Dwyer H, O'Sullivan P, Fitzgerald D, et al. The fat pad sign following elbow trauma in adults: its usefulness and reliability in suspecting occult fracture. J Comput Assist Tomogr 2004;28(4):562–565.

Pike JM, Athwal GS, Faber KJ, King GJ. Radial head fractures—an update. *J Hand Surg Am*. 2009;34(3):557–565.

Reuben AD, Benger JR, Beech F, Duston J. Elbow extension test to rule out elbow fracture: multicentre, prospective validation and observational study of diagnostic accuracy in adults and children. *BMJ*. 2008:337:a2428.

Ring D, Quintero J, Juperiter JB. Open reduction and internal fixation of fractures of the radial head. *J Bone Joint Surg JBJS*. 2002;84:1811–1815.

Ring D. *Fractures and Dislocations of the Elbow. Rockwood and Green's Fractures in Adults*. 6th ed. Philadelphia, PA: Lippincott Williams & Wilkins; 2006.

Rosenblatt Y, Athwal GS, Faber KJ. Current recommendations for the treatment of radial head fractures. *Orthop Clin North Am*. 2008;39(2):173–185, vi.

Shearman CM, El-Khoury GY. Pitfalls in the radiologic evaluation of extremity trauma: Part l. The upper extremity. *Am Fam Physician*. 1998;57(5):995–1005.

Teh J, Sukumar V, Jackson S. Imaging of the elbow. *Imaging*. 2003;15:193–204.

Tejwani N, Mehta H. Fractures of the radial head and neck: current concepts in management. *J Am Acad Orthop Surg*. 2007;15(7):380–387.

CHAPTER 34

Elbow Dislocations

George M. Bridgeforth, David S. Wellman, and Charles Carroll IV

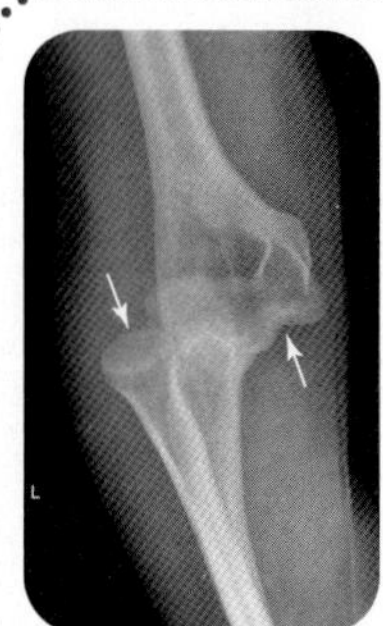

A 20-year-old man was wrestling and heard his arm "pop" while wrestling. He presents with severe elbow pain and cannot bend his arm.

Clinical Presentation

The elbow is a relatively stable hinge joint, and dislocation of this joint requires considerable force. Dislocation of the elbow is second in frequency to that of the shoulder. Athletic injuries account for up to 50% of elbow dislocations. Posterior dislocations are most common (90%) and may result from a fall onto an outstretched hand with a combination of axial, rotational, and varus (or valgus) force. For example, a person who is ice skating may fall backward and extend an arm to break his or her fall. Anterior dislocations occur much less frequently as a result of direct trauma to the flexed elbow. Associated fractures often occur with elbow dislocations.

An elbow dislocation is not difficult to diagnose; the elbow deformity is readily evident and is associated with a marked pain, swelling, and tenderness of the elbow. Impaired range of motion also occurs.

A plain radiographic workup should follow the initial physical examination (see section, "Radiographic Evaluation").

Finally, the clinician should evaluate the patient for evidence of the "terrible triad." This consists of an elbow injury with radiographic evidence of a radial head fracture and a coronoid fracture. The terrible triad occurs in approximately 10% of elbow dislocations and is more common with posterior dislocations. If the physician misses a terrible triad injury, the fracture of the coronoid may result in recurrent elbow subluxations due to hinge instability.

CLINICAL POINTS

- The majority of elbow dislocations involve posterior displacement.
- Some deformity may be present.
- It is important to examine the middle and distal forearm for an associated fracture.

A thorough physical examination is essential. The physician should:

- look for marked pain, swelling, tenderness, and deformity.
- check for limited range of motion with crepitus.

(Continued)

Radiographic Evaluation

A complete elbow series consists of anteroposterior, lateral, and oblique radiographs of the elbow, and these diagnose most dislocations and subluxations. The clinician should evaluate each film closely as a subluxation can be subtle. A view specifically centered on the radial head and capitellum can be obtained if there is concern about radial head or capitellum fracture/dislocations.

Dislocations can be simple or represent components of fracture dislocations with complex associated injuries. There may be fractures, dislocations, subluxations, and ligament injuries, all occurring in the same setting. A computed

CLINICAL POINTS (*Continued*)

- check for limited range of motion with crepitus.
- check for neurovascular impairment (i.e., cold limb, with diminished or absent radial, ulnar, and brachial pulses; dusky hue).
- check skin integrity.
- evaluate for ulnar nerve damage: weakness of the ulnar wrist flexors and interosseus muscles, as well as sensory impairment of the hypothenar eminence and the fourth (ulnar half) and the fifth finger.
- evaluate for median nerve damage: weakness of the radial wrist flexors and thumb interphalangeal joint flexion with a sensory impairment of the thenar eminence and the volar first, second, third, and radial half of the fourth fingers.

PATIENT ASSESSMENT

1. Pain, instability, and lack of range of motion
2. Possible effusion

NOT TO BE MISSED

- Elbow strains/contusions/dislocations
- Medial or lateral epicondylitis
- Olecranon fractures
- Olecranon bursitis
- Septic joint
- Triceps tears (inability to extend the arm in a horizontal plane)
- Gout
- Rheumatoid arthritis

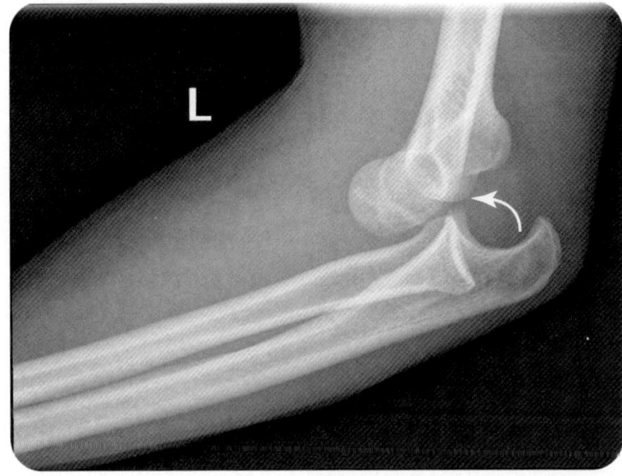

Figure 34.1 Lateral radiograph of the patient in the introductory case, showing a left elbow dislocation.

tomography (CT) scan or magnetic resonance imaging scan may be ordered to evaluate these injuries further and to assist with preoperative planning; however, the dislocated joint should be reduced first.

Elbow dislocations are best identified on the lateral view (Figs. 34.1 and 34.2). Elbow dislocations represent a progression of injuries to the elbow that allow for dislocation—the first stage represents an injury to the lateral collateral ligament, allowing for radiocapitellar subluxation. The examiner "draws" a longitudinal line down the anterior humeral cortex. A second line that bisects the long axis of the radius should intersect near the center (middle third) of the capitellum (Fig. 34.3). If there is any displacement of the intersection of these two lines, the examiner must suspect an elbow dislocation. Generally, the radius should line up with the capitellum on all views. As the injury progresses, subluxation and finally dislocation of the ulnohumeral joint become apparent.

One of the most important parts of the initial radiographic workup is determining whether the dislocation is simple or associated with other injuries. Fracture dislocations have several typical patterns of presentation:

- Posterior dislocation with radial head fracture
- Posterior dislocation with radial head and coronoid fracture (terrible triad injury)

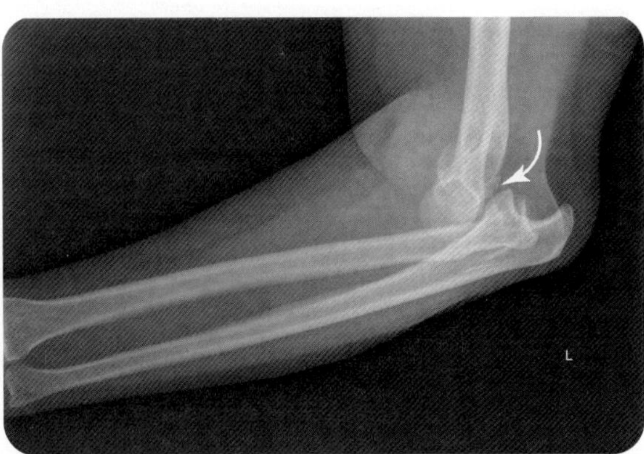

Figure 34.2 Lateral radiograph of the left elbow, demonstrating dislocation of the distal humerus from the radius and ulna.

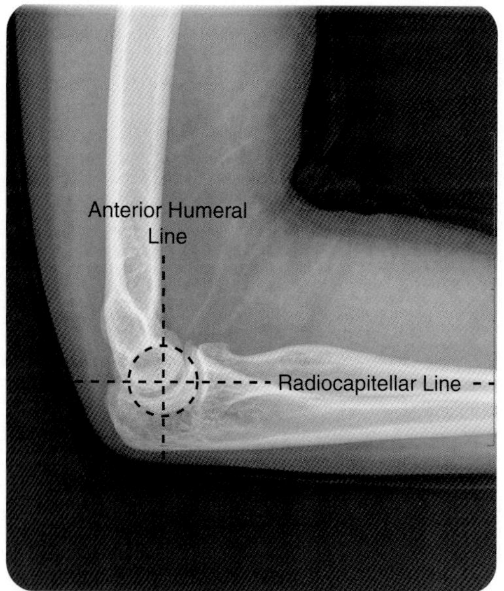

Figure 34.3 Normal lateral radiograph of the right elbow, demonstrating the anterior humeral and radiocapitellar lines that intersect the capitellum (*circle*).

- Varus posteromedial injury with coronoid fracture
- Olecranon fracture dislocation

Associated fractures can be quite subtle and usually represent injury patterns with gross instability. Therefore, identifying them early is essential to treatment. The examiner should check the lateral view carefully for displaced fat pads. Displacement of the anterior fat pad may indicate an underlying intraarticular fracture. The anterior fat pad forms a small dark (radiolucent) oblique triangle that extends from the distal humerus to the proximal radius. Enlargement of this radiolucency represents displacement of the soft tissue by the hemarthrosis. A second fat pad sign may be present posteriorly at the distal humerus. Small nondisplaced radial head fractures are notorious for not appearing on the initial radiographs, so it is important to always examine the fat pads (especially the anterior fat pad) carefully.

Treatment

Treatment of uncomplicated cases may involve closed reduction, which is usually followed by physical therapy in several days. Reduction of simple dislocations occurs under conscious sedation, usually in the emergency department setting. Before initiating treatment, it is necessary to perform a complete neurovascular examination and document the results. The physician should apply traction across the elbow with flexion held at 90 degrees. It helps to apply supination and correct medial/lateral displacement before applying traction. While palpating for any instability, the physician checks the range of motion in the elbow. A well-padded posterior mold splint placed at 90 degrees of flexion is necessary along with a repeat radiographic series taken to document postreduction joint alignment. A patient with a simple dislocation that is stable to postreduction range of motion testing should use the splint at 90 degrees for 1 to 2 weeks, after which range of motion is initiated. The physician can pronate the forearm for added stability. A postreduction neurovascular examination is necessary.

Severe cases may require an external fixation device. It should be noted that complicated cases with terrible triad injuries require an open reduction and internal fixation. The aim of surgical intervention is restoration of stability so that early range of motion can be initiated. Many surgical options exist and are beyond the scope of this chapter.

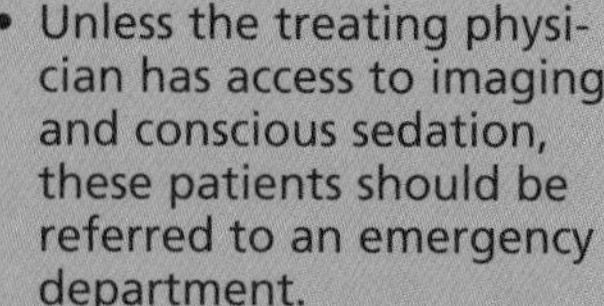

- Unless the treating physician has access to imaging and conscious sedation, these patients should be referred to an emergency department.
- Primary care physicians comfortable with elbow injuries can initiate the workup with radiographs and a reduction attempt.
- Any patient with postreduction instability or with complex fracture–dislocations should prompt immediate orthopaedic consult.
- All patients warrant close follow-up by an orthopaedic surgeon, because instability patterns are subtle and potentially devastating to the function of the elbow.

Suggested Readings

Beingessner DM, Dunning CE, Stacpoole RA, et al. The effect of coronoid fractures on elbow kinematics and stability. *Clin Biomech*. 2007;22(2):183–190.

Mathew PK, Athwal GS, King GJ. Terrible triad injury of the elbow: current concepts. *J Am Acad Orthop Surg*. 2009;17(3):137–151.

Morrey BF. Current concepts in the management of complex elbow trauma. *Surgeon*. 2009;7(3):151–161.

Morrey BF. Current concepts in the treatment of fractures of the radial head, the olecranon, and the coronoid. *JBJS*. 1995;77:316–327.

O'Driscoll SW, Morrey BF, Korinek S, An KN. Elbow subluxation and dislocation. A spectrum of instability. *Clin Orthop Relat Res*. 1992;(280):186–197.

Pugh DMW, Wild LM, Schemitsch EH, King GJW. Standard surgical protocol to treat elbow dislocations with radial head and coronoid fractures. *JBJS*. 2004;86:1122–1130.

Ring D. *Fractures and Dislocations of the Elbow. Rockwood and Green's Fractures in Adults*. 6th ed. Philadelphia, PA: Lippincott Williams and Wilkins; 2006.

Ring D, Harness N. *Elbow Trauma. Surgical Treatment of Orthopaedic Trauma*. New York, NY: Thieme; 2007.

Ring D, Jupiter JB, Zilberfarb J. Posterior dislocations of the elbow with fractures of the radial head and coronoid. *JBJS* 2002;84:547–551.

Shearman CM, El-Khoury GY. Pitfalls in the radiologic evaluation of extremity trauma: Part 1. The upper extremity. *Am Fam Physician*. 1998;57:995–1005.

Tashjian RZ, Katarinic JA. Complex elbow instability. *J Am Acad Orthop Surg*. 2006;14(5):278–286.

Teh J, Sukumar V, Jackson S. Imaging of the elbow. *Imaging*. 2003;15:193–204.

CHAPTER 35 Olecranon Fractures

George M. Bridgeforth, David S. Wellman, and Charles Carroll IV

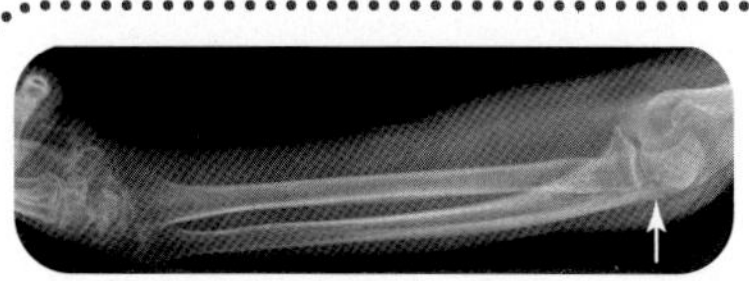

An 80-year-old woman lost consciousness and fell down the stairs. She sustains multiple injuries as a result.

Clinical Presentation

Olecranon fractures account for approximately 20% of all elbow fractures. These fractures are caused by direct or indirect forces. Direct force fractures tend to occur secondary to falls onto the elbow. Indirect force injuries are caused by forceful contraction of the triceps and are often simple transverse or oblique fractures. Olecranon fractures are characterized by acute swelling, pain, and tenderness. Patients usually exhibit painful range of motion as well. Following acute trauma, several conditions, including olecranon bursitis and pseudofractures can mimic the picture seen with olecranon fractures.

CLINICAL POINTS

- The majority of these fractures are isolated injuries.
- Either direct or indirect trauma may cause olecranon fractures.
- Olecranon bursitis may develop.

During the physical examination, the clinician should

- evaluate range of motion.
- check for skin integrity and swelling (bursitis) around the joint.
- perform a complete neurovascular examination focusing on the following nerves:

(Continued)

OLECRANON BURSITIS AND OLECRANON PSEUDOFRACTURES

Olecranon bursitis is a condition that can present simultaneously or independently of an olecranon fracture. It can be grossly categorized into septic and nonseptic presentations.

A septic bursitis is characterized by warm, tender, painful swelling of the olecranon. Immediate evaluation with aspiration, gram staining, culture, and cell counts/fluid analysis is necessary. Most penetrating infections are caused by gram-positive organisms such as *Staphylococcus aureus, Staphylococcus epidermidis,* and *Streptococcus*. Initial treatment consists of aspiration and antibiotics. Repeat aspirations may be necessary if fluid reaccumulates. The clinician should consider formal incision and drainage if a trial of aspiration and antibiotics fails, as the infection could spread into the elbow joint. Care must be taken, as rheumatiod arthritis and gout can produce a similar picture and masquerade as a bacterial infection.

A traumatic or idiopathic (nonseptic) olecranon bursitis is a golf ball–like swelling over the olecranon (Fig. 35.1). Chronic changes may result in a thickening of the overlying skin with a peau d'orange (orange peel) appearance. Treatment consists of aspiration, fluid culture, and analysis (to rule out septic bursitis and evaluate for crystals). The clinician should consider starting a nonsteroidal anti-inflammatory drug and giving a steroid injection, because researchers have hypothesized that both hasten recovery. It is sometimes necessary to perform a surgical bursectomy in refractory cases.

Patients with elbow spurs (syndesmophytes) at the olecranon may present with a pseudofracture of the olecranon and chronic (nonseptic) bursitis. Pseudofractures appear as a small translucent line in the syndesmophyte. Generally, these lines do not extend into the cortical margin of the olecranon.

CLINICAL POINTS (*Continued*)

- Median (opponens pollicis weakness with diminished grip strength associated with impaired sensation of the thenar eminence)
- Ulnar (decreased sensation and weakness of the ulnar wrist flexors, hypothenar eminence, fourth and fifth fingers)
- Radial (acute wrist drop or wrist extensor weakness with impaired sensation over the dorsal wrist and forearm)

- check for neurovascular compromise or compartment syndromes (swollen painful cyanotic limb with numbness and diminished or absent pulses), and document findings prior to treatment.
- check the wrist and shoulder for associated injuries.

PATIENT ASSESSMENT

1. Pain, swelling, and tenderness about the elbow
2. Pain-limited range of motion
3. Possible crepitation (displaced bone fragments) and palpable bone defects

NOT TO BE MISSED

- Elbow strains/contusions
- Elbow dislocations/other fractures around the elbow
- Medial or lateral epicondylitis
- Olecranon bursitis
- Septic joints
- Triceps tears
- Gout
- Rheumatoid arthritis

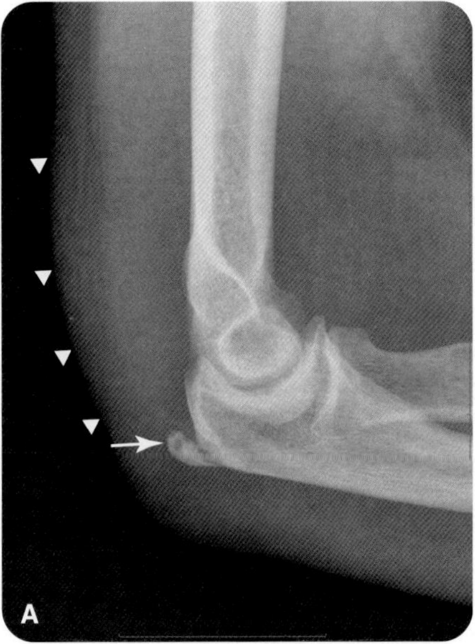

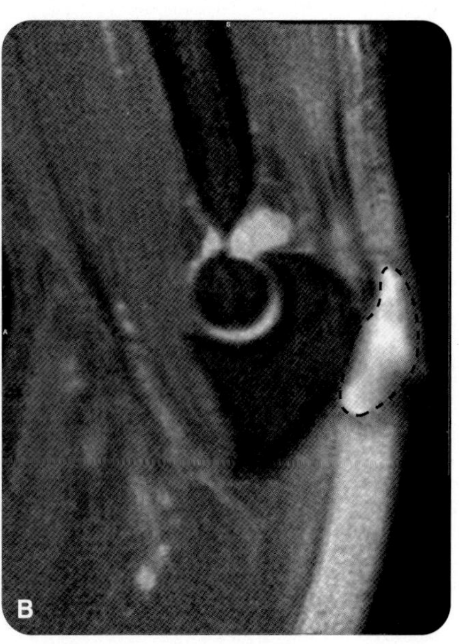

Figure 35.1 (A) Lateral radiograph of the left elbow in an 80-year-old man with 1 month of left elbow pain and swelling, which demonstrates a prominent olecranon spur at the insertion site of the triceps tendon (*arrow*) with soft tissue swelling posteriorly (*arrowheads*), suggesting olecranon bursitis. **(B)** A selected sagittal fluid-sensitive image of the left elbow in the same patient confirms abnormal fluid posterior to the olecranon (*outline*) compatible with olecranon bursitis. Fluid analysis should be performed to exclude an infectious etiology.

Pseudofractures commonly appear in syndesmophytes because of the poor quality of the porous bone in elbow spurs. Generally, they do not require any treatment, and management of the bursitis can proceed as described above.

TRICEPS TEARS

Triceps tears are uncommon injuries. However, the differential diagnosis of olecranon injuries may include rupture of the triceps muscle. Causes include an eccentric load on a contracting triceps muscle or direct impact. Patient with acute tears complain of "pop" followed by pain, swelling, and tenderness at the olecranon. In these cases, patients usually report pain with lifting heavy objects. The lateral radiograph shows soft tissue swelling. With complete tears, the patient lacks the ability to extend the arm because the triceps is the major extensor of the elbow through its attachment to the olecranon. Partial tears leave the patient with some ability to extend the arm.

If a triceps tear is suspected, it is better to test the triceps function in the horizontal plane (i.e., with the arm positioned across the body in front of the chest) with gravity eliminated. When triceps function is tested in the vertical plane (i.e., with the fist on the shoulder), the patient can give a false impression of intact triceps function by lowering their arm.

Historically, management varies. Treatment of partial tears of the triceps is conservative, and surgical repair is required for complete tears.

Radiographic Evaluation

Required radiographs include anteroposterior (AP), lateral (elbow flexed at 90 degrees), and oblique (arm extended) views (Fig. 35.2). Computed tomography (CT) scans are not necessary to work up an isolated olecranon fracture. However, olecranon fractures can be seen along with other fractures in the elbow

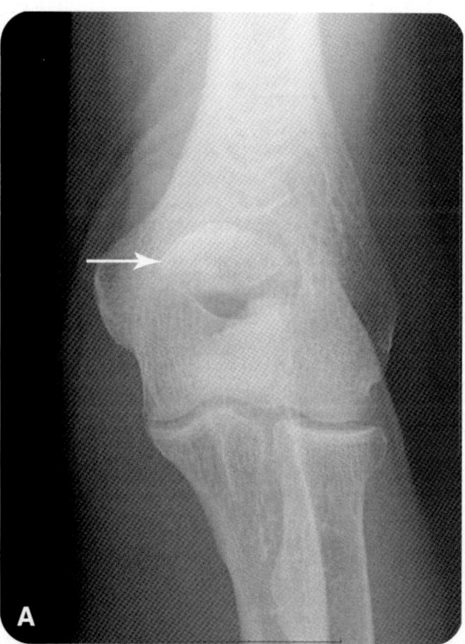

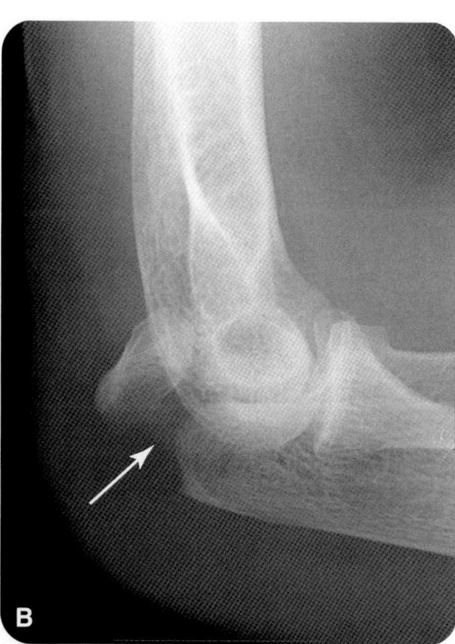

Figure 35.2 **(A)** Anterioposterior and **(B)** lateral radiographs of the left elbow demonstrating a displaced acute fracture of the olecranon.

with severe trauma, and CT scans are helpful to define these injuries. If a triceps tear is suspected, referral for a magnetic resonance imaging scan is necessary.

Olecranon fractures are best identified on the lateral view. Small nondisplaced fractures may appear as thin translucent lines that extend to the cortex. Like radial head fractures, olecranon fractures may cause bleeding into the joint capsule and may be associated with positive anterior and posterior fat pad signs (lucent areas anterior and posterior to the distal humerus from displaced fat pads). It is essential to take note of the displacement of the fracture fragments; this is one of the main characteristics of the injury that drives operative intervention.

It is also necessary to evaluate AP and lateral x-rays for associated injuries. The examiner should make sure to evaluate the integrity of the proximal radius and its association with the capitellum of the distal humerus (the radial head should be in line with the capitellum on all views). In addition, the examiner should also evaluate for subluxation or dislocation of the humerus and ulna.

Plain radiographs allow a gross estimate of the age of the fracture. Acute fractures are generally associated with radiographic evidence of soft tissue swelling and well-defined fracture lines. Old fractures demonstrate sclerotic, smooth fracture lines, and normal appearing soft tissue.

Treatment

The overall goals of treatment of olecranon fractures are to reestablish joint congruity, promote anatomic bone healing, and initiate early range of motion exercises to prevent posttreatment stiffness. Both operative and conservative treatment strategies exist to meet these goals, and the characteristics of the injury help guide the decision of which type of treatment to offer.

Nonoperative treatment is appropriate for closed, nondisplaced, and minimally displaced (<2 mm) fractures. Typically, placement of a well-padded posterior-based splint at 45 to 90 degrees of flexion occurs in the acute setting. It is important not to place a circumferential cast immediately after the injury, because casts do not allow for swelling. Once swelling has subsided, a transition from a splint to a full cast may occur, for a total immobilization time of approximately 4 weeks. At this point, active-assisted range of motion exercise to prevent stiffness begins, often in consultation with a physical therapist. It is necessary to delay resistance exercise until the 8-week mark to allow for healing of the bony fragments. It is necessary to tell patients to expect some loss of range of elbow motion.

Surgeons pursue operative treatment for displacement exceeding 2 mm, open injury, and injury to the triceps extensor mechanism. Surgical options include plate/screw construct, pin/wire constructs, and fragment excision.

WHEN TO REFER

- Patients with open fractures, neurovascular injuries, compartment syndromes, impaired extensor function, or displaced fractures should be referred immediately.
- Uncomplicated nondisplaced fractures may be referred at the discretion of the primary care physician, especially if the physician is not experienced in fracture management.
- Partial or complete triceps tears should be referred to an orthopedist quickly for management.

Suggested Readings

Cain EL, Dugas JR, Wolf RS, Andrews JR. Elbow injuries in throwing athletes: a current concepts review. *Am J Sports Med*. 2003;31(4):621–635.

Hak DJ, Golladay GJ. Olecranon fractures: treatment options. *J Am Acad Orthop Surg*. 2000;8(4):266–275.

Kijowski R, Tuite M, Sandford M. Magnetic resonance imaging of the elbow. Part II: abnormalities of the ligaments, tendons and nerves. *Skeletal Radiol*. 2005;34(1):1–18.

Lindehovius AL, Brouwer KM, Doornberg JN, et al. Long-term outcome of operatively treated fracture-dislocations of the olecranon. *J Orthop Trauma*. 2008;22(5):325–331.

Ly JQ, Sanders TG, Beall DP. MR imaging of the elbow: a spectrum of common pathologic conditions. *Clin Imaging*. 2005;29(4):278–282.

Mair SD, Isbell WM, Gill TJ, Schlegel TF, Hawkins RJ. Triceps tendon ruptures in professional football players. *Am J Sports Med*. 2004;32(2):431–434.

Newman SD, Mauffrey C, Krikier S. Olecranon fractures. *Injury*. 2009;40(6):575–581.

Nork SE, Jones CB, Henley MB. Surgical treatment of olecranon fractures. *Am J Orthop*. 2001;30(7):577–586.

O'Dwyer H, O'Sullivan P, Fitzgerald D, et al. The fat pad sign following elbow trauma in adults: its usefulness and reliability in suspecting occult fracture. *J Comput Assist Tomogr*. 2004;28(4):562–565.

Potter HG, Ho ST, Alcheck DW. Magnetic imaging of the elbow. *Semin Musculoskelet Radiol*. 2004;8(1):5–16.

Ring D. *Fractures and Dislocations of the Elbow. Rockwood and Green's Fractures in Adults*. 6th ed. Philadelphia, PA: Lippincott Williams &Wilkins; 2006.

Ring D, Harness N. *Elbow Trauma. Surgical Treatment of Orthopaedic Trauma*. New York, NY: Thieme; 2007.

Safran MR. Elbow injuries in athletes. A review. *Clin Orthop Relat Res*. 1995;310:257–277.

Safran M, Ahman CS, Elattrache NS. Ulnar collateral ligament of the elbow. *Arthroscopy*. 2005;21(11): 1381–1395.

Schmeling GJ, Maciolek LJ. *Olecranon Fractures: Open Reduction Internal Fixation. Master Techniques in Orthopaedic Surgery: Fractures*. 2nd ed. Philadelphia, PA: Lippincott Williams &Wilkins; 2006.

Stell IM. Septic and non-septic olecranon bursitis in the accident and emergency department—an approach to management. *J Accid Emerg Med*. 1996;13(5):351–353.

Veilette CJ, Steinmann SP. Olecranon Fractures. *Orthop Clin North Am*. 2008;39(2):229–236.

CHAPTER 36 Forearm Fractures

Joan Williams, George M. Bridgeforth, and Charles Carroll IV

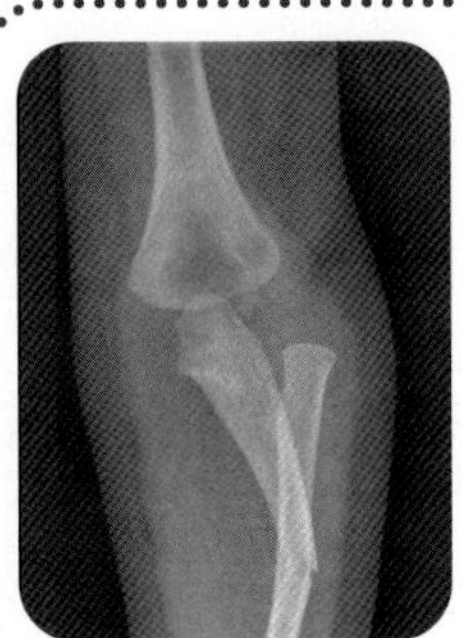

A 2-year-old male infant fell from his high chair. He acts as if his left arm, which is swollen and tender, hurts.

Clinical Presentation

Nearly 50% of fractures affect the arm. Fractures of the forearm are most often due to direct blows, although they may also occur with falls onto an outstretched hand. It is important to recognize that the forearm, which consists of the radius and ulna, acts as a ring and that dissipation of energy results in fractures or dislocations of both bones in most cases. These fractures may be classified according to their occurrence on the proximal, middle, or distal shafts of the radius and ulna. With forearm fractures, associated injuries may occur in the elbow and wrist.

MONTEGGIA FRACTURE

A Monteggia fracture is a fracture of the proximal ulna with an associated radial head dislocation (Fig. 36.1). The majority (60%) of these injuries involve anterior dislocation of the radial head. Anterior and lateral dislocations are seen primarily in children. Posterior dislocations are seen primarily in adults.

GALEAZZI FRACTURE

A Galeazzi fracture is a fracture of the radial diaphysis at the junction of the middle and distal thirds (Figs. 36.2, 36.3). Also known as a reverse Monteggia fracture, it is associated with disruption of the distal radioulnar joint (DRUJ).

NIGHTSTICK FRACTURE

A nightstick fracture is an isolated fracture of the ulnar shaft, most often due to direct trauma to the ulna (Fig. 36.4). The forearm is usually held in protection across the face (Fig. 36.5).

Radiographic Evaluation

Radiographs to order include anteroposterior (AP) and lateral films of the forearm. If necessary, the examiner may obtain oblique views of the forearm for

CLINICAL POINTS

- Causes include sports and trauma.
- A fracture of the proximal (or middle ulna) is associated with a dislocation of the radial head.
- Forearm fractures are often open fractures.

  During physical examination for patients with all types of forearm injuries, the physician should
- palpate the wrist, elbow, and shoulder to assess for associated injuries, because often these fractures are a result of high-speed injury.

(*Continued*)

CLINICAL POINTS (*Continued*)

- conduct a thorough neurovascular examination. It is important to pay special attention to the radial, ulnar, and median nerves, including evaluation of the anterior interosseous and posterior interosseous nerve branches. With neurovascular damage, the patient will manifest diminished or absent pulses. Moreover, the extremity will be cold. Motor strength will be severely affected and will be absent or pain limited. In addition, accompanying sensory abnormalities which are characterized by decreased pinprick and light touch are common findings as well. Neurovascular impairment may occur as the result of a compartment syndrome or from direct trauma to the neurovascular structures. The damaged extremity usually demonstrates pallor in fair-skinned individuals. However, this may not be present in dark-skinned patients. It is essential to document the neurovascular examination carefully.
- evaluate for compartment syndrome. The most sensitive clinical test for this is pain with passive extension of the fingers. There is marked swelling of the arm. The increased pressure inside the forearm is diminishing the blood flow to the extremities. The presence of a radial pulse does not rule out compartment syndrome; capillary blood flow ceases at a pressure lower than arterial blood flow.
- Check for open wounds on the forearm, because these injuries are frequently open fractures.

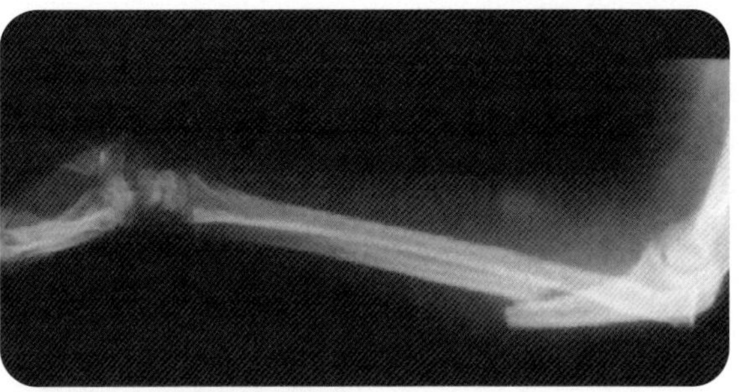

Figure 36.1 Type II Bado fracture with a posterolateral dislocation of the radial head in a 26-year-old woman. (From Bucholz RW, Heckman JD. *Rockwood and Green's Fractures in Adults*. 5th ed. Philadelphia, PA: Lippincott, Williams & Wilkins, 2001.)

further fracture definition. Elbow and wrist films of the injured extremity are important to obtain, because forearm radiographs are not adequate for ruling out associated wrist and elbow injuries.

MONTEGGIA FRACTURE

In both the AP and lateral views, the radial head should be in line with the capitellum. A vertical line drawn along the anterior border of the humerus on

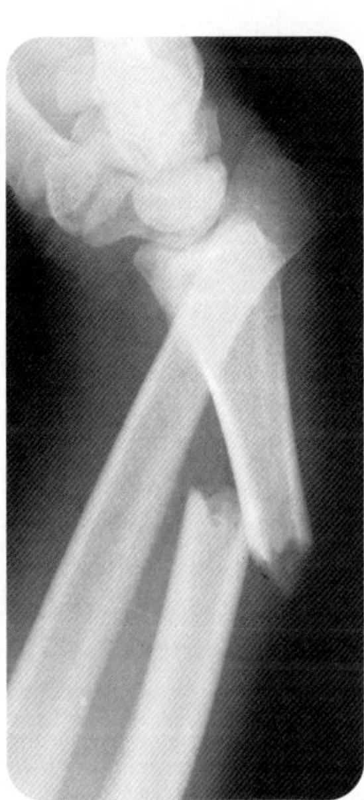

Figure 36.2 Severely displaced Galeazzi fracture–dislocation in lateral projection. The distal radioulnar dislocation (*open arrow*) is secondary to the marked shortening of the radius caused by the severe ulnar displacement and dorsal angulation of the distal radial fragment. (From Harris JH Jr, Harris WH. *The Radiology of Emergency Medicine*. 3rd ed. Philadelphia, PA: Lippincott-Raven; 2000:390, with permission.)

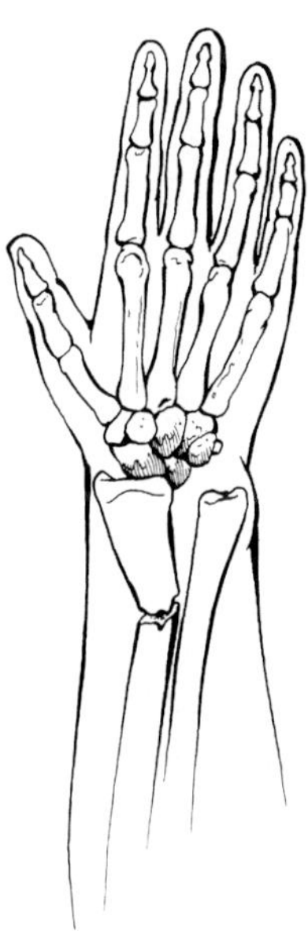

Figure 36.3 Galeazzi fracture–dislocation. (From Harwood-Nuss A, Wolfson AB, et al. *The Clinical Practice of Emergency Medicine*. 3rd ed. Philadelphia, PA: Lippincott Williams & Wilkins; 2001.

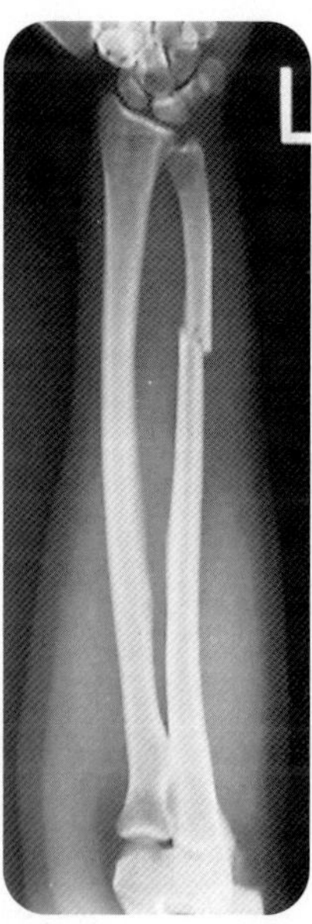

Figure 36.4 Nightstick fracture. Minimally displaced oblique fracture of the ulna without associated fracture of the radius (L, left). (From Eisenberg RL. *An Atlas of Differential Diagnosis*. 4th ed. Philadelphia, PA: Lippincott Williams & Wilkins; 2003.

PATIENT ASSESSMENT

1. Gross deformity of the forearm
2. Pain, swelling, and loss of hand and forearm function

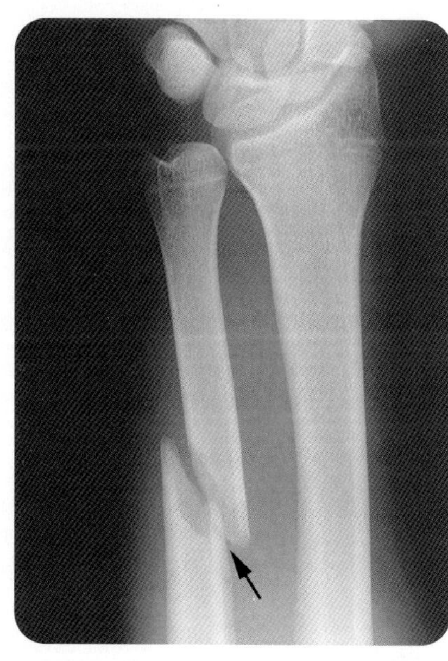

Figure 36.5 Nightstick fracture: ulnar fracture. Note the fracture of the distal ulna. COMMENT: This type of ulnar fracture can be associated with an attempt at self-protection of the head during an assault with a handheld object. Because assaults often occur at night and a stick may be used as the attack weapon, this fracture has been called a nightstick fracture. (From Yochum TR, Rowe LJ. *Yochum and Rowe's Essentials of Skeletal Radiology*. 3rd ed. Philadelphia, PA: Lippincott Williams & Wilkins; 2004.)

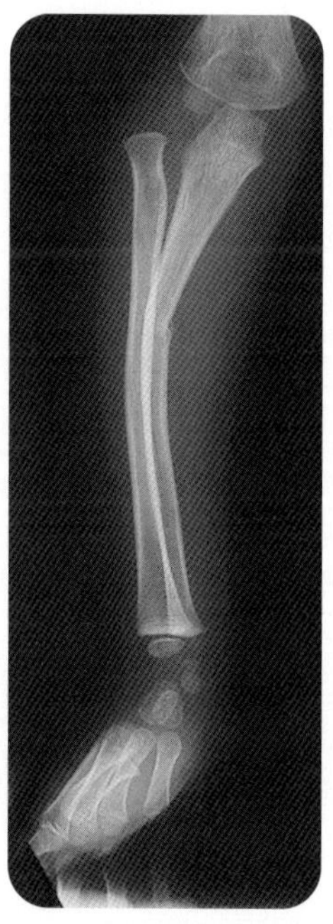

Figure 36.6 Monteggia fracture/dislocation. A 4-year-old boy fell off his bike. The ulna is fractured and angulated, and a line through the radius clearly does not pass through the center of the capitellum. (Courtesy of Dr. Andrew Capraro.) (From Fleisher GR, Ludwig S, Baskin MN. *Atlas of Pediatric Emergency Medicine*. Philadelphia, PA: Lippincott Williams & Wilkins; 2004.)

NOT TO BE MISSED

- Radial head dislocations (most important element of fracture management)
- Disruption of the DRUJ
- Neurovascular impairment
- Compartment syndrome

the lateral view should intersect a horizontal line that bisects the long axis of the radius at the middle third of the capitellum. The absence of these relationships indicates a dislocation of the radial head (Fig. 36.6).

The examiner should also be aware of the following points:

- To rule out injuries to the distal radius or ulna, the examiner should always include radiographs of the ipsilateral wrist.
- Often, if the ulnar fracture is angulated, the direction of angulation correlates with the direction of the radial head dislocation.
- Not all radial head dislocations are Monteggia fractures. If the ulnohumeral joint is also disrupted, this is not a Monteggia fracture as previously described.

GALEAZZI FRACTURE

Signs of DRUJ disruption on radiography include a fracture at the base of the ulnar styloid, widening of the disruption of the DRUJ on an AP film; radial shortening of 5 mm or greater; and subluxation of the ulna on the lateral film (Figs. 36.7, 36.8). It should be noted that there may be variants in which fractures occur at any point along the radius with DRUJ disruption.

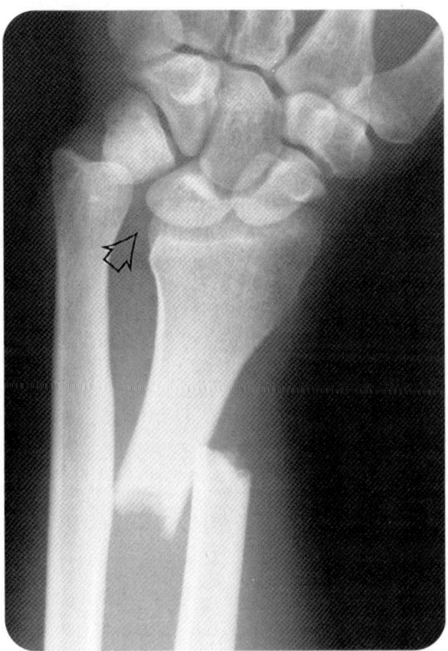

Figure 36.7 Severely displaced Galeazzi fracture–dislocation in frontal projection. The distal radioulnar dislocation (*open arrow*) is secondary to the marked shortening of the radius caused by the severe ulnar displacement and dorsal angulation of the distal radial fragment. (From Harris JH Jr, Harris WH. *The Radiology of Emergency Medicine.* 3rd ed. Philadelphia, PA: Lippincott-Raven; 2000:390, with permission.)

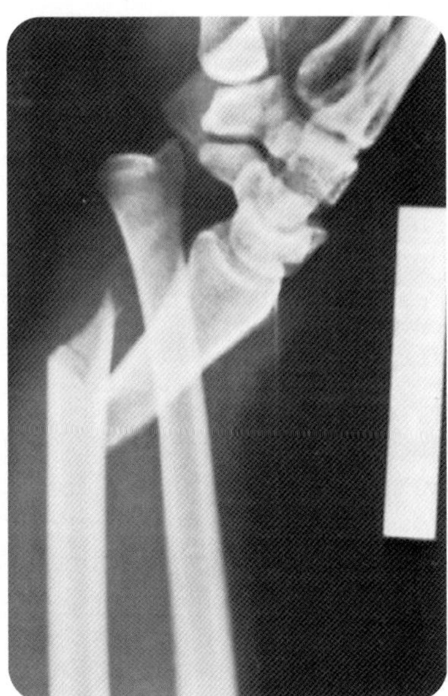

Figure 36.8 Galeazzi fracture. A lateral projection shows the dorsally angulated distal radial fracture and the obvious disruption of the distal radioulnar joint. The ulna is intact. (From Eisenberg RL. *An Atlas of Differential Diagnosis.* 4th ed. Philadelphia, PA: Lippincott Williams & Wilkins; 2003.

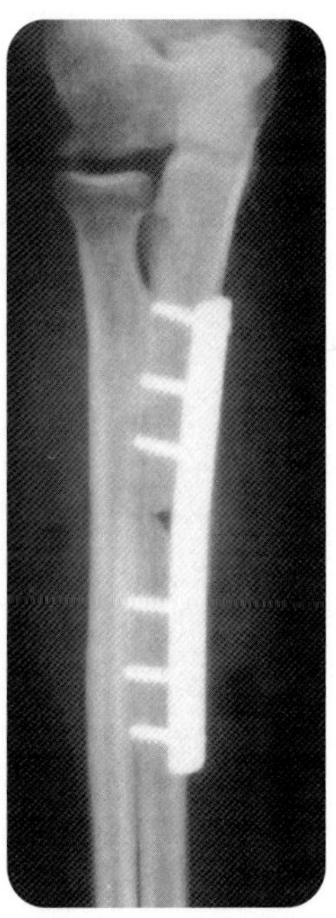

Figure 36.9 The ulna was fixed with a seven-hole dynamic compression plate, and the radial head was closed and reduced with satisfactory stability to permit early motion at 7 days. (From Bucholz RW, Heckman JD. *Rockwood & Green's Fractures in Adults.* 5th ed. Lippincott, Williams & Wilkins; 2001.)

NIGHTSTICK FRACTURE

Examiners should obtain views of ipsilateral wrist and elbow to rule out associated injuries along with AP and lateral views of the forearm.

WHEN TO REFER

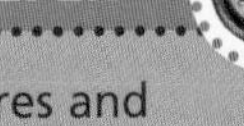

- Open fractures and displaced fractures
- Nondisplaced fractures at the examiners discretion
- Fractures with neurovascular impairment
- Acute dislocation of a major extremity
- Suspected Monteggia fractures, especially in children. If follow-up is greater than 1 week after the injury and they have a recurrent dislocation, the opportunity for nonoperative management of the fracture may have been lost or may be more difficult.

Treatment

MONTEGGIA FRACTURE

These fractures require surgical intervention involving open reduction and internal fixation of the ulnar fracture and closed reduction of the radial head (Fig. 36.9). When seen in the emergency department or office setting, any open wounds should be washed out with sterile saline. A tetanus shot should be given if the patient has not had one within the past 10 years. Most importantly, the radial head should be reduced, because prolonged dislocation of the radial head can lead to an increased incidence of posttraumatic arthritis.

After providing adequate anesthesia, the reduction maneuver for this fracture depends on the direction of the radial head dislocation. In all types of dislocations, medial or lateral displacement should be corrected first. For anterior dislocations, gentle longitudinal traction on the forearm, with elbow flexion and manual reduction of the radial head is typically effective. For posterior dislocations, longitudinal traction on the forearm, flexion of the elbow, supination, and manual reduction of the radial head is suggested. Postreduction imaging should be obtained to ensure that the radial head is in place.

These fractures may be splinted in a posterior mold splint with the elbow in 90 degrees of flexion and neutral rotation.

GALEAZZI FRACTURE

These fractures require surgical fixation, because nonoperative management is often associated with a high failure rate. Emergency department or office management should consist of temporary stabilization of the forearm with a posterior mold or sugar tong splint. Attempts at reduction should be made in order to restore the length of the radius, if possible.

NIGHTSTICK FRACTURES

Nondisplaced or minimally displaced fractures may be treated with a sugar-tong splint for 7 to 10 days, followed by functional bracing or sling immobilization with active range of motion exercises for the elbow, wrist, and hand. Studies have shown that patients treated with functional bracing tended to have better forearm range of motion and significantly better wrist range of motion when compared with patients treated with a long arm cast.

Unstable fractures are defined as having greater than 10 degrees of angulation in any plane, greater than 50% displacement of the shaft of the ulna, or involvement of the proximal third of the ulna. Displaced fractures require surgical management to preserve forearm supination and pronation.

Suggested Readings

Bruce HE, Harvey JP, Wilson JC. Monteggia Fractures. *J Bone Joint Surg JBJS*. 1974;56:1563–1576.

Davis KW. Names and Numbers in Musculoskeletal Radiology. University of Wisconsin Radiology. Unpublished document. Query: Kirdland W. Davis. Accessed July, 2009.

Eathiraju S, Mudgal CS, Jupiter JB. Monteggia fracture–dislocations. *Hand Clin*. 2007;23(2):165–177.

Giannoulis FX, Sotereanos DG. Galeazzi fractures and dislocations. *Hand Clin*. 2007;23:153–163.

Konrad GG, Kundel K, Kreuz PC, Oberst M. Monteggia fractures in adults: long-term results and prognostic factors. *J Bone Joint Surg JBJS*. 2007:889-B(3):354–360.

Morgan WJ, Breen TF. Complex fractures of the forearm. *Hand Clin*. 1994;10(3):375–390.

Nicolaidis SC, Hildreth DH, Lichtman DM. Acute injuries of the distal radioulnar joint. *Hand Clin*. 2000;16(3):449–459.

Ring D, Jupiter JB, Simpson NS. Monteggia fractures in adults. *J Bone Joint Surg JBJS* 1998;80(12):1733–1744.

Ring D, Rhim D, Carpenter C, Jupiter JB. Isolated radial shaft fractures are more common than galeazzi fractures. *J Hand Surg Am*. 2006;31(1):17–21.

Ring D, Jupiter JB, Waters PM. Monteggia fractures in children and adults. *J Am Acad Orthop Surg JAAOS*. 1998;6:215–224.

Sauder DJ, Athwal GS. Management of isolated ulnar shaft fractures. *Hand Clin*. 2007;23:179–184.

Shearman CM, El-Khoury GY. Pitfalls in the radiologic evaluation of extremity trauma: Part l. The upper extremity. *Am Fam Physician*. 1998;57(5):995–1005.

SECTION 8

Wrist

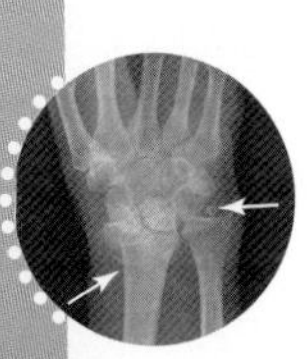

Chapter 37 Distal Radial and Ulnar Fractures

George M. Bridgeforth, Joan Williams, and Charles Carroll IV

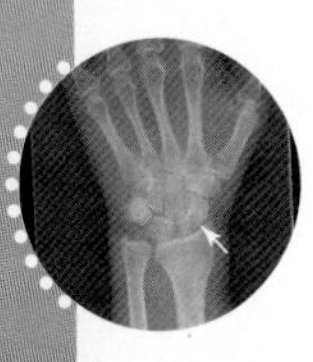

Chapter 38 Scaphoid Fractures

George M. Bridgeforth, Thomas Hearty, and Charles Carroll IV

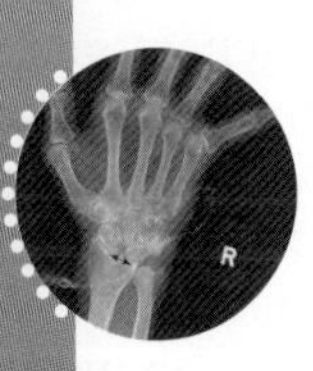

Chapter 39 Scapholunate Dissociation

George M. Bridgeforth, Thomas Hearty, and Charles Carroll IV

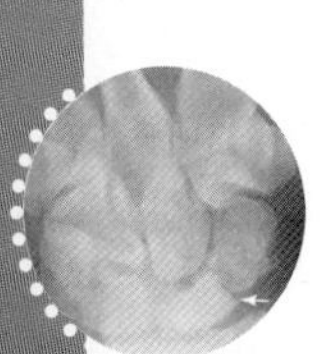

Chapter 40 Avascular Necrosis (Scaphoid)

George M. Bridgeforth, Thomas Hearty, and Charles Carroll IV

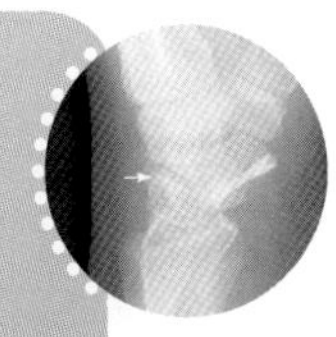

Chapter 41 Avascular Necrosis of the Lunate (Kienböck's Disease)

George M. Bridgeforth, Kathryn J. McCarthy, and Charles Carroll IV

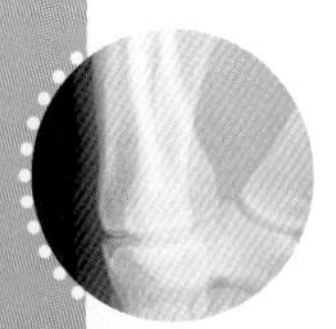

Chapter 42 Perilunate Dislocation

George M. Bridgeforth, Kathryn J. McCarthy, and Charles Carroll IV

Functional Anatomy

The wrist is a complex ellipsoid joint that has three degrees of freedom: one for flexion–extension, one for supination–pronation, and one for radioulnar deviation. It is composed of eight carpal bones (the Latin *carpus* means wrist), which are linked by fibrous carpal ligaments to create a semirigid intercalated ring structure. Each carpal bone can be identified by its position and anatomical configuration.

The carpal bones are divided into two rows (Fig. 1). The first (proximal) row consists of the scaphoid (navicular), the lunate, the triquetrum, and the overlying volar pisiform. The scaphoid, which has an oblong boat-shaped configuration, lies distal to the radius. It makes up the floor of the anatomic snuffbox. The crescent-shaped lunate, which received its name because the head of the capitate fits inside its semilunar concave-shaped configuration, lies at the ulnar border of the scaphoid (just distal to the ulna). The triquetrum, or the three cornered, lies on the ulnar border of the lunate and slightly distal. It is easy to recognize the triquetrum because the overlapping pea-shaped pisiform lies on its volar surface. The pisiform protects the flexor carpal ulnaris tendon by helping to anchor it, thus preventing its displacement during wrist movement.

The second (distal) carpal row consists of the trapezium, trapezoid, the capitate, and the hamate (Fig. 2). These bones all articulate with the metacarpals, which are numbered one through five, beginning with the thumb. The trapezium joins with the first metacarpal to form the saddle joint of the thumb. The trapezoid articulates with the ulnar border of the trapezium. Distally, it connects with the base of the second metacarpal. The capitate lies at the center of the wrist (mnemonic: **c**apitate at the **c**enter). It articulates proximally with the scaphoid and the lunate and distally with the bases of the third and fourth metacarpals. The hamate, which is located next to the ulnar border of the capitate, joins the bases of the fourth (sharing the base of the fourth metacarpal with the neighboring

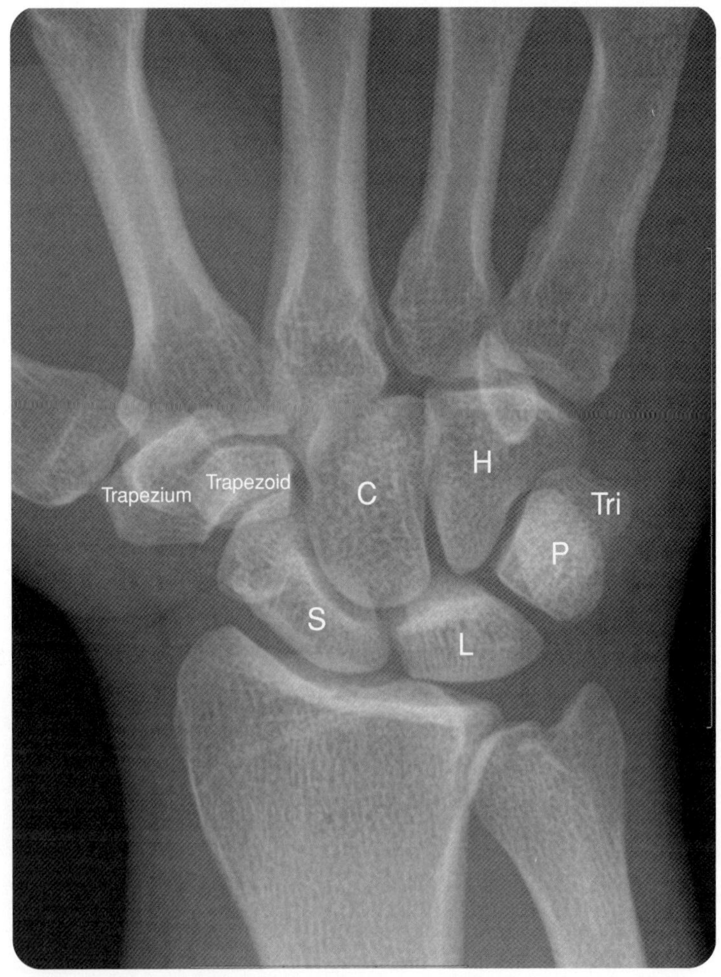

Figure 1 AP view of the carpal bones. The proximal row comprises the scaphoid (S), lunate (L), triquetrum (Tri), and pisiform (P). The distal row comprises the hamate (H), capitate (C), trapezoid, and trapezium.

capitate) and fifth metacarpals. Easily recognized, the hamate has a characteristic hook on its volar surface. The hook of the hamate and the more proximal pisiform help form Guyon's canal. This fibro-osseous tunnel containing the ulnar nerve and the ulnar artery runs along the ulnar border of the wrist.

The distal radius and ulna constitute the distal radioulnar joint (DRUJ). Technically, the DRUJ is not part of the wrist; rather, it is part of the distal forearm. The DRUJ is the larger, broader, distal styloid of the radius that limits wrist extension and radial deviation by approximately 10 degrees (compared with wrist flexion and ulnar deviation). Ulnar deviation is greater because the ulna does not articulate directly with the carpal bones.

The triangular fibrocartilage complex (TFCC), which has a triangular shape, extends from the ulnar notch of the radius to the fovea (eye) of the ulnar styloid process. The TFCC consists of the meniscus homologue, dorsal and volar radiocarpal ligaments, sheath of the extensor carpi ulnaris tendon, dorsal and palmar ulnocarpal ligaments, ulnar collateral ligament, and triangular fibrocartilage. The TFCC is largely responsible for stabilization of the DRUJ during wrist movement, helping to anchor the distal radius and ulna. Along the TFCC's ulnar border lies the meniscus homologue, a fibrocartilaginous disc that is interposed between the distal ulna and the triquetrum. The meniscus homologue provides a load (weight)-bearing cushion for the ulna. Approximately 80% of a weight-bearing load is carried by the radius, and the other 20% is carried by the ulna.

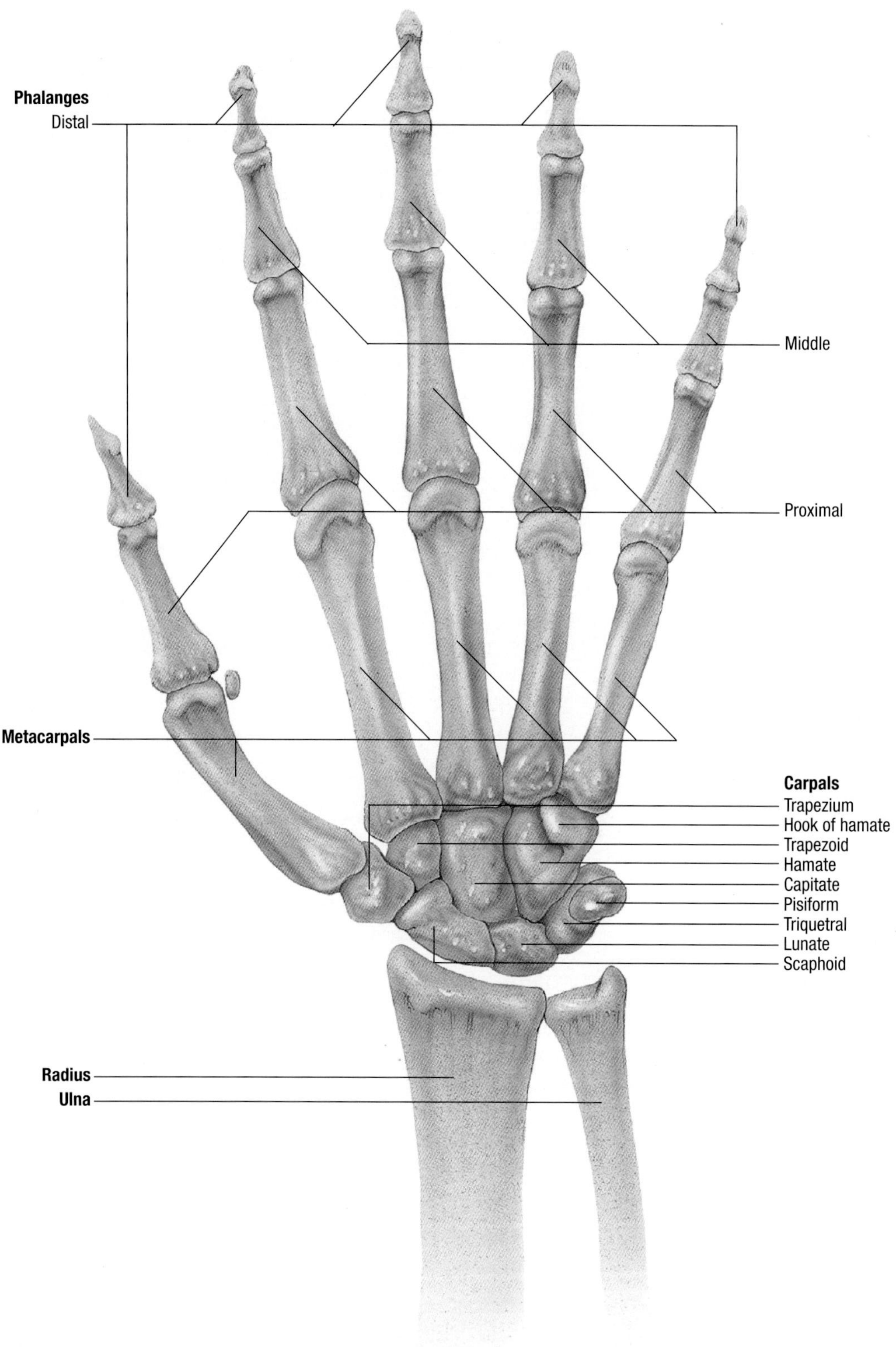

Figure 2 Wrist and hand bones: palmar view. Asset provided by Anatomical Chart Co.

CHAPTER 37 Distal Radial and Ulnar Fractures

George M. Bridgeforth, Joan Williams, and Charles Carroll IV

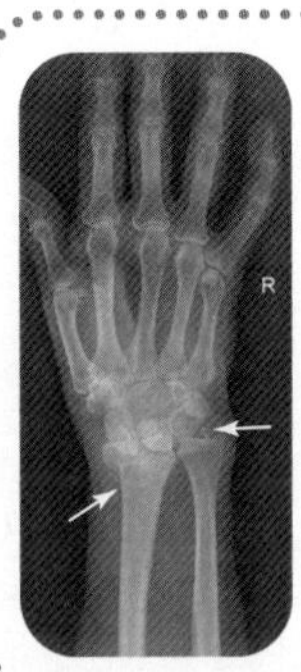

A 83-year-old woman fell in her kitchen and tried to break her fall with her right hand.

Clinical Presentation

Distal radial fractures account for approximately 17.5% of all fractures. The most common mechanism of injury is a fall onto outstretched hand usually with the wrist in dorsiflexion. In younger individuals, fractures may result from higher energy traumas.

Other injuries from falls unto the outstretched hand are more commonly missed. Scaphoid fractures occur almost as commonly as distal radial fractures (see Chapter 39, "Scapholunate Dissociation"). Clinically, distal radial fractures are characterized by pain, swelling, and tenderness of the anatomic snuffbox and scaphoid region just distal to the radius.

A dislocation of the carpal ligaments may occur following a fall, and the clinician may easily miss this. Usual characteristics include moderate-to-marked pain and soreness between the scaphoid and the lunate at the center of the proximal wrist. Patients may complain of clicking. A Watson shift test may reveal a subluxating scaphoid. The test is performed by stabilizing the patient's wrist with one hand and placing the patient's wrist in ulnar deviation. The examiner stabilizes the wrist with the opposite hand and places his or her thumb over the volar scaphoid. He or she then places the patient's wrist in extension with ulnar deviation and then applies pressure as the wrist is flexed and radially deviated repeatedly. A scapholunate dislocation with a rotating subluxating scaphoid produces a noticeable click. However, other injuries such as a perilunate dislocation or a TFCC tear (distal ulna) may cause clicking of the wrist as well.

Radial and ulnar styloid fractures may be characterized by focal tenderness and pain with limited range of motion. Examiners can easily miss them on radiographs. In fact, the presence of an ulnar fracture should prompt reexamination of the radiographs for an associated radial fracture. Patients with persistent pain and soreness over the wrist who do not have a scaphoid or distal radius fracture may develop de Quervain's tendonitis. In the absence of a fracture, it is a tendonitis of the extensor and abductor tendons of the thumb. A positive Finkelstein's test (pain over the anatomic snuffbox with ulnar deviation of the wrist) is characteristic. Treatment includes analgesics, spica splints, cold packs, physical therapy, and steroid injections.

Finally, falls on the ulnar wrist with the hand pronated may result in damage to the ulnar nerve as it passes through Guyon's canal. Although these injuries are not common, they can be disabling. It is important to check for tenderness over

CLINICAL POINTS

- A triangular fibrocartilage complex (TFCC) tear may present with pain and soreness along the distal ulna.
- Pain with torquing (i.e., opening jars or turning keys) is common.
- Patients may present with clicking with wrist movement.
- Triangular fibrocartilage tears may present with pain and soreness along the distal ulna.
- Carpal tunnel symptoms often occur with distal radius fractures.

PATIENT ASSESSMENT

1. Pain, swelling, and tenderness of the wrist
2. Pain-limited range of motion and grip strength

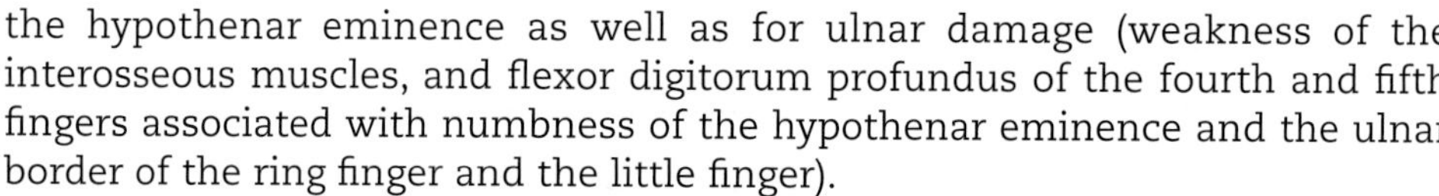

NOT TO BE MISSED

- Scaphoid and other carpal fractures
- Perilunate dislocation
- Hypothenar pain
- Ulnar nerve palsy from damage to Guyon's canal

the hypothenar eminence as well as for ulnar damage (weakness of the interosseous muscles, and flexor digitorum profundus of the fourth and fifth fingers associated with numbness of the hypothenar eminence and the ulnar border of the ring finger and the little finger).

When performing the physical examination, the physician should:

- palpate the distal radius, ulna, scaphoid, and interosseous region for focal tenderness and bony displacement.
- evaluate the ipsilateral elbow and shoulder for associated injuries.
- perform careful neurovascular assessment, paying particular attention to the median nerve. Carpal tunnel symptoms are common with distal radius fractures due to traction during hyperextension or increased compartment pressure secondary to swelling.
- check for clicking (subluxated carpal bone or a TFCC tear).
- check neurovascular status (cold cyanotic limb with diminished or absent pulses)
- check for ganglion cysts.
- check the hypothenar eminence for ulnar nerve injuries (hypothenar numbness with numbness and weakness of the fourth and fifth fingers). Evaluate for hypothenar pain; look for fractures in the hook of the hamate and hamate, as well as pisiform and triquetral fractures.

COLLES AND SMITH FRACTURES

A Colles fracture is the most common form of distal radius fracture, accounting for 90% of distal radius fractures. Most of these fractures can be recognized by the marked swelling, pain, and tenderness of the wrist. In addition, the dorsally displaced distal fragment causes a characteristic deformity of the distal forearm, known as the "dinner fork" deformity. Wrist range of motion is pain limited.

A Smith fracture, sometimes known as a reverse Colles fracture, is another type of fracture of the distal radius. This type of injury is typically unstable. It is characterized by volar (ventral) displacement of the distal radius. (In a Colles fracture, the displacement is dorsal.) The volar displacement may be caused by a fall on a flexed wrist.

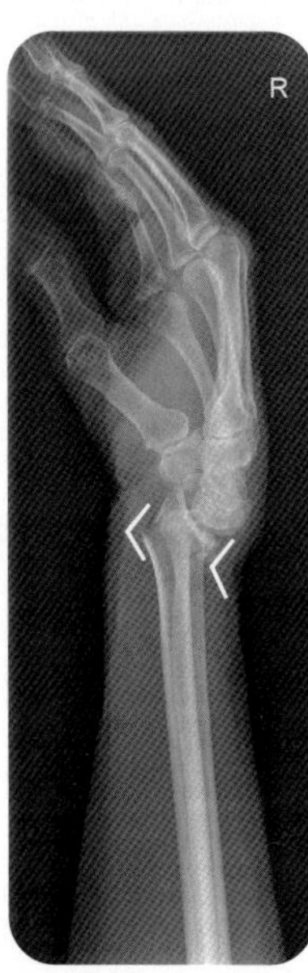

Figure 37.1 Lateral radiograph of the right wrist of the patient in the introductory case, demonstrating acute fracture of the right distal radius and ulnar styloid.

BARTON FRACTURES

Barton fractures, which are uncommon, are fractures involving the volar or palmar rim (articulation) of the distal radius. They occur as the result of the carpal bones shearing against the volar or dorsal lip of the radial articular surface. Although Barton fractures may appear stable, they can be associated with torn carpal ligaments and carpal instability. In addition, radial styloid fractures are often seen in association with these fractures. (Radial styloid fractures are commonly linked with intercarpal ligamentous injuries such as scapholunate dissociation or perilunate dislocation.)

Radiographic Evaluation

It is necessary to obtain posteroanterior (PA) and lateral views (Fig. 37.1) of the wrist, along with oblique views for further fracture definition, if needed. Optional tests include

- traction views, which may be obtained by specialists, to help determine if the fracture is intra-articular;
- contralateral wrist films, which may be obtained by specialists, to compare normal ulnar variance and scapholunate angle;

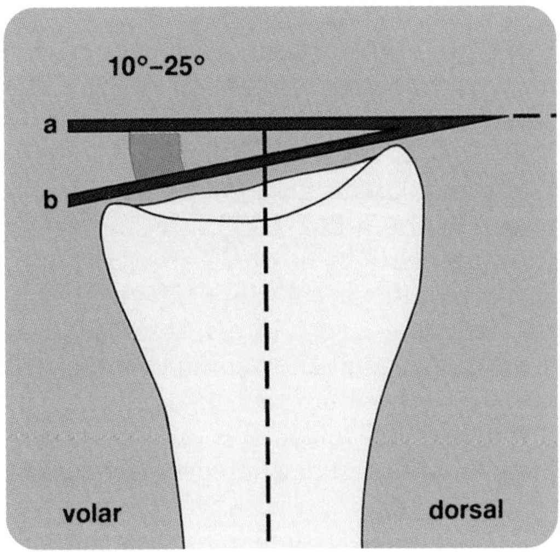

Figure 37.2 Palmar (volar tilt) measured on the lateral radiograph has a normal range from 10 to 25 degrees. Measurements outside of this range may be seen with anatomic abnormalities or displaced fractures. (From Greenspan A. *Orthopedic Imaging: A Practical Approach*. 4th ed. Philadelphia, PA: Lippincott Williams & Wilkins; 2004.)

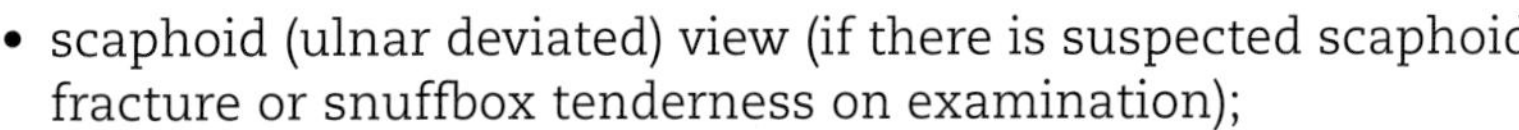

- scaphoid (ulnar deviated) view (if there is suspected scaphoid fracture or snuffbox tenderness on examination);
- computed tomography scan to assess intra-articular involvement in trauma cases that may require surgical intervention; and
- possible magnetic resonance imaging (MRI) or MRI arthrogram to check for Barton fracture, a fracture of the palmar segment of the distal radius. As previously stated, it is important to remember that many radial and ulnar fractures do not appear on routine films, and they may not be visible using MRI. A closed MRI arthrogram or a direct arthroscopic examination may be necessary.

Normally, distal radial fractures have the following radiographic characteristics:

- Radial inclination of 15 to 25 degrees: this is measured on the PA view as the angle formed by constructing a line across the distal radial articular surface and a second line across the width of the distal radius (omitting the radial styloid). The second line is constructed perpendicular to the long axis (i.e., shaft) of the radius. The two lines intersect to form an angle near the distal radial ulnar region.
- Radial height of 11 mm: measured on the PA view as the distance between two lines. Some observers prefer to draw two parallel lines that are perpendicular to the long axis of the radial shaft. The distal line is constructed across the width of the distal radial ulnar joint (DRUJ) at the radial styloid. The proximal line is constructed across the width of the DRUJ across the articular surface of the distal radius (just proximal to the scaphoid and lunate articulations), omitting the radial styloid. A decreased radial height may be seen with impaction injuries.

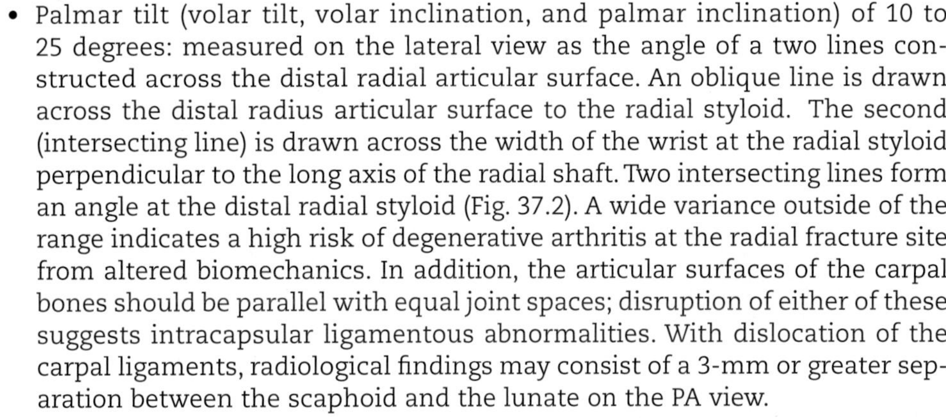

- Palmar tilt (volar tilt, volar inclination, and palmar inclination) of 10 to 25 degrees: measured on the lateral view as the angle of a two lines constructed across the distal radial articular surface. An oblique line is drawn across the distal radius articular surface to the radial styloid. The second (intersecting line) is drawn across the width of the wrist at the radial styloid perpendicular to the long axis of the radial shaft. Two intersecting lines form an angle at the distal radial styloid (Fig. 37.2). A wide variance outside of the range indicates a high risk of degenerative arthritis at the radial fracture site from altered biomechanics. In addition, the articular surfaces of the carpal bones should be parallel with equal joint spaces; disruption of either of these suggests intracapsular ligamentous abnormalities. With dislocation of the carpal ligaments, radiological findings may consist of a 3-mm or greater separation between the scaphoid and the lunate on the PA view.

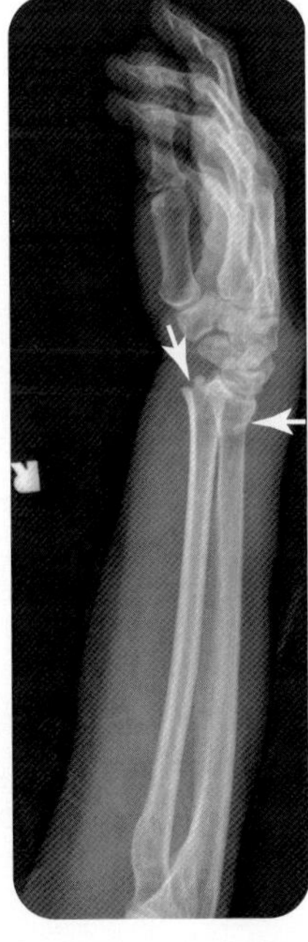

Figure 37.3 Radiograph from a 74-year-old woman who fell and sustained a Colles fracture of her right wrist.

In Colles fractures, dorsal angulation, dorsal displacement, radial shortening, and radial shift are evident (Fig. 37.3). In Smith fractures, the volar displacement of the distal radius is best appreciated on the lateral view. In Barton fractures, it is important to note that even slight displacement of the radial styloid (as little as 3 mm) may be associated with a scapholunate dislocation. In addition, look for evidence of buckling or carpal displacement on the lateral view or gaps (>3 mm) between the carpal bones on the PA view. These clues may indicate associated carpal instability. Finally, it is easy to miss intra-articular fractures of the radius. Innocent-appearing fractures with slight (1 mm) displacement of the articular surface may require operative intervention. In addition, intra-articular radial fractures have a high rate of posttraumatic osteoarthritis.

Treatment

Initially, close reduction is appropriate for all fractures of the distal radius. The reduction maneuver depends on the fracture pattern seen on radiographs. In general, the surgeon should recreate the original deforming forces (i.e., hyperextending the distal fragment in a dorsally angulated fracture). The application of longitudinal traction should then restore the radial height. A sugar-tong splint is necessary, with the wrist in neutral or slight flexion. Patients should avoid extreme wrist flexion, because it can lead to carpal tunnel syndrome.

Research has shown that fractures with 1 to 2 mm of displacement can lead to degenerative osteoarthritis. In addition, radial shortening or increased dorsal tilt of the hand on the wrist can alter the amount of axial load that is distributed through the ulnar shaft. If fractures are left in this amount of displacement without surgical intervention, patients can develop decreased wrist motion, decreased grip strength, and carpal subluxation with wrist instability. The goals of treatment, therefore, are to restore the articular surface through anatomic reduction and allow early motion and rehabilitation.

Some risk factors for secondary instability after initial reduction have been shown to include dorsal tilt greater than 2 degrees, significant comminution, intra-articular involvement, associated ulnar fractures, and age older than 60 years. With nonsurgical management, follow-up with weekly radiographs and shifting from a splint to a cast after 1 to 2 weeks is necessary.

WHEN TO REFER

- Patients with the following injuries require referral:
  - Open fractures
  - Displaced fractures
  - Fractures with neurovascular impairment
  - Fractures that involve the joint surface
  - Perilunate and displaced dislocations
- Patients with fractures that involve suspected TFCC/carpal tears merit further evaluation and referral.
- Uncomplicated nondisplaced fractures may be referred at the examiner's discretion and are dependent on the primary care physician's experience with fracture management

Suggested Readings

American College of Emergency Physicians, Tintinalli J, eds. *Emergency Medicine*. 6th ed. New York, NY: McGraw-Hill; 2004:1682–1687.

Bozentka DJ, Beredjiklian PK, Westawski D, Steinberg DR. Digital radiographs in the assessment of distal radius fracture parameters. *Clin Orthop Relat Res CORR*. 2002;397:409–413.

Cooney WP. Fractures of the distal radius. *Orthop Clin North Am*. 1993;24(2):211–216.

Eiff MP, Hatch RL, Calmbach WL. *Fracture Management for Primary Care*. 2nd ed. Philadelphia, PA: Saunders; 2003:116–122.

Greenspan A. *Orthopedic Imaging*. 4th ed. Philadelphia, PA: Lippincott Williams & Wilkins; 2004:170–174.

Harris J, Harris W, Noveline R. *The Radiology of Emergency Medicine*. 3rd ed. Baltimore, MD: Williams & Wilkins; 1993:385–407.

Simic PM, Weiland AJ. Fractures of the distal aspect of the radius: changes in treatment over the past two decades. *J Bone Joint Surg JBJS Am*. 2003;85:552–564.

Trumble TE, Culp R, Hanel DP, Geisselr WB. The American Academy of Orthopaedic Surgeons—Intra-articular fractures of the distal aspect of the radius. *J Bone Joint Surg JBJS* 1998;80:582–600.

Wulf CA, Ackerman DB, Rizzo M. Contemporary evaluation and treatment of distal radius fractures. *Hand Clin*. 2007;23(2):209–226.

CHAPTER 38

Scaphoid Fractures

George M. Bridgeforth, Thomas Hearty, and Charles Carroll IV

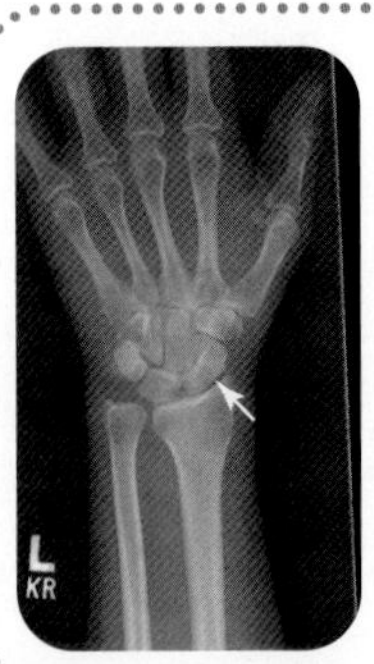

A 40-year-old man injured himself in a moped accident, where he fell onto his outstretched hand. He now presents with pain and swelling of the wrist.

Clinical Presentation

As stated in the previous chapter, scaphoid fractures are the second most common fracture to the distal forearm/wrist (behind radial fractures). Fractures of the carpal bones account for approximately 6% of all fractures, and the scaphoid is the carpal bone fractured most often. Scaphoid fractures are most likely to occur in men who are 20 to 30 years of age. Like Colles fractures, scaphoid (navicular) fractures are usually caused by a fall onto an outstretched hand with the wrist in hyperextension, but they can result in other ways.

Pain, swelling, and tenderness (as well as bruising when present) are characteristic signs that point the examiner to the fracture. The combination of snuffbox tenderness, scaphoid tubercle tenderness, and pain with axial compression is 100% sensitive for a scaphoid fracture.

Note that patients with both Colles fractures and scaphoid fractures may present with pain with limited range of motion. However, in the case of scaphoid fractures, the pain-limited range of motion may be out of proportion to the injury unless the examiner specifically palpates for scaphoid tenderness at the anatomic snuffbox and proximal radial surface of the wrist. It is also necessary to check neurovascular status (cold cyanotic fingers, diminished or absent pulses, delayed capillary refill of over 4 seconds in fingertips) carefully. In addition, another key clinical clue helps differentiate a scaphoid fracture from a Colles fracture. Patients with Colles fractures usually have a characteristic dorsal deformity of the distal segment of the radius, whereas patients with scaphoid fractures do not.

Other injuries can mimic a scaphoid fracture. It is always important to check the distal radius for a small radial styloid fracture or a nondisplaced distal radial fracture (which appears as a small dark line which extends to the cortex) (see section, "Radiographic Evaluation"). Patients who complain of constant clicking with wrist movement may have a subluxating scaphoid or lunate. Those with persistent pain and soreness of the anatomic snuffbox (in the absence of a fracture/dislocation) should be evaluated and treated for de Quervain's tendonitis. This is a tendonitis affecting the extensor and abductor tendons of the thumb. De Quervain's tendonitis may be seen with overuse injuries or following acute trauma.

CLINICAL POINTS

- Injury often involves a fall onto an outstretched hand.
- The scaphoid bone is located on the thumb side of the wrist.
- Untreated scaphoid fractures may lead to instability, premature degenerative arthritis, and necrosis of the proximal scaphoid.

PATIENT ASSESSMENT

1. Pain and swelling of the wrist
2. Tenderness of the scaphoid
    - Anatomic snuffbox (inaccurate finding if in isolation)
    - Scaphoid tubercle
3. Pain with axial compression
4. Pain-limited range of motion

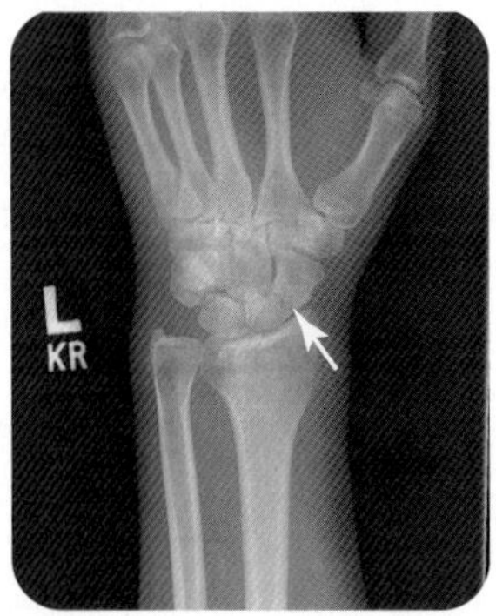

Figure 38.1 An oblique radiograph of the left hand of the patient in the introductory case demonstrating an acute fracture through the scaphoid.

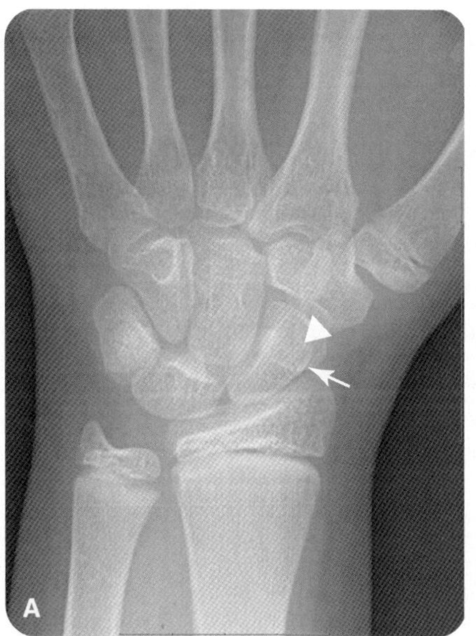

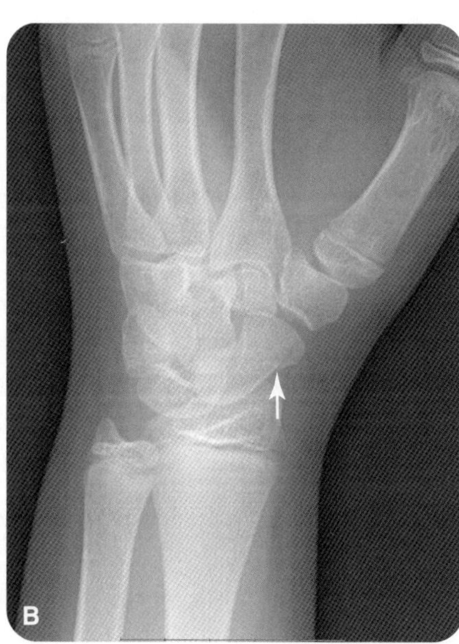

Figure 38.2 **(A)** An AP radiograph of the left wrist demonstrates a subtle overhanging edge (*arrow*) and dense overlapping fracture line (*arrowhead*) along the ulnar aspect of the scaphoid. **(B)** An oblique radiograph of the same patient, which better demonstrates the acute scaphoid fracture without distraction (*arrow*).

Radiographic Evaluation

In patients who present with acute swelling, pain, focal tenderness with limited range of motion, radiographs should be strongly considered. It is necessary to obtain a posteroanterior (PA) view of the wrist with the hand in a fist; a lateral view of the wrist, to look primarily on for perilunate dislocation; and oblique views (Fig. 38.1), including a radial oblique view (a supinated PA view of the wrist) and an ulnar oblique view (a pronated PA view of the wrist). It is optional to check the contralateral wrist for comparison and to view the scaphoid with a PA view with ulnar deviation (Fig. 38.2). Other imaging involves:

- Magnetic resonance imaging (MRI) scan: most sensitive and specific for occult fractures
- MRI arthrogram: suspected carpal ligament tears
- Computed tomography (CT) scan: good for characterization of fracture but poor at diagnosing occult fractures (Fig. 38.3).

Nondisplaced fractures of the scaphoid appear as dark lines that usually extend to the cortex. In the introductory case, the fracture is identifiable on both the PA view and the scaphoid (ulnar-deviated) view. However, it is easy to miss scaphoid fractures, and it is not uncommon for scaphoid fractures to appear on the scaphoid view only. Approximately 30% of all scaphoid fractures may not present acutely on standard radiographs; these are termed occult fractures. The majority of scaphoid fractures, 80%, occur at the waist (the narrowed middle third) of the scaphoid.

Scapholunate dislocations, which may accompany fractures, exhibit a 3-mm or greater separation between the scaphoid and the lunate (positive Terry Thomas [British comedian] or David Letterman sign). If the examiner does not look specifically for this gap, he or she may miss it.

Unrecognized scaphoid fractures may develop nonunion. Over time, these injuries may lead to carpal instability and premature degenerative arthritis of the wrist. The retrograde blood supply of the scaphoid makes it susceptible to avascular necrosis after fractures, particularly if they are displaced. Revascularization

NOT TO BE MISSED

- Other fractures of carpals, distal radius, and/or ulna
- Perilunate dislocation
- Wrist sprain or contusion
- Scaphoid avascular necrosis
- De Quervain's tendonitis
- Degenerative arthritis of the carpometacarpal joint
- Kienböck's disease (osteonecrosis of the lunate)
- Rheumatoid arthritis
- Gout

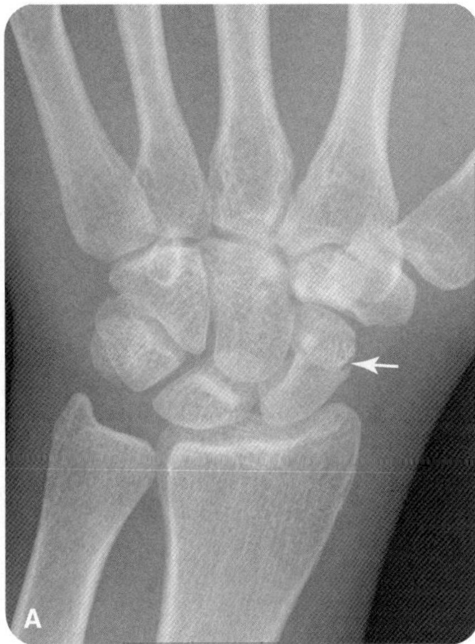

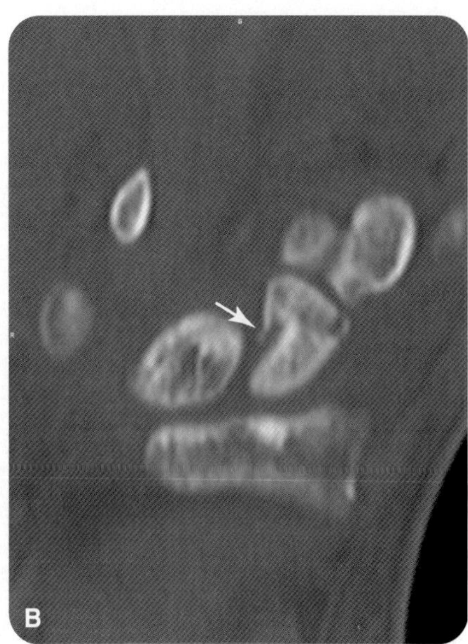

Figure 38.3 **(A)** AP radiograph of the right wrist demonstrates an acute scaphoid fracture (*arrow*). **(B)** Coronal CT image performed 4 months later demonstrates the scaphoid fracture with better detail regarding the degree of impaction (*arrow*)

occurs with healing: 100% of distal fractures, whereas 80% to 90% of waist fractures heal and only 60% to 70% of proximal fractures heal.

Preexisting avascular necrosis is characterized by a small, sclerotic, pellet-like appearance of the proximal fractured scaphoid segment. As the proximal fracture scaphoid bone becomes necrotic, it implodes over time and adopts a pellet-like appearance. However, the bony necrosis leads to carpal instability and premature arthritis.

WHEN TO REFER 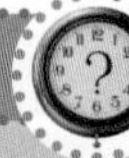

- Immediate referral: open fractures, displaced fractures, or fractures with neurovascular compromise
- Prompt referral: nondisplaced scaphoid fractures
- Other indications
  - Persistent pain in wrist after immobilization despite no evidence of fracture. (A negative MRI or MRI arthrogram may not completely rule out torn carpal ligaments.)
  - Subluxating scaphoid or lunate (hand specialist)

Treatment

The physician should assume that snuffbox and scaphoid tubercle pain and tenderness without radiologic evidence of fracture may indicate an occult scaphoid fracture or a De Quervain's tendonitis. Analgesics and treatment with a thumb spica cast for 10 to 14 days are warranted. After this time, it is necessary to remove the cast and repeat the radiographs. If the symptoms persist and the radiographs are still negative, the physician should strongly consider an MRI, with referral to a specialist. The cast should be reapplied.

Nondisplaced scaphoid fractures require treatment with a spica cast and proper radiological follow-up. If there is any doubt regarding displacement of a fracture, a CT scan is necessary. A short arm spica cast should be sufficient, and some specialists have shown that a forearm cast without thumb immobilization is adequate. This requires at least 4 to 6 weeks of immobilization.

It is essential to immobilize any displaced scaphoid fracture in a long arm thumb spica splint. This injury will likely require surgical intervention.

Suggested Readings

Alho A, Kankaanpaa U. Management of fracture scaphoid bone: a prospective study of 100 fractures. *Acta Orthop Scand*. 1975;46:737–743.

Barton NJ. Twenty questions about scaphoid fracture. *J Hand Surg*. 1992;17-B:289–310.

Boles C. Wrist, Scaphoid Fractures and Complications. www.medscape.com. Accessed July, 2009.

Brydie A, Raby N. Early MRI in the management of clinical scaphoid fracture. *Br J Radiol*. 2003;76:296–300.

Burroughs KE, Eiff P, Grayzel J. Overview of Carpal Fractures. Up to Date. Query: uptodate.com. Accessed July 14, 2009.

Clay NR, Dias JJ, Costigan PS, et al. Need the thumb be immobilized in scaphoid fractures? A randomized prospective trial. *JBJS*. 1991;73B:828–832

Forman TA, Forman SK, Rose NE. A clinical approach to diagnosing wrist pain. *Am Fam Physician*. 2005;72(9):1753–1758.

Gaebler C. Fractures and dislocations of the carpus. In: Bucholz RW, Heckman JD, Court-Brown C, eds. *Rockwood and Green's Fractures in Adults*. Philadelphia, PA: Lippincott-Raven, 2006:857–908.

Gaebler CH, Kukla CH, Breitenseher MJ, et al. Diagnosis of occult scaphoid fractures and other wrist injuries: are repeated clinical examinations and plain radiographs still state of the art. *Langenbeck's Arch Surg*. 2001;386:150–154.

Gaebler C, Kukla C, Breitenseher M, et al. Magnetic resonance imaging of occult scaphoid fractures. *J Trauma*. 1996;41:73–76.

Goldfarb CA, Yin Y, Gilula LA, Fisher AJ. Wrist fractures: what the clinician wants to know. *Radiology*. 2001;219:11–28.

Greenspan A. *Orthopedic Imaging*. 4th ed. Philadelphia, PA: Lippincott Williams & Wilkins; 2004:188–189.

Haims AH, Schweitzer ME, Morrison WB, Deely D. Limitations of MR imaging in the diagnosis of peripheral tears of the triangular fibrocartilage of the wrist. *AJR*. 2002;178:419–422.

Hobby JL, Dixon AK, Bearcroft WP, Tom BDM. MR imaging of the wrist: effect on clinical diagnosis and patient care. *Radiology*. 2001;220:589–593.

Mann FA, Wilson AJ, Gilula L. Radiographic evaluation of the wrist: what does the hand surgeon want to know? *Radiology*. 1992;184:15–24.

Mazet R, Hohl M. Fractures of the carpal a navicular: an analysis of ninety-one cases and review of the literature. *JBJS*. 1963;45:82–112.

Parvizi J, Wayman J, Kelly P, et al. Combining the clinical signs improves diagnosis of scaphoid fractures. A prospective study with follow up. *J Hand Surg*. 1998;23–B:324–327.

Phillips TG, Reibach AM, Slomiany P. Diagnosis and management of scaphoid fractures. *Am Fam Physician* 2004;70:879–884.

Ring D, Jupiter JB, Herndon JH. Acute fractures of the scaphoid. *J Am Acad Orthop Surg*. 2000;8(4):225–231.

Zanetti M, Linkous D, Giula LA, Hodler J. Characteristics of triangular fibrocartilage defects in symptomatic and contralateral asymptomatic wrists. *Radiology*. 2000;216:840–845.

CHAPTER 39

Scapholunate Dissociation

George M. Bridgeforth, Thomas Hearty, and Charles Carroll IV

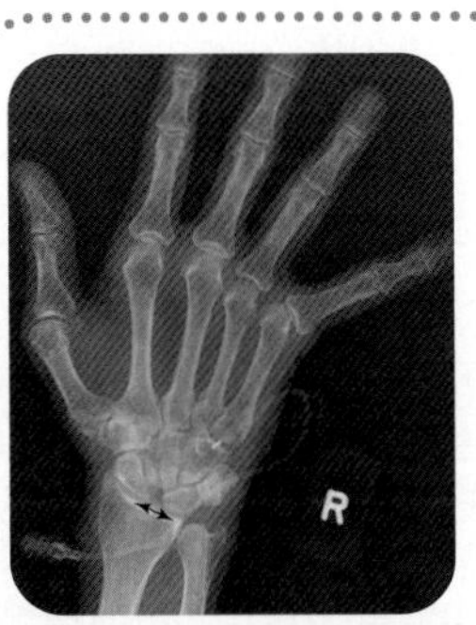

A 81-year-old woman fell down 20 steps. She complains of marked pain and soreness with an inability to move her wrist.

Clinical Presentation

The scapholunate joint is essential to carpal function. A scapholunate dissociation (SLD), which progresses through several stages, finally ends as a perilunate dislocation. The injury can be completely ligamentous or can be a combined fracture and ligamentous injury. SLD is one of the most common types of carpal instability. Often overlooked, it may lead to weakness and arthritis. Associated with torsion injuries to the wrist with an axial load, SLD is usually caused from a fall on an outstretched hand with the wrist extended, ulnarly deviated, and the forearm pronated.

Patients may exhibit pain and swelling over the proximal carpus near the center of the wrist. Limited range of motion occurs. Clicking from a rotation scaphoid or lunate may be present. To test for wrist stability, the examiner performs a Watson test (scaphoid shift test). The examiner stabilizes the wrist with both hands and places his or her thumb over the volar aspect (palm side) of the scaphoid. While holding the wrist in ulnar deviation and moving it radially, the flexing scaphoid subluxes dorsally, causing a reproducible "click." There may be a painful "clunk" as the scaphoid reduces back into the radial scaphoid fossa when the thumb pressure is removed. A recurrent click is diagnostic of carpal subluxation. The physician should also check neurovascular status carefully (cold cyanotic fingers with absent or diminished pulses and delayed capillary refill greater than 4 seconds in fingertips).

The differential diagnosis includes the following: wrist contusion, radial styloid fracture, scaphoid fracture, scapholunate dislocation, ulnar fracture, triangular fibrocartilage complex (TFCC) tear, perilunate dislocation, and gonococcal septic arthritis, as well as rheumatological conditions and other carpal fractures. It should be noted that SLD is associated with distal radial fractures in more than 50% of cases. Patients with marked pain and swelling of the proximal carpus who do not have any radiological evidence of a distal forearm or wrist fracture may have a TFCC tear. The TFCC, which attaches the ulnar border of the distal radius to the ulna, consists of the radioulnar ligaments, the articular disc, ulnar collateral ligament, the extensor carpi ulnaris tendon, and the meniscus homolog. These structures help stabilize the distal radius and ulna with the neighboring carpals. The mechanism of injury is similar to that of scapholunate dislocations (torsion injuries and falls), and TFCC tears can be misdiagnosed as a more common wrist contusion.

CLINICAL PRESENTATION

- Patients may complain of a tear or a "pop."
- Long-standing cases may present with deformity and/or degenerative arthritis due to carpal instability.
- Clicking may be present with recurrent subluxation during motion.

PATIENT ASSESSMENT

1. Pain, swelling, and soreness over the scaphoid lunate area
2. Pain-limited range of motion
3. Increased pain with resisted torsion (supination and pronation)
4. Possible obvious deformity at the wrist, if there is a perilunate dislocation
5. Median nerve dysfunction associated with carpal dislocation

With a TFCC tear, patients can complain of pain, swelling, and tenderness over the distal ulna and proximal wrist. Painful, limited range of motion, especially with torsion (pronation and supination), and particularly with ulnar deviation, may be present. A positive press test—marked wrist pain when the patient tries to use the affected wrist to lift himself or herself up from an examination table or chair—may indicate a TFCC tear. In addition, fractures of the distal ulna, ulnar styloid, or distal radius are associated with TFCC tears.

Radiographic Evaluation

In patients who present with acute swelling, pain, focal tenderness, and limited range of motion, the physician should strongly consider the use of radiographs. It is necessary to take posteroanterior (PA) views with a clenched fist for provocation. Lateral views may also be required. Optional radiographs include a:

- scaphoid view (ulnar deviation): to rule out scaphoid fracture,
- PA with traction, and
- contralateral wrist for comparison.

In addition, a magnetic resonance imaging (MRI) scan or an MRI arthrogram for evaluation of ligament disruption may be helpful.

For an SLD, the primary radiographic finding is a 3-mm or greater separation between the scaphoid and the lunate on the PA view. This gap is indicative of a SLD secondary to a torn carpal ligament. It is known as the "Terry Thomas sign," after the British comedian who had a small gap in his front teeth, and it has also been called the David Letterman sign for similar reasons. Any separation between the carpal bones that is 3 mm or greater is suspicious for a carpal dissociation, and a gap larger than 5 mm is diagnostic (Figs. 39.1 and 39.2). It is important to check a contralateral radiograph to rule out an anatomic variant, and a clenched fist PA view may create the separation not seen on a standard PA view.

NOT TO BE MISSED

- Scaphoid fractures
- Radial styloid fractures
- Other wrist/carpal fractures
- Wrist sprain/contusions
- Perilunate dislocation
- De Quervain's tendonitis
- Ganglion cyst
- Degenerative arthritis of the carpometacarpal joint
- Kienböck's disease (osteonecrosis of the lunate)
- Rheumatoid arthritis
- Gout

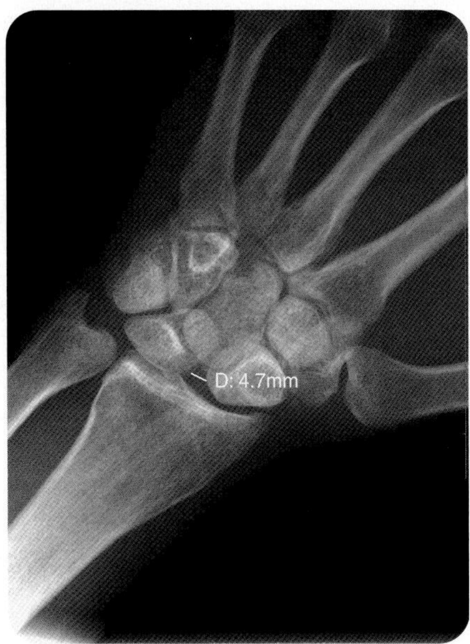

Figure 39.1 AP view of the left wrist in a 20-year-old man with left wrist pain after a fall demonstrates widening of the scapholunate space by approximately 5 mm suspicious for scapholunate dissociation.

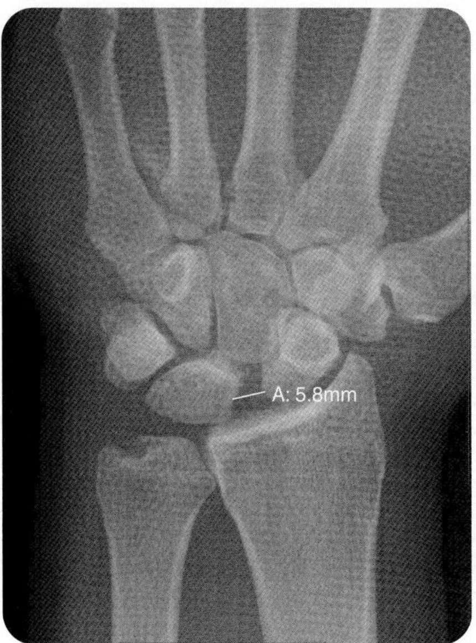

Figure 39.2 AP view of a casted left wrist after reduction of a lunate dislocation demonstrates widening of the scapholunate space by approximately 6 mm.

On the lateral view, scaphoid flexion is suspicious of a SLD. This rotational displacement of the scaphoid is indicative of a torn scapholunate ligament. Normally, on the lateral view, the long axis of the scaphoid should lie at an angle of 30 to 60 degrees to the long axis formed by the radius, lunate, and the capitate. Sometimes, the rotation of the scaphoid may result in a rounded sclerotic density, which is the proximal head of the scaphoid rotating rostrally (i.e., flipped upward). This may appear on the PA films as a rounded sclerotic ring–like structure; this rounded density is known as a "signet ring sign." The rotated head of the scaphoid resembles the imprint from a signet ring. Although signet ring signs are uncommon, their presence is pathognomonic for a scaphoid lunate disruption.

Scapholunate subluxations and TFCC tears are misdiagnosed as wrist contusions. Patients complain of increased pain with physical therapy. Radiological findings may be absent, but the injury should be suspected in patients with displaced ulnar styloid fractures or fractures of the ulnar styloid base. An MRI may be helpful, but there is some evidence that it offers a limited evaluation of lesions affecting the extensor ulna region. An MRI arthrogram or direct arthroscopic evaluation may be more helpful.

For perilunate dislocations, arcuate lines of the wrist should be examined on the PA view. This association is covered in the chapter on lunate dislocations. Briefly, the first arcuate line is constructed along the proximal concave borders of the first carpal row (i.e., the proximal scaphoid, lunate, and triquetrum). The second arcuate line is constructed along the concave-shaped distal borders of the same structures. The third arcuate line is constructed along the proximal concave borders of the capitate and the hamate. On a PA view, three curved arcs maintain a parallel relationship. Any disruptions in a single arc or in the parallel relationship among the three arcs are indicative of a displaced carpal fracture or dislocation secondary to ruptured carpal ligaments and/or fracture. It is critically important to always examine the relationship among these three arcs very carefully. With perilunate dislocations, the normal appearing quadrangular bone may appear triangular in shape on the PA view.

However, it should be noted that with a TFCC tear, radiographs do not show a gap between the scaphoid and the lunate. TFCC tears may be misdiagnosed as wrist sprains. In addition, patients with TFCC tears may feel a "pop" or a "tear" at the time of the initial injury and present with recurrent clicking inside the wrist. TFCC tears may be confirmed with an MRI arthrogram or direct arthrosopic examination by a specialist.

Treatment

WHEN TO REFER

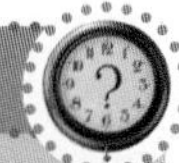

- Immediate referral: open wrist fractures or fractures with neurovascular impairment, compartment syndromes, and perilunate dislocations
- Prompt referral
  - Uncomplicated SLDs (for arthroscopic evaluation)
  - Suspected TFCC tears

Treatment practices may vary according to the experience of the treating specialist. Less severe cases of SLD may warrant nonsurgical therapy consisting of splinting, rest, pain control, and therapy for several weeks. More severe cases of SLD may require a closed (nonsurgical) reduction with percutaneous pinning or an open reduction (surgical) and internal fixation of fractures and/or ligament reconstruction. Most TFCC tears respond to conservative care (splinting and analgesic medication) for several weeks. Patients should be advised to avoid any heavy lifting with the affected extremity.

For patients who fail to respond to conservative treatment, surgery may be considered. Patients who are surgical candidates should discontinue nonsteroidal anti-inflammatory drugs (NSAIDs) for at least 10 days prior to surgical care. NSAIDs may cause bleeding at the surgical site. Patients who cannot tolerate NSAIDs may be treated with other analgesics.

Suggested Readings

Cassidy C, Ruby LK. Carpal Instability. *Instr Course Lect.* 2003;52:209–220.

Daniels JM, Zook EG, Lynch JM. Hand and wrist injuries: Part I. Nonemergent evaluation. *Am Fam Physician.* 2004;69:1941–1949.

Daniels JM, Zook EG, Lynch JM. Hand and wrist injuries: Part II. Emergent evaluation. *Am Fam Physician.* 2004;69:1949–1956.

Goldfarb CA, Yuming Y, Gilula LA, et al. Wrist fractures: what the clinician wants to know. *Radiology.* 2001;219:11–28.

Green DP, Hotchkiss RN, Pederson WC, Wolfe SW, eds. *Green's operative Hand Surgery*. 5th ed. Philadelphia, PA: Churchill Livingston; 2005:557

Green DP, O'Brien ET. Classification and management of carpal dislocations. *Clin Orthop Relat Res.* 1980;149:55–72.

Hobby JL, Dixon AK, Bearcroft WP, et al. MR imaging of the wrist: effect on clinical diagnosis and patient care. *Radiology*. 2001;220:589–593.

Mayfield JK, Kilcoyne RK, Johnson RP. Carpal dislocations: pathomechanics and progressive perilunate instability. *J Hand Surg.* 1980;5:226–241.

Morawa LG, Ross PM, Schock CC. Fractures and dislocations involving the navicular–lunate axis. *Clin Orthop Relat Res.* 1976:118:48–53.

Murray P. Dislocations of the wrist: carpal instability complex. *J Hand Surg.* 2003;3:88–99.

Panting AL, Lamb DW, Noble J, Haw CS. Dislocations of the lunate with and without fractures of the scaphoid. *J Bone Joint Surg JBJS.* 1984;66(3):391–395.

Prosser AJ, Brenkel IJ, Irvine GB. Articular fractures of the distal scaphoid. *J Hand Surg.* 1998;19B:87–91.

Side D, Laorr A, Greenspan A. Carpal scaphoid: radiographic pattern of dislocation. *Radiology.* 1995;195(1): 215–216.

CHAPTER 40

Avascular Necrosis (Scaphoid)

George M. Bridgeforth, Thomas Hearty, and Charles Carroll IV

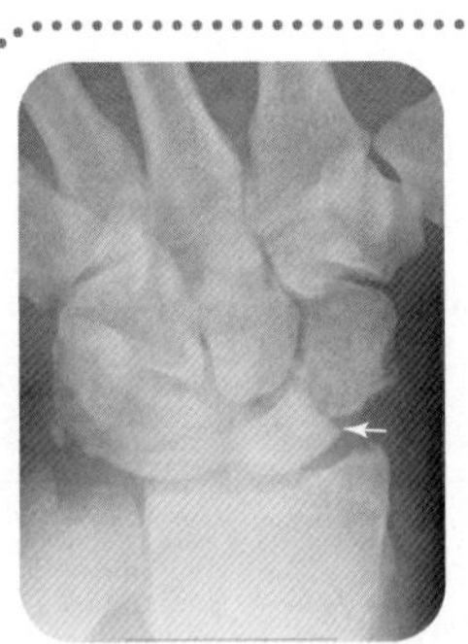

A 42-year-old man presents with left wrist pain after an injury that occurred 4 months ago.

CLINICAL POINTS

- A poor blood supply may be associated with a higher risk of AVN.
- Lack of blood to the scaphoid may lead to arthritis.
- Many patients with long-standing degenerative arthritis of the wrist may have had chronic instability from a preexisting wrist injury (i.e., unstable fracture or ligament tear) several years earlier.

Clinical Presentation

Avascular necrosis (AVN) is the death of bone tissue due to a lack of blood. There may be poor retrograde blood flow from the distal to the proximal scaphoid. This can result in tiny breaks in the bone and the bone's eventual collapse.

The scaphoid is the most frequently fractured wrist bone (see Chapter 38, "Scaphoid Fractures"), and AVN is the most common complication of a scaphoid fracture, occurring in 15% to 30% of cases. Trauma leading to displaced scaphoid fractures is the most likely cause of AVN. Much less common is an idiopathic osteonecrosis of the scaphoid. The risk of AVN depends on the location of the fracture. The proximal one-third has the highest incidence of AVN. The middle one-third, the most frequent fracture site, is associated with a moderate risk of AVN, and fracture in the distal one-third rarely leads to AVN. The proximal segment is most susceptible to damage because of the retrograde vascular supply, making the proximal vascularity the most tenuous. Acute AVN is more likely to follow a displaced scaphoid fracture greater than 1 mm, usually at the middle (waist), or an acute fracture involving the proximal pole. In addition, a poor blood supply, as occurs in diseases such as diabetes, may increase the risk.

Long-standing cases of AVN of the scaphoid may result in a degenerative arthritis of the wrist; this complication is caused by longstanding carpal instability. Patients present with unilateral involvement and complaints of joint pain; stiffness, with decreased range of motion; pain with activities such as lifting or gripping; and hypertrophy. Other carpal fractures or dislocations may also cause long-term instability and a degenerative arthritis.

Other conditions may cause arthritis of the wrist. The presence of bilateral acute wrist pain or recurrent wrist pain is more likely secondary to a rheumatoid arthritis. Flare-ups consist of signs of recurrent acute inflammation, including pain, redness, swelling, tenderness, and warmth. Rheumatoid arthritis usually has a bilateral distribution, and other joints such as the knee, metacarpals, and proximal interphalangeal joints may be affected.

Gout may present as an oligoarthropathy affecting the wrist. Most patients have signs of acute inflammation characterized by marked acute swelling, redness, warmth, and tenderness. Moreover, a prior history of gouty attacks, which usually affect the great toe, knee, or ankle, may indicate this diagnosis.

PATIENT ASSESSMENT

1. Pain, swelling, and tenderness over the scaphoid at the anatomic snuffbox
2. Pain-limited range of motion
3. Possible clicking with recurrent subluxation during motion

Psoriasis may also lead to an oligoarthritis that affects the wrist. Patients usually have clinical manifestations of psoriasis—salmon-colored plaques with silver reticuli over the knees, elbows, lower back, and gluteal regions. In addition, there may be pitting of the nails (very small groups of indentations) as well.

To evaluate for AVN of the scaphoid, the clinician should palpate the scaphoid; the oblong-shaped scaphoid makes up the floor of the anatomical snuffbox. It is also important to determine whether clicking instability of the scaphoid is present (positive Watson shift test; see Chapter 39, "Scapholunate Dissociation" for details). Finally, it is necessary to check for neurovascular compromise (cold cyanotic fingers with diminished or absent pulses and delayed capillary refill).

Radiographic Evaluation

It is necessary to order various radiograph, including posteroanterior (PA), lateral, scaphoid (PA with ulnar deviation), and oblique (45–60 degrees of pronation from PA) views (Fig. 40.1). Optional radiographs include

- views of the contralateral wrist for comparison and
- PA view with clenched fist to check carpal separation from torn ligaments

Other tests that may be necessary are

- magnetic resonance imaging (MRI) scan: used prior to any surgery for scaphoid nonunion to differentiate AVN from nonunion,
- MRI arthrogram: used to examine for torn carpal ligaments, and
- computed tomography scan: can aid in surgical planning and characterization of osseous structure and nonunion.

The examiner should look for a fracture of the scaphoid, primarily in the neck where 80% of fractures occur. As previously stated, patient with proximal fractures have the highest risk of AVN. Early AVN may be characterized by a poorly defined diminishing proximal segment; therefore, it may not

NOT TO BE MISSED

- Wrist contusions sprains
- Distal radial/ulnar fractures
- Scaphoid (other carpal) fractures
- Perilunate dislocations
- De Quervain's tendonitis
- Degenerative arthritis of the carpometacarpal joint
- Kienböck's disease (osteonecrosis of the lunate)
- Rheumatoid arthritis
- Gout

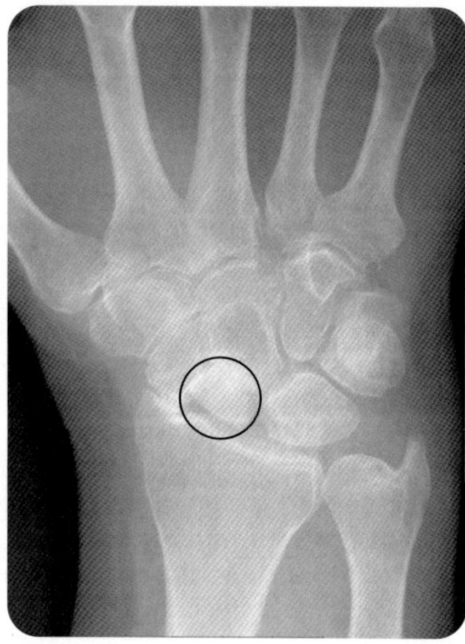

Figure 40.1 Chronic scaphoid waist fracture with sclerosis of the proximal fragment compatible with avascular necrosis. There is impaction of the proximal scaphoid into the proximal capitate with sclerosis of the adjacent bone at their articulation.

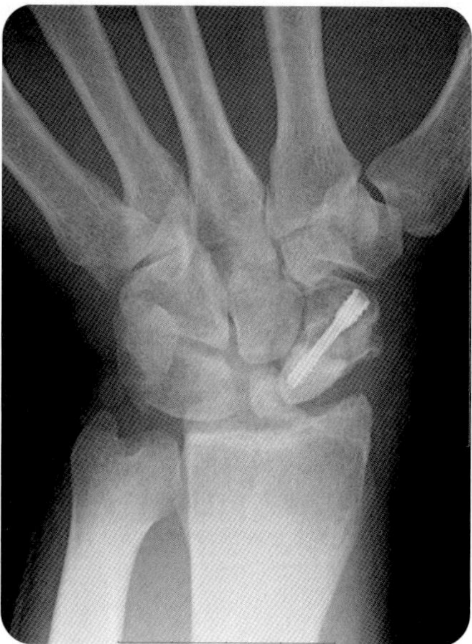

Figure 40.2 AP view of the left wrist of the patient in the introductory case demonstrating surgical pinning of the scaphoid.

WHEN TO REFER

- Early cases of AVN should be seen promptly
- Chronic cases of AVN (underlying carpal instability may lead to arthritis)
- High-risk patients (e.g., those with diabetes) with acute scaphoid fractures

appear on the initial films. Eventually, radiographic features of AVN include collapse and fragmentation. When bone dies, it collapses and implodes. AVN is also characterized by sclerotic and cystic changes. With time, the necrotic bone diminishes in size and becomes more sclerotic; it adapts a dense, pellet-like appearance.

Treatment

The patient should be placed in a spica-type splint and referred to a specialist for a surgical evaluation. Therapy depends on health, age, and extent of use of the upper extremity. In addition, the area and the amount of the scaphoid damage may affect therapeutic decisions. Nonoperative treatment consists of splinting, pain control, and physical therapy. Operative treatment consists of drilling, curettage, allograft replacement, vascularized bone grafting, excision, and/or fusion of the wrist (Fig. 40.2). The patient should not use the affected hand at work until he or she receives clearance from a specialist.

Suggested Readings

Cassidy C, Ruby LK. Carpal instability. *Instr Course Lect*. 2003;52:209–220.

Daniels JM, Zook EG, Lynch JM. Hand and wrist injuries: Part I. Nonemergent evaluation. *Am Fam Physician*. 2004;69:1941–1949.

Daniels JM, Zook EG, Lynch JM. Hand and wrist injuries: Part II. Emergent evaluation. *Am Fam Physician*. 2004;69:1949–1956.

Ferlic DC, Morin P. Idiopathic avascular necrosis of the scaphoid: Preiser's disease. *J Hand Surg Am*. 1989;14:13–16.

Gaebler C. Fractures and dislocations of the carpus. In: Bucholz RW, Heckman JD, Court-Brown C, eds. *Rockwood and Green's Fractures in Adults*. Philadelphia, PA: Lippincott-Raven; 2006:857–908.

Goldfarb CA, Yuming Y, Gilula LA, et al. Wrist fractures: what the clinician wants to know. *Radiology*. 2001; 219:11–28.

Green DP, O'Brien, ET. Classification and management of carpal dislocations. *Clin Orthop Relat Res*. 1980; 149:55–72.

Hobby JL, Dixon AK, Bearcroft WP, et al. MR imaging of the wrist: effect on clinical diagnosis and patient care. *Radiology*. 2001;220:589–593.

Morawa LG, Ross PM, Schock CC. Fractures and dislocations involving the navicular–lunate axis. *Clin Orthop Relat Res*. 1976:118:48–53.

Panting AL, Lamb DW, Noble J, Haw CS. Dislocations of the lunate with and without fractures of the scaphoid. *J Bone Joint Surg JBJS*. 1984;66(3):391–395.

Side D, Laorr A, Greenspan A. Carpal scaphoid: radiographic pattern of dislocation. *Radiology*. 1995;195(1): 215–216.

Trumble TE, Salas P, Barthes T, Robert KQ. Management of scaphoid nonunions. *J Am Acad Orthop Surg*. 2003;11:380–391.

Avascular Necrosis of the Lunate (Kienböck's Disease)

George M. Bridgeforth, Kathryn J. McCarthy, and Charles Carroll IV

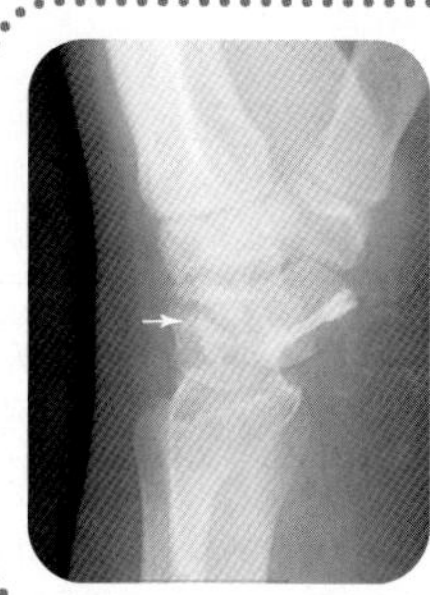

A 33-year-old man complains of persistent wrist pain with limited range of motion. He notes moderate soreness with swelling of the left wrist. He has a history of left wrist injury and scaphoid fracture 10 months ago.

Clinical Presentation

Kienböck's disease is a disorder that involves the fragmentation and collapse of the lunate as a result of vascular insufficiency and avascular necrosis. The disease usually affects men between 20 and 40 years of age. It is more common in patients with negative ulnar variances (the ulna is shorter than the distal radius). It is thought that the short ulna does not provide adequate structural support to the neighboring lunate; however, the exact etiology is not clear. Kienböck's disease is usually unilateral. Bilateral disease is very rare, which indicates that other factors such as the biomechanical stresses on the dominant hand and wrist come into play.

Pain and soreness over the lunate are characteristic of Kienböck's disease. The pain and soreness occur just distal to the radius over a bony area at the center of the wrist (in line with the middle finger). Decreased grip strength in the hand may also be present. Physicians often misdiagnose acute cases as acute wrist sprains or contusions.

Associated findings include pain-limited range of motion. Moreover, patients with instability may complain of recurrent clicking. It is necessary to check neurovascular status carefully (cold cyanotic limb with numbness and diminished or absent pulses).

In Kienböck's disease, the necrotic lunate characterized can lead to joint instability, hypermobility of the surrounding structures, and premature degenerative arthritis. The premature development of the arthritis results from carpal instability. Characteristics of the degenerative arthritis include joint hypertrophy, tenderness, stiffness, and pain-limited range of motion.

It is important to point out that patients who fall on the hypothenar eminence, the ulnar half of the palm, can sustain a fracture to the ulna, the triquetrum, the pisiform, or the hamate. Moreover, in an occupational setting, workers who use tools to strike objects can sustain fractures to the pisiform or the hook of the hamate. Patients often complain of pain, soreness, and swelling along the hypothenar eminence. Associate complaints are swelling and inability to grasp objects. Damage to Guyon's canal (a tunnel formed by the pisiform and the hook of the hamate) may produce ulnar nerve damage. Patients report hypothenar pain and swelling associated with numbness of the hypothenar region, the fourth and the fifth fingers.

CLINICAL POINTS

- Kienböck's disease is characterized by avascular necrosis of the lunate.
- The cause of the disease is not known.
- Degenerative arthritis may develop because of carpal instability.

PATIENT ASSESSMENT

1. Pain, swelling, and tenderness over the lunate
2. Pain-limited range of motion
3. "Clicking" with carpal instability

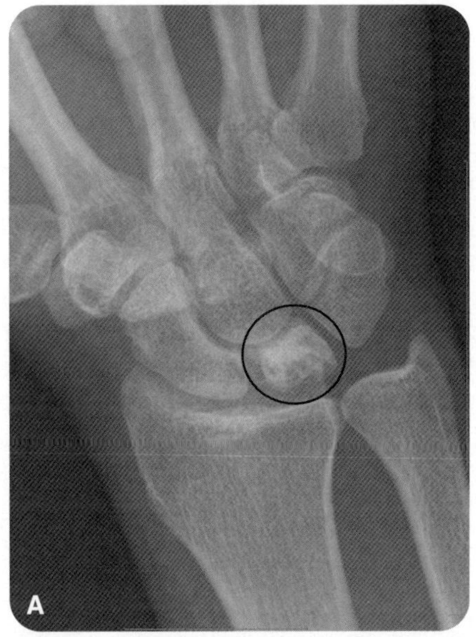

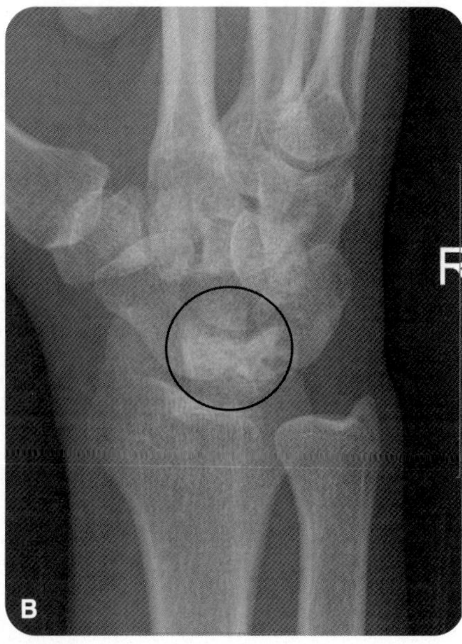

Figure 41.1 (A) AP and (B) oblique views of the right wrist in a 22-year-old man with persistent right wrist pain without history of trauma demonstrates avascular necrosis of the lunate (*circle*).

Radiographic Evaluation

It is necessary to order various radiographs, including posteroanterior (PA), lateral, and oblique views. Kienböck's disease is best appreciated on the PA view (Fig. 41.1).

The avascular necrosis causes a sclerotic collapse of the lunate. Initial radiographs may be normal. With time, the lunate can adopt a rounded dense pellet-like appearance. The examiner should look a poorly defined lunate; chronic cases have a small sclerotic lunate. If the patient complains of nonresolving wrist pain, then computed tomography (CT) or magnetic resonance imaging (MRI) scans may reveal the initial damage to the lunate.

As previously stated, Kienböck's disease is more common in patients with a negative ulnar variance (short ulnas). Ulnar variance is measured by

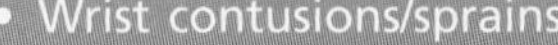

NOT TO BE MISSED

- Wrist contusions/sprains
- Distal radial/ulnar fractures
- Scaphoid (other carpal) fractures
- Scaphoid lunate dislocations
- Perilunate dislocations
- De Quervain's tendonitis
- Triangular fibrocartilage complex tear
- Degenerative arthritis of the carpometacarpal joint
- Rheumatoid arthritis and other rheumatoid diseases
- Gonococcal arthritis
- Gout

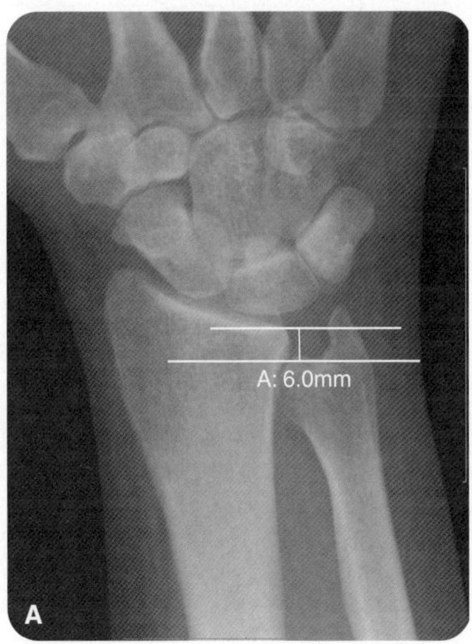

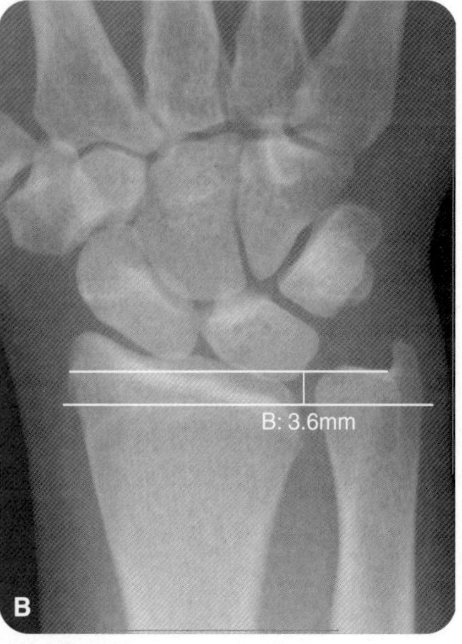

Figure 41.2 Ulnar variance: (A) negative ulnar variance and (B) positive ulnar variance.

constructing a transverse across the distal ulna. This line is compared with a second transverse line drawn across the distal radius. A negative ulnar variance is defined by an ulnar line that is proximal to the distal radius. A positive ulnar variance exists when the distal ulna extends past the distal radius. A variance does not exist when the distal ulna and distal radius are equal (Fig. 41.2).

The radiological differential diagnosis includes over types of carpal fractures (scaphoid injuries were discussed in Chapters 38 and 39). Fractures involving the pisiform or the hook of the hamate are very subtle. On standard PA films, there may be a very subtle effacement of the pisiform or the hook of the hamate. In patients who complain of traumatic injuries to the hypothenar eminence, effacement of the small eyelet of the pisiform or the hook of the hamate is an important but subtle clue to the presence of an underlying fracture. Moreover, in patients with traumatic hypothenar injuries, a carpal view may be helpful. This view allows the examiner to identify subtle fractures of the pisiform or the hamate. For patients who complain of severe pain and swelling of the hypothenar eminence with suspicious radiographic findings, a CT or MRI scan is warranted (Fig. 41.3).

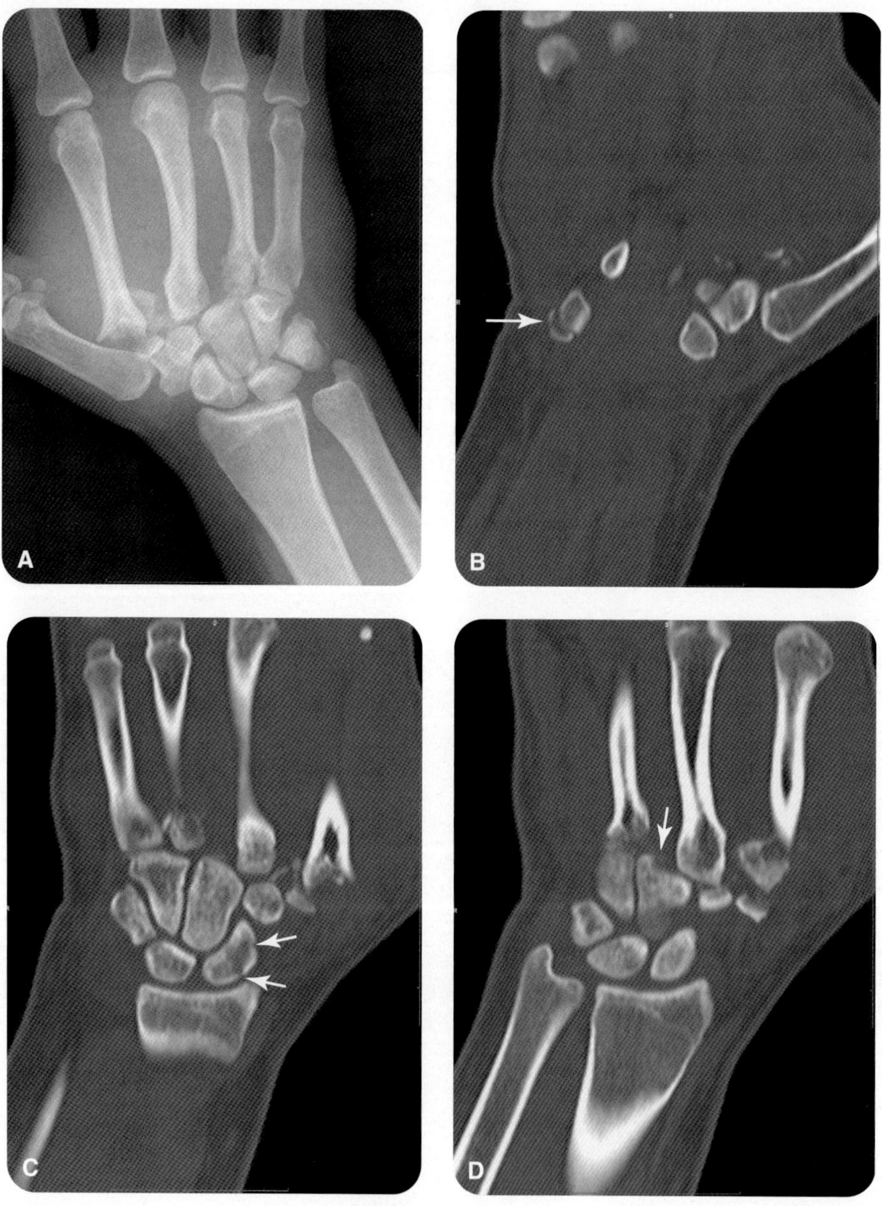

Figure 41.3 **(A)** AP radiograph of the right hand of a 21-year-old man after a crush injury to his right hand demonstrates multiple carpal and metacarpal fractures. CT was performed, and it demonstrated acute fractures of the **(B)** pisiform, **(C)** scaphoid, and **(D)** capitate (*arrows*).

WHEN TO REFER

- Referral is warranted for all patients for:
  - surgery and
  - degenerative arthritis

Treatment

The patient should be placed in an O-ring type of wrist splint and referred for a surgical evaluation. Depending on stage of disease presentation, surgical intervention may be warranted. The corrective surgical procedure may vary on a case-by-case basis. In early disease, procedures designed to decrease compressive load on the lunate are the goal. These include radial shortening, ulnar lengthening, and capitate–hamate fusion, as well as scaphotrapeziotrapezoid fusion with a scaphocapitate fusion. In late disease, procedures may include proximal row corpectomy or wrist arthrodesis.

With advancing Kienböck's disease, the patient has progressive instability of the wrist. Over time, the patient may develop a progressive degenerative disabling arthritis.

Fractures of the body of the hamate and pisiform fractures are generally treated with short arm casts for 4 to 6 weeks. However, hook of the hamate fractures that are unstable should be evaluated for surgical excision immediately.

Suggested Readings

Allan CH, Joshi A, Lichtman DM. Kienböck's disease: diagnosis and treatment. *J Am Acad Orthop Surg.* 2002;9(2):128–136.

Bassem E, Shin AY. Management of wrist arthritis secondary to advanced Kienböck disease. *Tech. Orthop.* 2009;24(1):27–31.

Becktnbaugh RD, Shives TC, Dobyns JH, Linscheid RL. Kienböck's disease: the natural history of Kienböck's disease and consideration of lunate fractures. *Clin Orthop Relat Res.* 2005;439:98–106.

Beredjiklian PK. Kienböck's disease. *J Hand Surg Am.* 2009;34(1):167–175.

Bonzar M, Firrel JC, Hainer M, et al. Kienböck disease and negative ulnar variance. *J Bone Joint Surg JBJS.* 1998;80:1154–1157.

Greenspan A. *Orthopedic Imaging.* 4th ed. Philadelphia, PA: Lippincott Williams & Wilkins; 2004:196–202.

McKiniis L. *Fundamentals of Orthopedic Radiology.* Philadelphia, PA: F.A. Davis; 1997:402–403.

Schuind F, Eslami S, Ledoux P. Kienböck's disease. *J Bone Joint Surg JBJS (Br).* 2008:90-B(2):133–139.

Szabo RM, Greenspan A. Diagnosis and clinical findings of Kienböck's disease. *Hand Clin.* 1993;9(3):399–498.

Taeisnik J. Carpal instability. *J Bone Joint Surg JBJS.* 1988;70:1262–1268.

Wagner JP, Chung KC. A historical report on Robert Kienböck (1871–1953) and Kienböck's disease. *J Hand Surg JHSA.* 2005;30(6):1117–1121.

CHAPTER 42 Perilunate Dislocation

George M. Bridgeforth, Kathryn J. McCarthy, and Charles Carroll IV

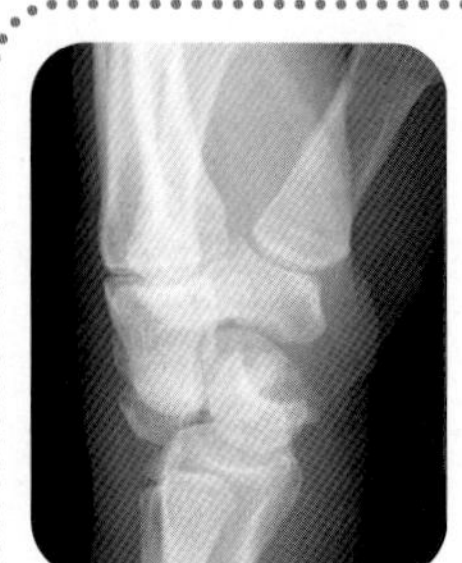

A 36-year-old man who fell from a ladder presents with right wrist pain.

Clinical Presentation

Perilunate dislocation occurs when the lunate remains in a normal position with respect to the distal radius while other carpal bones are dislocated posteriorly. The lunate may be forced into the carpal canal. A relatively rare injury, a perilunate dislocation is commonly associated with scaphoid and transscaphoid wrist fractures. The most common mechanism of injury is a fall onto an outstretched hand. Motor vehicle accidents can also cause volar dislocations of the lunate (Fig. 42.1).

In addition, the volar skin can become ischemic as a result of pressure from the volar radius. Patients may present with arterial compromise or compartment syndrome. As with any acute traumatic injury of the wrist, it is important to check and document the neurovascular status carefully (coldness, pallor, diminished or absent pulses, sensory impairment).

CLINICAL POINTS

- Pronounced subluxation or dislocation results in a palpable deformity.
- Vascular damage may occur.
- Long-standing cases may lead to degenerative arthritis due to carpal instability.

Radiographic Evaluation

It is necessary to order posteroanterior (PA), lateral (Fig. 42.2), and oblique radiographs.

With a perilunate dislocation, the examiner should look for an overlapping of the dorsal displaced capitate, which partially overlies the volar subluxed lunate (PA view). The space between the capitate and lunate is obliterated. The overlapping region has a triangular configuration that is known as a "piece of pie" sign.

Normally, on the lateral view, the alignment of the radius, lunate, and capitate should be within 10 degrees and is shaped like three sequential "C"s (Fig. 43.3). The examiner can think of it as three "C"s in a row. If the middle "C" is displaced volarly, the examiner should suspect a perilunate dislocation. With a lunate dislocation, there is a volar subluxation of the middle "C" (the lunate). The subluxed lunate resembles a tipped teacup that is spilling tea onto the palm. The three "C"s are the concave surface of the distal radius, the lunate (the middle "C"), and the concave surface of the capitate. There is a gap between the radius and capitate (in that gap lies the volar displaced lunate).

If there is a volar subluxation of the lunate (spilled teacup sign), the condition is a lunate dislocation (Fig. 42.3). In these cases, the lunate shows volar displacement beneath a horizontal line constructed through the long axis of

PATIENT ASSESSMENT

1. Marked swelling, pain, and soreness of the capitate and lunate
2. Pain-limited range of motion
3. Possible "clicking" with lunate subluxations

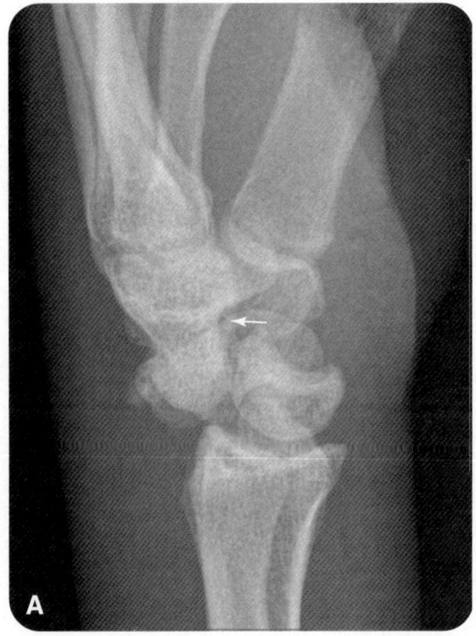

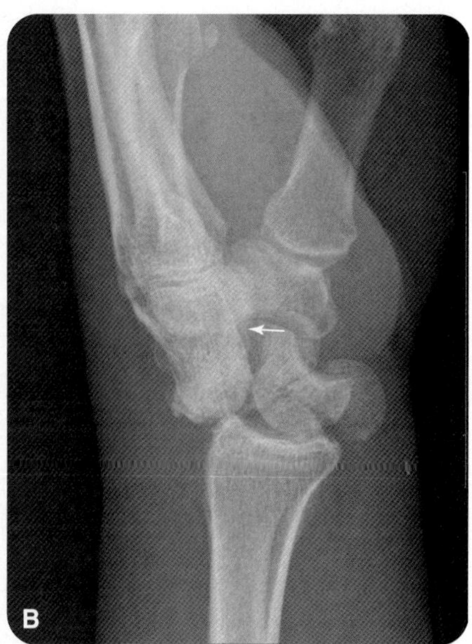

Figure 42.1 Various examples of perilunate dislocations. **(A)** A 26-year-old man with left wrist pain after falling demonstrates volar displacement of the carpal bones (*arrow*) relative to the normally positioned lunate. **(B)** A 62-year-old male with unspecified trauma demonstrates a perilunate dislocation. He also sustained a fracture to the scaphoid, not clearly shown.

the radius and through the middle of the articulating lunate and capitate. Essentially, the middle "C" (the concave surface of the lunate) is beneath this axis, tipped over and pointed downward toward the palm. This finding is best appreciated on the lateral view. However, if there is a dorsal subluxation of the capitate (the third "C") onto the volar subluxed lunate, so that the capitate subluxation is more pronounced, this condition is referred to as a perilunate dislocation. However, the capitate subluxes dorsally and sits on top of the lunate disrupting the almost straight-line relationship of the three "C"s anatomical

NOT TO BE MISSED

- Wrist contusions/sprains
- Compartment syndrome of hand
- Distal radial and ulnar fractures
- Scaphoid (other carpal) fractures
- Scapholunate dislocation
- Triangular fibrocartilage complex tear
- De Quervain's tendonitis
- Degenerative arthritis of the carpometacarpal joint
- Kienböck's disease (see prior chapter—lunate pain usually with a negative ulnar variance)
- Rheumatological disease (rheumatoid arthritis, gout, psoriatic arthritis)
- Gonococcal arthritis

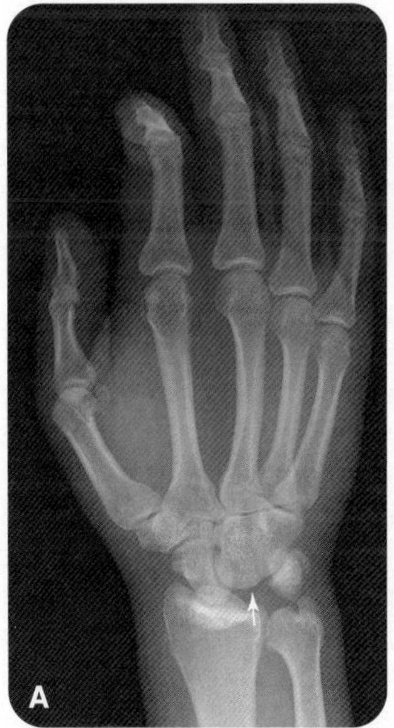

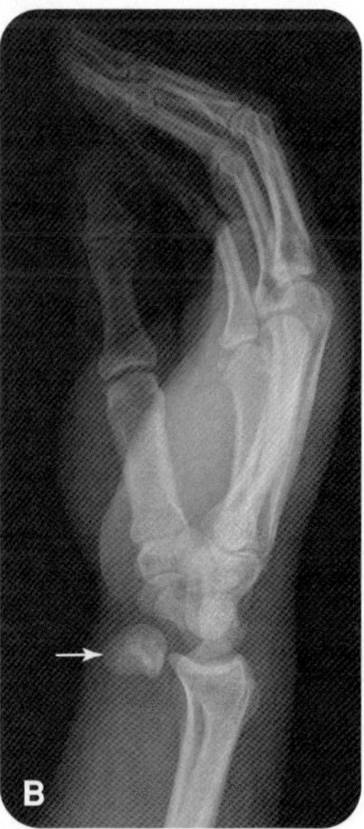

Figure 42.2 A 28-year-old man fell from a bike onto his right wrist. He complains of a sprained wrist. **(A)** AP and **(B)** lateral radiographs of the right wrist demonstrate ventral dislocation of the lunate to the carpal row (*arrow*), a lunate dislocation.

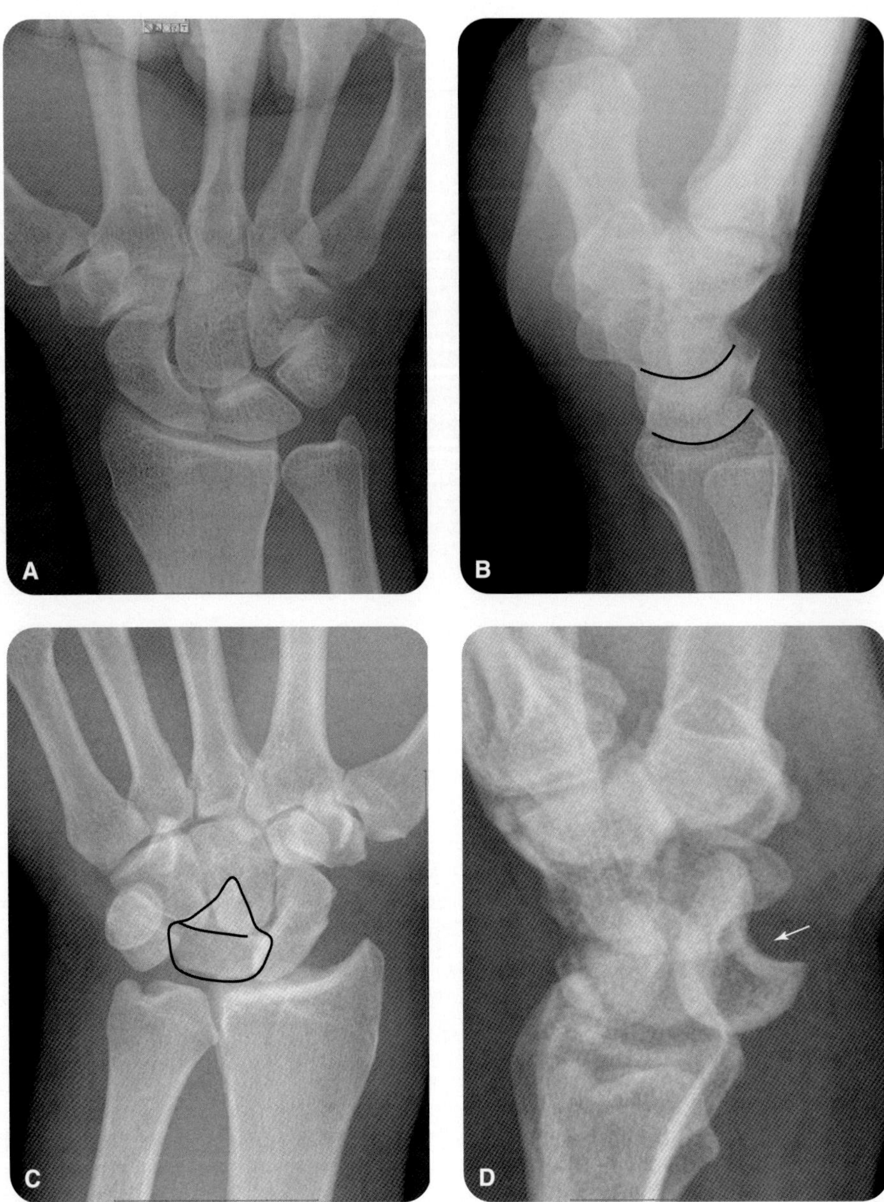

Figure 42.3 **(A and B)** Normal wrist position of the lunate on an AP and lateral x-ray of the wrist in a 27-year-old man with tendonitis. **(C)** AP view of ventral lunate dislocation demonstrating the "piece of pie" configuration (*outline*). **(D)** Lateral view of the patient in part (B) demonstrating the "spilled teacup" configuration of the dislocated lunate (*arrow*).

disruption may be identified on the lateral view. Although the linear radiolunate axis appears to be maintained (on the lateral view), there may be an associated disruption of the scapholunate ligament.

When identifying carpal injuries, the examining physician must evaluate the relationship of the three carpal arcs of the wrist. The first arc is constructed by drawing a curved line that delineates the proximal border of the proximal carpal bones; a line is drawn along the proximal concave surfaces of the scaphoid, the lunate, and the triquetrum. The second arc is constructed by drawing a curved line across the concave distal borders of the same bony structures. The third arc is constructed by drawing a curved line across the concave proximal borders of the capitate and the hamate (from the distal row). The trapezium and the trapezoid are omitted. On a normal PA view, the parallel relationship between these three arcs is maintained. However, if this relationship is disrupted, then the physician should look very closely for a fracture or a dislocation. With small nondisplaced fractures, the relationship of the three arcs may remain intact.

In addition, when examining the carpal arcs on the PA view, the two rows of carpal bones should be separated by 1 to 2 mm. Any overlap or separation of 3 mm or more is suspicious for a subluxation.

WHEN TO REFER

- Immediate referral

Treatment

Reduction, open or closed, is necessary. The patient should remain immobilized in at volar wrist splint until seen by hand specialist. Reduction maneuvers require adequate sedation with optimization of muscle relaxation. Therefore, if the index of suspicion is high for dislocation that will require sedation as part of the treatment, it is necessary to give the patient nothing by mouth until evaluated by a specialist. Maneuver is traction with forced flexion after clearing the carpal row over the lunate. After the procedure, the patient is immobilized with a sugar tong splint with monitoring of swelling.

Suggested Readings

Brant WE, Helms CA. *Fundamentals of Diagnostic Radiology*. 3rd ed. Philadelphia, PA: Lippincott Williams & Wilkins; 2007:1114–1115.

Eiff MP, Hatch RL, Calmbach WL. *Fracture Management for Primary Care*. Philadelphia, PA: Saunders; 2003: 112–114.

Gelberman RH, Cooney WP III, Szabo RM. Carpal instability. *J Bone Joint Surg JBJS*. 2000;82(4):578.

Greenspan A. *Orthopedic Imaging: A Practical Approach*. Philadelphia, PA: Lippincott Williams & Wilkins; 2004:200–203.

Harris JH, Harris WH, Novelline RA. *The Radiology of Emergency Medicine*. 3rd ed. Baltimore, MD: Williams & Wilkins; 1993:408–411.

Herzberg G, Comtet JJ, Linscheid RL, et al. Perilunate dislocations and fracture- dislocations: a multicenter study. *J Hand Surg Am*. 1993;18(5):768–779.

Knoll VD, Allan C, Trumble TE. Trans-scaphoid perilunate fracture dislocations: results of screw fixation of the scaphoid and lunotriquetral repair with a Dorsal approach. *J Hand Surg Am*. 2005;30(6):1145–1152.

Kozin SH. Perilunate injuries: diagnosis and treatment. *J Am Acad Orthop Surgeons JAAOS*. 1998;6:114–120.

Linscheid RL, Dubyns JH, Beabout JW, Bryan RS. Traumatic instability of the wrist. *JBJS*. 1972;54:1612–1632.

Murray PM. *Perilunate Fracture Dislocation: Treatment*. Updated July 10, 2009. www.edmedicine.com. Accessed September 20, 2009.

Rosen P, Doris PE, Barkin RM, Barkin SZ, Markovchick VJ. *Diagnostic Radiology in Emergency Medicine*. Saint Louis, MO: Mosby Year Book; 1992:173–175.

SECTION 9

Hand

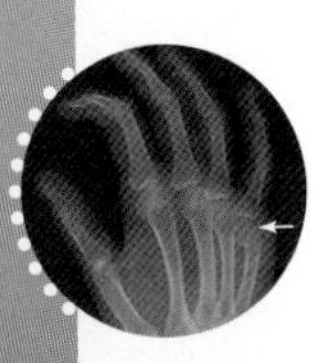

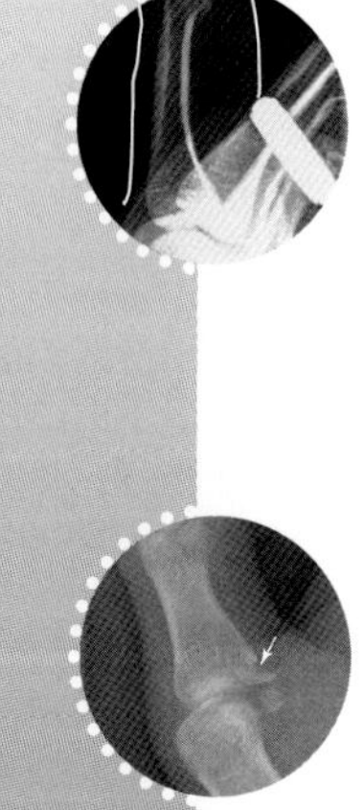

Chapter 47 Mallet Finger

George M. Bridgeforth, David Roberts, and Charles Carroll IV

Chapter 48 Thumb Fractures

George M. Bridgeforth, Brian Weatherford, and Charles Carroll IV

Functional Anatomy

The human hand consists of four digits attached to a palm, plus an opposable thumb. It is the ability of the volarly placed opposable thumb that enables humans to perform movement and very fine motor skills. This evolutionary modification separates us from other primates. The fingers are numbered one through five, beginning with the thumb. The index finger (second finger), middle finger (third finger), ring finger (fourth finger), and little finger (fifth finger) have three phalanges each: proximal, middle, and distal (Fig. 1). The articulations of each finger, from proximal to distal, are the metacarpophalangeal (MCP) joint, the proximal interphalangeal (PIP) joint, and the distal interphalangeal (DIP) joint. Each of these joints is a hinge joint. The range of motion of the DIP and PIP joints is approximately 0 to 90 degrees (flexion, with one degree of freedom). The MCP joint is a condyloid joint (two degrees of freedom). In the second, third, and fourth fingers, the MCP joint has a similar range of flexion but allows for some limited extension, adduction (fingers approximated together), and abduction (fingers spread apart).

The dorsal extensor tendon separates into a fork-like central slip whose function is to extend the PIP joint (Fig. 2). The central slip continues as two lateral bands that insert into the distal phalanx to extend the DIP joint. The flexor tendons, which run along the volar (palmar) surface of the phalanges, comprise the flexor digitorum superficialis and the flexor digitorum profundus.

The flexor digitorum profundus tendon runs between the flexor digitorum superficialis and the volar surface of the proximal phalanx. The flexor digitorum superficialis tendon attaches to the volar surface of the middle phalanx. It exerts a pulley-like action that flexes the PIP joint. Prior to its insertion into the base of the middle phalanx, the flexor digitorum superficialis tendon has a small opening that allows for the passage of the flexor digitorum profundus tendon.

The flexor digitorum profundus tendon attaches to the volar surface of the distal phalanx. It, too, exerts a pulley-like action that flexes the DIP joint. Moreover, the flexor tendons are anchored by a series of fibrous bands to create a pulley system. Each finger has five circumferential annular bands (A1 through A5 [named from the proximal to distal phalanx]) and three x-shaped criss-crossing fibrous bands (C1 through C3), which are located between the A2 through A5 pulleys. These bands help stabilize the flexor tendons during flexion and extension and prevent their displacement. The

Dorsal view

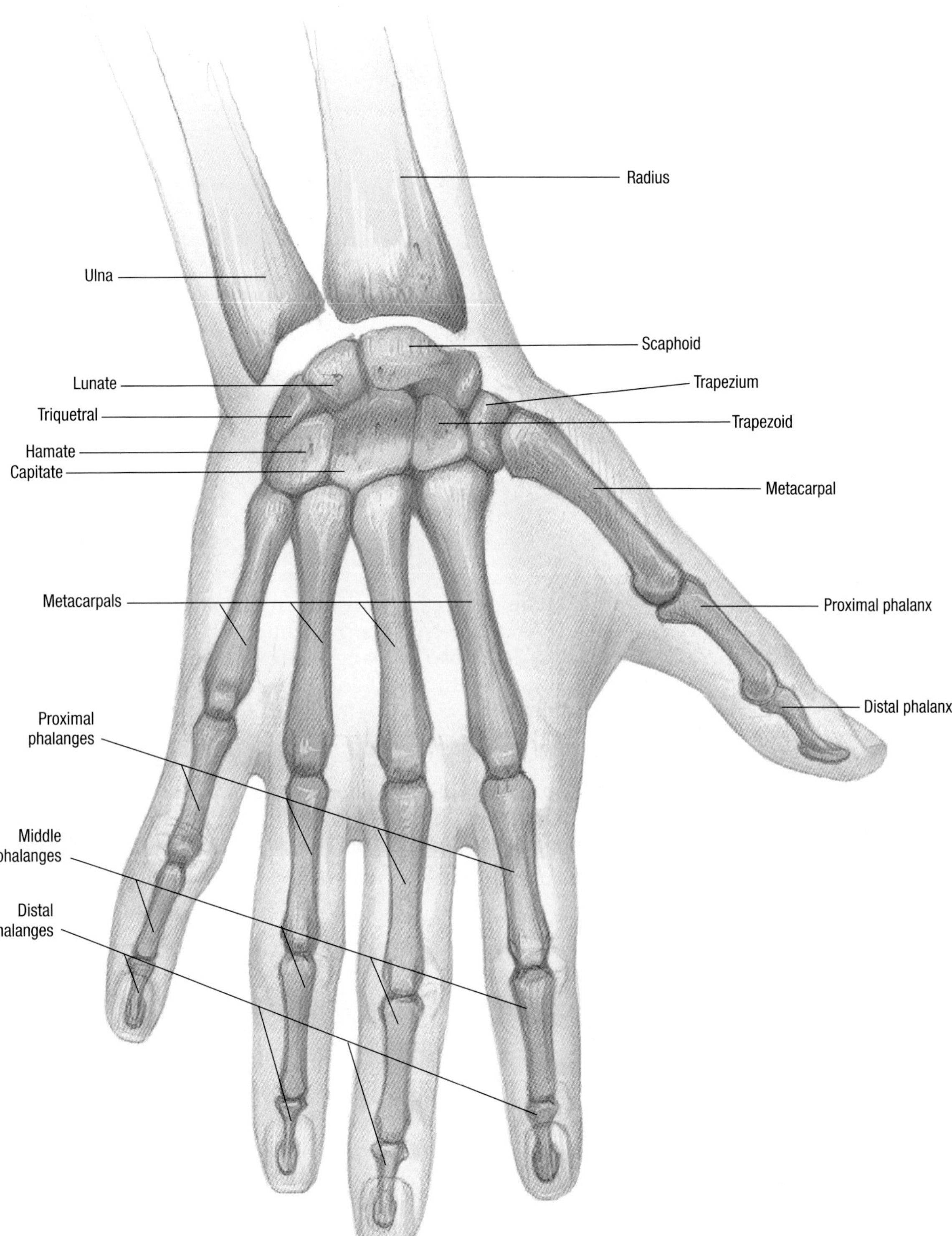

Figure 1 Wrist and hand bones. Dorsal view. Asset provided by Anatomical Chart Co.

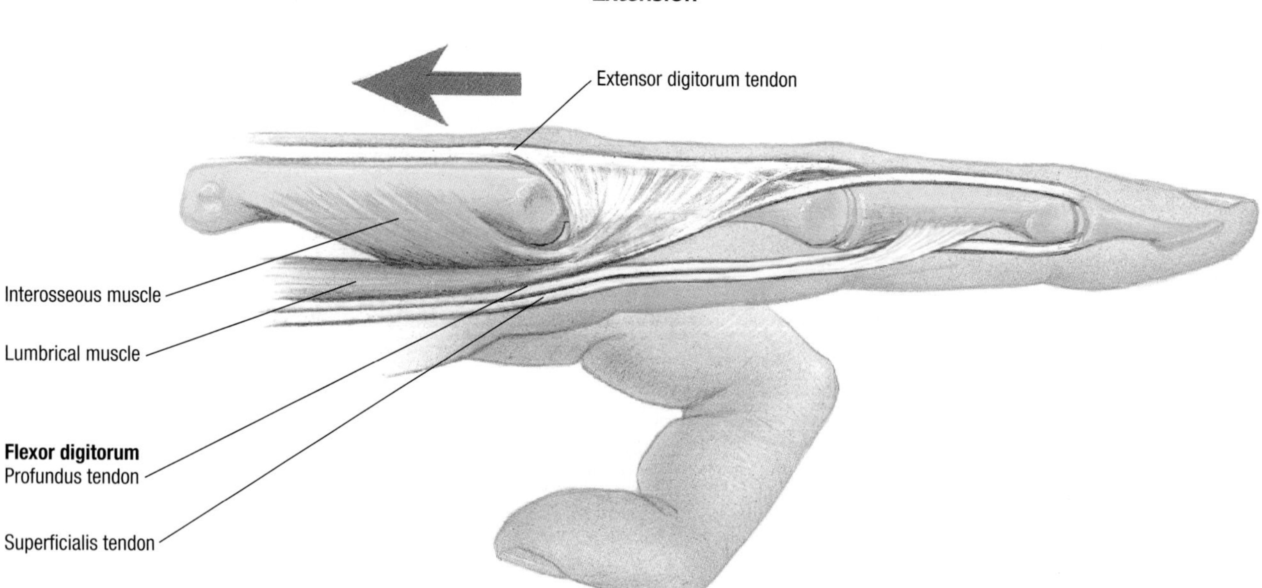

Figure 2 Finger muscles and tendons. Extension. Asset provided by Anatomical Chart Co.

pulleys approximate during finger flexion to form a protective tunnel. A protective fibrous sheath also encases the tendons.

The thumb contains two phalanges: proximal and distal. The first MCP joint of the thumb is a camplex saddle joint that is capable of multi-planar movement including: (i.e., in three planes): flexion (bending the thumb toward the palm), extension (extending the thumb into a hitchhiking position), adduction (placing the thumb next to the index finger), abduction (raising the extended thumb upward against gravity), opponens function (placing the tips of the thumb and one of the other fingers to form a circle), and circumduction (clockwise or counterclockwise rotation of the thumb at the saddle joint).

CHAPTER 43

Boxer's Fractures

George M. Bridgeforth, Jessica Peelman, and Charles Carroll IV

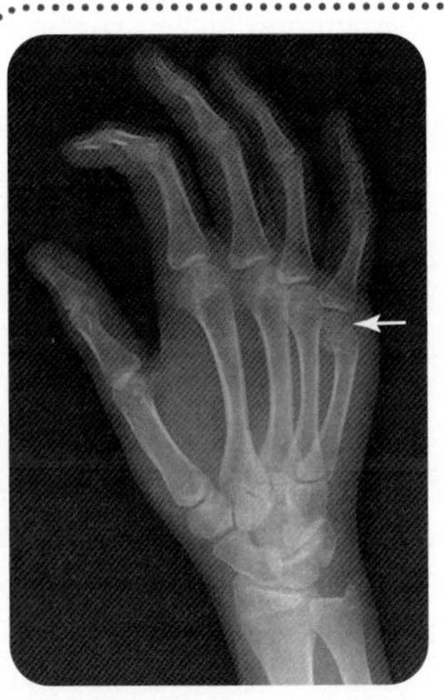

A 15-year-old female adolescent punches a wall. She complains of severe pain, swelling, and tenderness of her right hand, with pain-limited range of motion.

Clinical Presentation

Boxer's fractures are fractures of the metacarpal neck, usually the fourth or fifth metacarpal heads—the ring and small metacarpals most frequently. Fifth metacarpal injuries are more common. The fourth and fifth metacarpal bones are smaller in diameter than the other metacarpal bones in the hand, and thus they are more vulnerable to injury. Boxer's fractures follow a 10% rule: 10% of all fractures affect the hand and 10% of all hand fractures affect the fifth metacarpal. Therefore, 1% of all fractures are Boxer's fractures of the fifth metacarpal. These fractures are characterized by the volar (palmar) displacement of the metacarpal head. The mechanism of injury generally is direct trauma—after throwing a punch or striking an object with one's fist. However, they can also result from heavy objects striking the hand.

Clinically, patients present with marked pain, swelling, and tenderness at the fracture site. In addition, because of the volar displacement of the metacarpal head, there is a depression deformity (sunken knuckle) at the fracture site. Moreover, the depression deformity is accentuated when the patient tries to make a fist. Usually, there is pain-limited range of motion and pain-limited grip strength. It is not uncommon for the patient to hold the injured hand with the opposite hand.

It is important to assess the neurovascular status (warmth, capillary refill, and sensation of fingers) carefully. The physician should also check for rotational deformities of the metacarpals (each finger should point to the scaphoid when the fist is clenched). Normally, when a patient makes a fist, the fingers should be uncrossed and each finger should point to the scaphoid. If the fingers cross or "scissor," there is a rotational deformity of the metacarpals. In addition, it is necessary to inspect the hand thoroughly for open wounds or human ("fight bite") marks. Untreated human bites may lead to serious infections (see section, "Treatment"). Patients with diabetes warrant very close monitoring.

Associated hamate fractures are uncommon but are characterized by wrist tenderness proximal to the fifth metacarpal. The neurovascular examination with an associated hamate injury should document any ulnar nerve damage because it passes through Guyon's canal.

CLINICAL POINTS

- Most commonly, the ring and/or small metacarpals are affected.
- Volar (palmar) displaced metacarpal heads may produce a depression at the knuckles and palpable metacarpal head in the palm.

PATIENT ASSESSMENT

1. Marked pain, swelling, and tenderness at the fracture site (usually at the necks of the ring and/or small metatarsals)
2. Range of motion and grip strength limited by pain
3. Possible inability to make a fist

NOT TO BE MISSED

- Associated carpal fracture with severe injuries, especially the hamate
- Dislocation of the metacarpophalangeal or carpometacarpal joints
- Open fractures or bite marks ("fight bite") (high risk of infection)

Radiographic Evaluation

Necessary radiographs include a posteroanterior (PA) view of the hand, as well as lateral and oblique views. Boxer's fractures are characterized by a fracture at the metacarpal neck with volar (palmar) displacement of the metacarpal heads (Fig. 43.1). The fractures of the metacarpal necks can be appreciated on the PA view. However, the volar (palmar) displacement of the metacarpal heads is best appreciated on the lateral view (Figs. 43.2 and 43.3).

Boxer's fractures can be classified as simple or complex. In simple fractures, there is fracture but no displacement. In complex fractures, the bones have been displaced and/or rotated.

With severe impact trauma, there may be associated fractures of the body of the hamate, because the fourth and the fifth metacarpals articulate with the hamate. These fractures of the body of the hamate may occur as a result of impact injuries or direct trauma (i.e., falling objects, crush injuries). Although they may appear on the PA view, fractures of the hook of the hamate may not appear on standard radiographs (PA, lateral, and oblique views). If a carpal tunnel view fails to identify a fracture of the hook of the hamate, a magnetic resonance imaging (MRI) scan or a computed tomography (CT) scan should be obtained. If a hook of a hamate fracture is suspected, the American College of Radiology's Committee on Appropriateness Criteria (Expert Panel on Musculoskeletal Imaging) recommends a CT scan over an MRI scan for detecting this type of fracture.

Treatment

Manual reduction is appropriate for most Boxer's fractures with minor displacement. Closed reduction (nonsurgical realignment) and casting are sufficient. The ring and small metacarpal necks can tolerate significant angulation without affecting hand function (approximately 30 to 45 degrees). Physicians who are familiar with treating Boxer's fractures generally place the patient in a gutter-type

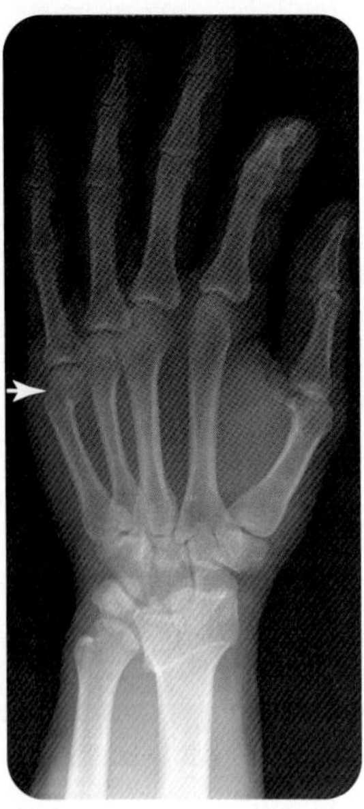

Figure 43.1 Oblique radiograph of the left in a 24-year-old man who punched a wall demonstrates an acute boxer's fracture of the fifth metacarpal.

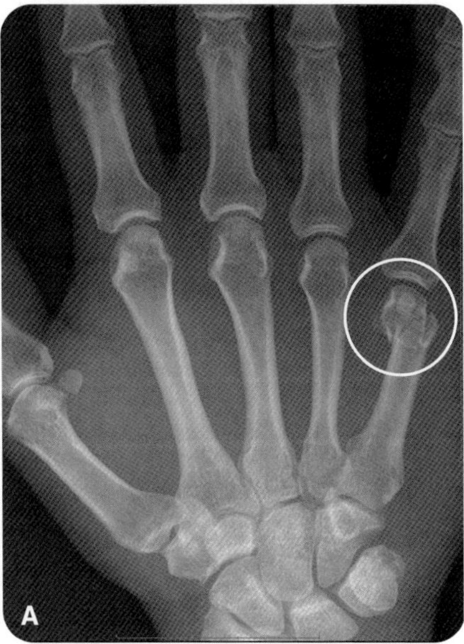

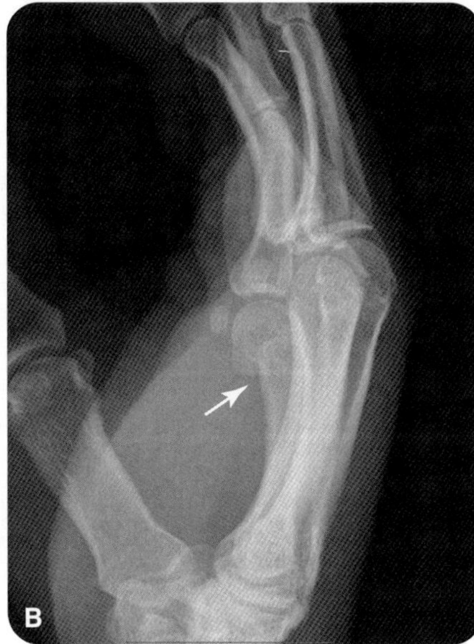

Figure 43.2 **(A)** AP and **(B)** lateral radiographs of the right hand in a 43-year-old man who caught his hand between the wall and dresser demonstrates an acute comminuted fracture of the distal fifth metacarpal (*circle*) with volar displacement (*arrow*).

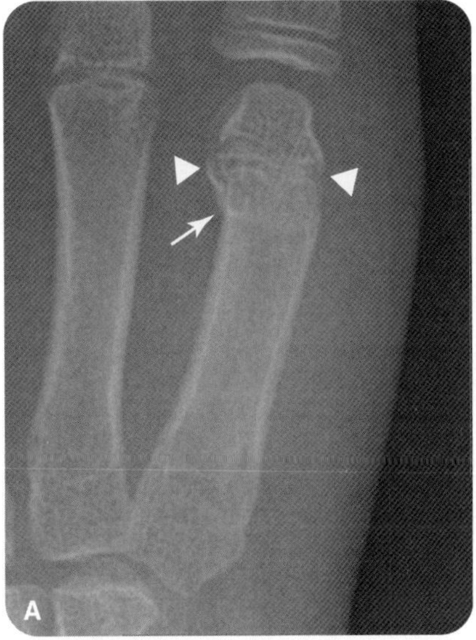

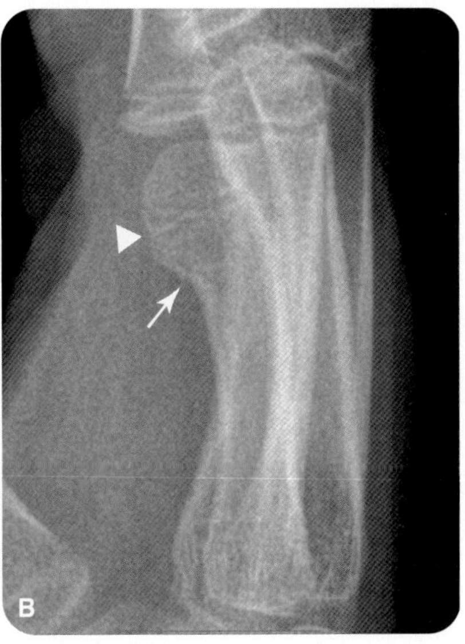

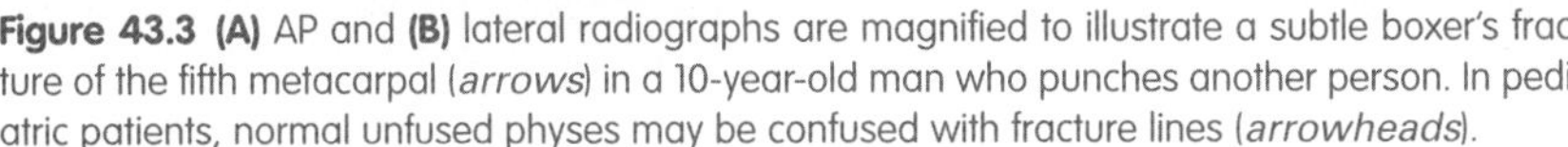

Figure 43.3 **(A)** AP and **(B)** lateral radiographs are magnified to illustrate a subtle boxer's fracture of the fifth metacarpal (*arrows*) in a 10-year-old man who punches another person. In pediatric patients, normal unfused physes may be confused with fracture lines (*arrowheads*).

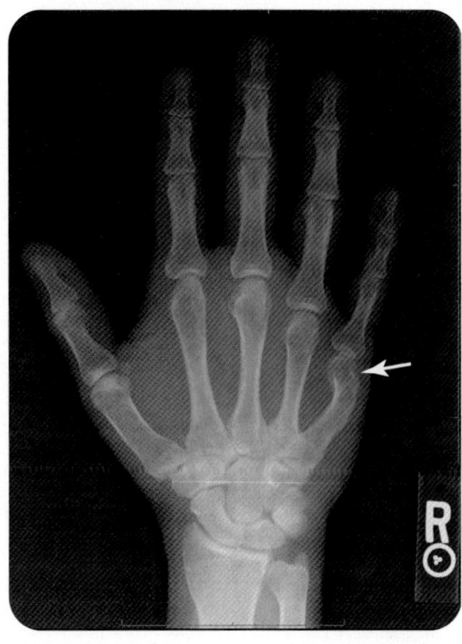

Figure 43.4 AP radiograph of the right hand demonstrates a healed fracture deformity of the fifth metacarpal (*arrow*).

WHEN TO REFER

- All Boxer's fractures warrant treatment by a specialist
- Open fractures and "fight bite" injuries require urgent treatment

or Burkhalter-type splint for a 3- to 4-week period. More complex fractures with displacement may warrant percutaneous pinning. Severely angulated, malrotated, comminuted, unstable, and open fractures require surgical treatment (Fig. 43.4).

"Fight bite" injuries, in which a tooth pierces the soft tissue and metacarpophalangeal joint capsule, require surgical debridement and treatment with antibiotics to prevent severe infection. Patients with open wounds also require prompt treatment with antibiotics. Gram-positive organisms such as staphylococcal and streptococcal species are common. If the patient is not allergic to penicillin, amoxicillin–clavulanic acid (Augmentin) or cefadroxil can be used. If the patient is allergic to penicillin, a combination such as trimethoprim–sulfamethoxazole and clindamycin may be considered.

Suggested Readings

Carlsen BT, Moran SL. Thumb Trauma: Bennet fractures, Rolando fractures and ulnar collateral ligament injuries. *J Hand Surg Am*. 2009;34(5):945–952.

Eiff MP, Hatch RL, Calbach WL. *Fracture Management for Primary Care*. 2nd ed. Philadelphia, PA: Saunders; 2003:71–74.

Freeland AE, Geissler WB, Weiss APC. Operative treatment of common displaced and unstable fractures of the hand. *J Bone Joint Surg JBJS*. 2001;83:928–945.

Greenspan A. *Orthopedic Imaging: A Practical Approach*. 4th ed. Philadelphia, PA: Lippincott Williams & Wilkins; 2004:207–208.

Harris JH, Harris WH, Novelline RA. *The Radiology of Emergency Medicine*. 3rd ed. Baltimore, MD: Williams & Wilkins 1993;440–444.

Henry MH. Fractures of the proximal phalanx and metacarpals in the hand: preferred methods of stabilization. *J Am Acad Orthop Surg*. 2008;16(10):586–595.

Kozin SH, Thoder JJ, Lieberman G. Operative treatment of metacarpal and phalangeal shaft fractures. *J Am Acad Orthop Surg*. 2000;8(2):111–121.

Lee SG, Jupiter JB. Phalangeal and metacarpal fractures of the hand. *Hand Clin*. 2000;16(3):323–332.

Morgan WJ, Slowman LS. Acute hand and wrist injuries in athletes: evaluation and management. *J Am Acad Orthop Surg*. 2001;9(6):389–400.

Peterson JJ, Bancroft LW. Injuries of the fingers and thumb in the athlete. *Clin Sports Med*. 2006;25(3):527–542.

Rosen P, Doris PE, Barkin RM, Barkin SZ, Markovchick VJ. *Diagnostic Radiology in Emergency Medicine*. Saint Louis, MO: Mosby Year Book; 1992:178–180.

Theeuwen GA, Lemmens JA, Van Niekerk JL. Conservative treatment of boxer's fracture: a retrospective analysis. *Injury*. 1991;22(5):394–396.

CHAPTER 

Volar Plate Fractures

George M. Bridgeforth, Jessica Peelman, and Charles Carroll IV

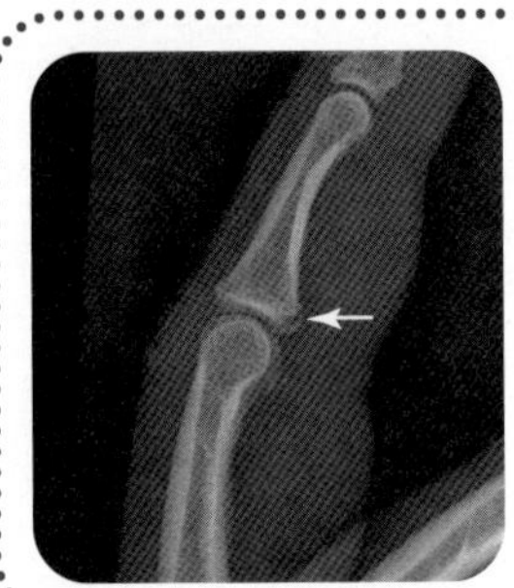

A 15-year-old girl complains of pain in the second digit of her right hand after jamming her finger while catching a baseball.

Clinical Presentation

Volar plate fractures usually involve the proximal interphalangeal (PIP) joint, the most commonly injured area of the hand. The volar plate, a dense band, forms a portion of the capsule (Fig. 44.1). An intact volar plate helps stabilize the joint and prevent hyperextension. The thick ulnar and radial collateral ligaments of the PIP joint combine with the volar plate to supply lateral stability. The PIP joint is especially vulnerable to either ligamentous injury or intra-articular fracture (with or without subluxation or dislocation). Often, there is a small fragment of bone avulsed from the volar aspect of the base of the proximal phalanx.

In volar plate fractures, the mechanism of injury is generally hyperextension or "jamming" of the finger. Volar plate injury may occur with dislocation of the PIP joint.

Clinical signs of a possible volar plate fracture include

1. a history of hyperextension to the injured finger,
2. moderate-to-marked swelling at the PIP joint,
3. tenderness at the volar plate (undersurface of the PIP joint), and
4. pain-limited range of motion.

Examination reveals clues to possible abnormalities. Thorough inspection and palpation of the area and localization of the tenderness is important. It is also necessary to check for marked tenderness at the volar (plate) surface of the PIP joint. Maximal tenderness occurs at the volar aspect of the affected joint. In addition, the clinician should test for full flexion and extension by asking the patient to open and close his or her fist. Lateral stressing of the joint evaluates collateral ligament stability.

The differential diagnosis consists of other finger injuries, including finger fractures and contusions. A tenosynovitis (trigger finger) is characterized by diffuse swelling along the fibrous tunic surrounding the finger. Moreover, trigger fingers commonly have decreased range of motion associated with snapping or locking of the finger. The snapping or locking is usually caused by a small fibrous nodule in the flexor tendon. Dislocations of the PIP joint are characterized by marked pain, swelling, and tenderness. Patients not only have impaired range of motion but also a pronounced step-off deformity from the dislocated PIP joint.

CLINICAL POINTS

- Volar plate injuries are hyperextension injuries to the finger that are commonly diagnosed as finger sprains.
- Many volar plate fractures are misdiagnosed as finger sprains.
- A history of mechanism and direction of injury aids in the diagnosis.

PATIENT ASSESSMENT

1. Pain and swelling at the pip joint
2. Moderate-to-marked tenderness at the volar plate (palmar surface of the PIP)
3. Usually associated with decreased range of motion at the PIP joint

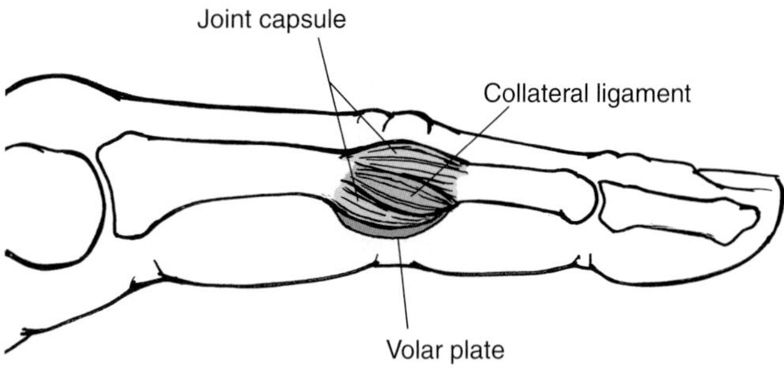

Figure 44.1 The supporting structures of the IP joints of the fingers. The supporting structures of the IP joints of the fingers include the capsule, collateral ligaments, and the volar plate. (From Oatis CA. *Kinesiology—The Mechanics and Pathomechanics of Human Movement*. Baltimore, MD: Lippincott Williams & Wilkins; 2004.)

NOT TO BE MISSED

- Finger sprains and/or contusions
- Finger dislocations with or without a fracture
- Subungual hematoma
- Nail avulsions
- Tenosynovitis (trigger finger): swelling, decreased range of motion, snapping, or locking
- Paronychia
- Felon (infection of the finger pad)
- Central slip finger injury (inability to extend the finger at the DIP joint)
- Mallet finger (avulsion of the extensor tendon with inability to extend the DIP joint)
- Jersey finger (avulsion of the flexor tendon with inability to flex the DIP joint)
- Osteoarthritis
- Cellulitis
- Psoriatic arthritis, rheumatoid arthritis
- Gout

Patients with a damaged flexor digitorum superficialis tendon are not able to flex the injured finger at the PIP joint. Patients with a damaged flexor digitorum profundus tendon lack finger flexion at the DIP joint. Damage to the lateral bands at the PIP joint results in varus or valgus instability. Normally, when the proximal phalanx is stabilized with hand, the middle phalanx should not bend internally (varus instability) or externally (valgus instability) when resistance is applied by the examiner. It is essential to check for signs of neurovascular impairment (coldness, cyanosis, impaired pulses or diminished capillary refill of the nail bed, decreased or absent sensation).

Patients with an active cellulitis following a traumatic injury have sign of acute inflammation. The finger is swollen, warm (calor), red (rubor), and tender (dolor). Usually, the examiner can identify a neighboring laceration or puncture wound as the portal of entry that resulted in the infection.

Patients with psoriatic arthritis may present with acutely inflamed swollen finger ("sausage digits"). Rheumatoid arthritis usually affects other joints as well. Most commonly are the wrists, the metacarpals, the knees, and other small joints of the hands. Gout may present as an oligoarthritis, but usually it affects other areas such as the great toe, knee, or ankle.

Radiographic Evaluation

Patients should receive posteroanterior (PA), lateral, and oblique radiographic views. If the injury is isolated to one finger, there is better resolution with a finger radiograph (Fig. 44.2). If the injury involves multiple fingers or the hand, then hand radiographs are a more appropriate choice.

On the lateral radiograph, the examiner should look very carefully for a small avulsion (chip) fracture at the base of the middle phalanx or signs of instability (i.e., an inverted V-shaped configuration of the finger indicates PIP joint subluxation) (Fig. 44.3). The fracture is usually located on the volar (palmar) surface near the PIP. It is generally appreciated best on the lateral or the oblique view. A larger fracture fragment, a V-shaped deformity, or a comminuted fracture may indicate an unstable joint (Fig. 44.4).

Treatment

Most volar plate fractures respond to conservative treatment (i.e., splinting or buddy taping). Stable injuries require splinting for no longer than 1 week to prevent stiffness, and then mobilization with buddy taping may follow. The most common complication of volar plate injuries is chronic stiffness and PIP flexion contracture. Signs of instability may include

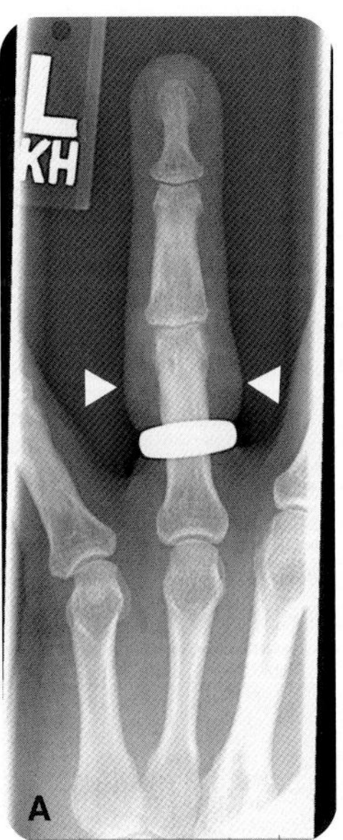

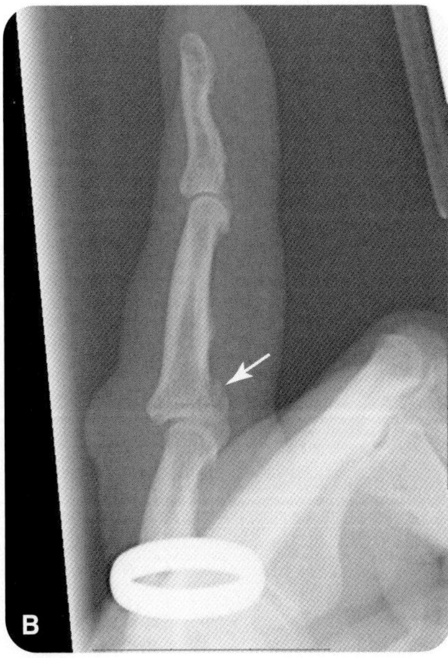

Figure 44.2 **(A)** AP view of the left fourth digit in a 51-year-old man who fell from a ladder demonstrates significant soft tissue swelling (*arrowheads*) such that the wedding ring could not be removed. **(B)** A lateral radiograph of the left fourth digit demonstrates an acute volar plate fracture (*arrow*).

1. a volar plate fracture involving at least 20% to 40% of the articular surface.
2. an unstable joint with dorsal subluxation (positive "V" sign) following reduction.
3. a bone fragment that blocks reduction and impairs range of motion.
4. a pilon (comminuted) type of fracture that extends to the articular surface of the joint.

Left untreated, unstable volar plate fractures may result in a permanent swan neck deformity of the finger. Swan neck deformities are characterized by hyperextension of the PIP joint and flexion of the distal interphalangeal joint.

WHEN TO REFER

- Unstable volar plate fractures (positive "V" signs, fractures extending to the articular surface, large fracture fragment [involving more than 20% and 40%]), a bone fragment that blocks range of motion, signs of neurovascular impairment, and open fractures require immediate referral.
- Stable fractures may warrant referral to a specialist if the primary physician is not familiar with treating them.

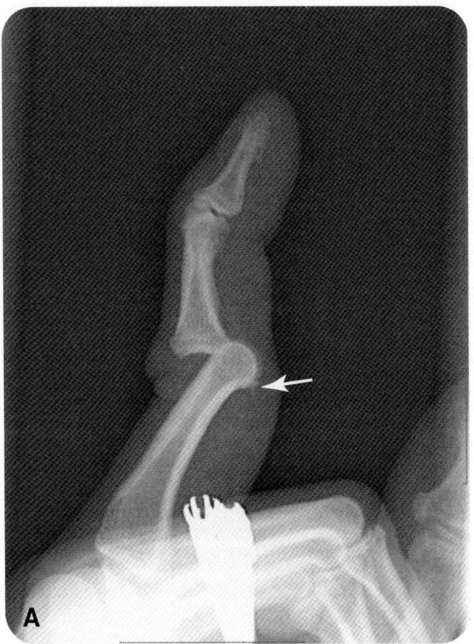

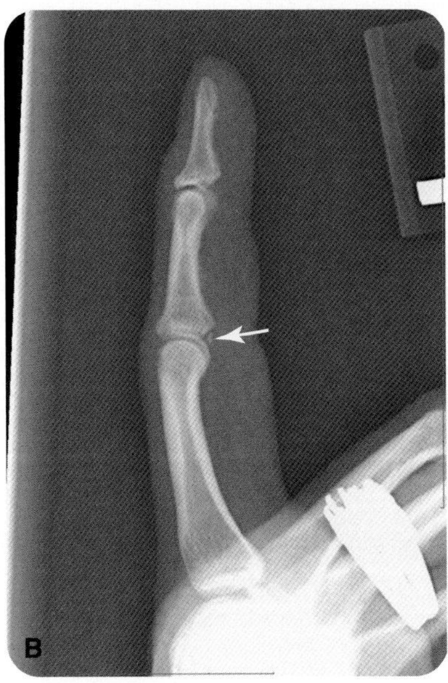

Figure 44.3 A 45-year-old woman fell off a horse and jammed her left index finger. **(A)** Lateral radiograph demonstrates an acute dorsal dislocation of the second PIP joint with a tiny bone fragment anterior to the distal aspect of the second proximal phalanx (*arrow*) suspicious for a volar plate avulsion. **(B)** After closed reduction, the second PIP joint is relocated and the volar plate fracture is more readily apparent (*arrow*).

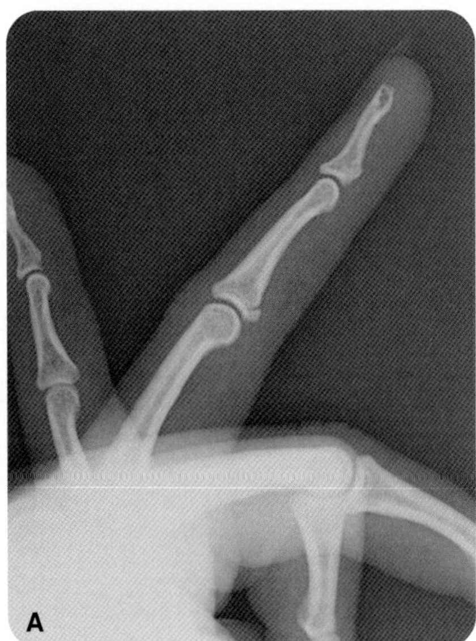

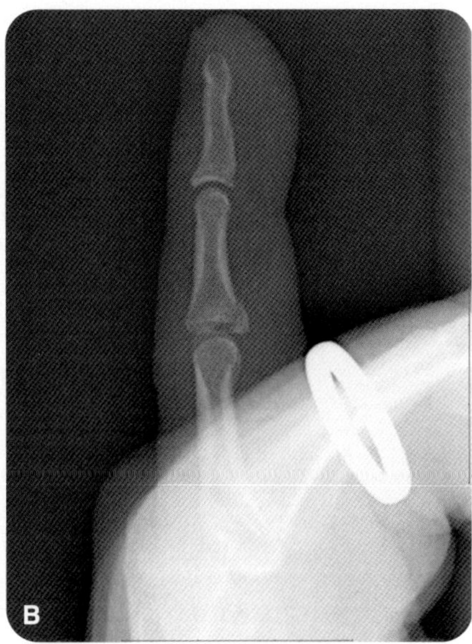

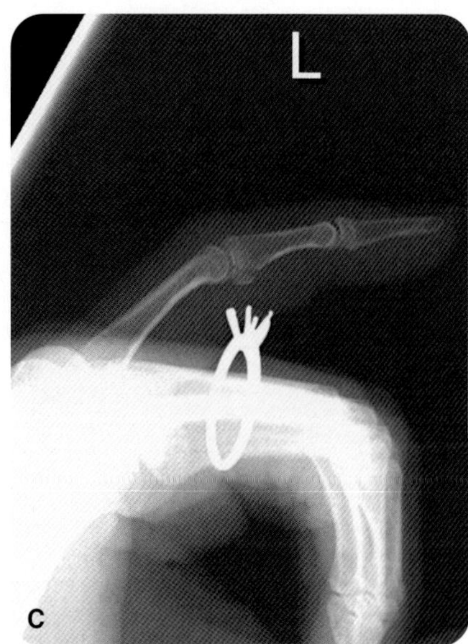

Figure 44.4 (A–C) Additional examples of volar plate fractures in three different patients on lateral radiographs.

Suggested Readings

Blazar PE, Steinberg DR. Fractures of the proximal interphalangeal joint. *J Am Acad Orthop Surg.* 2000; 8(6):383–390.

Bowers WH. The proximal interphalangeal joint volar plate. II: A clinical study of hyperextension injury. *J Hand Surg Am.* 1981;6(1):77–81.

Eiff MP, Hatch Rl, Calmbach WL. *Fracture Management for Primary Care.* 2nd ed. Philadelphia, PA: Saunders; 54–60.

Glickel SZ, Barron OA. Proximal interphalangeal joint fracture dislocation. *Hand Clin.* 2000;16(3):333–344.

Harris JH, Harris WH, Novelline RA. *The Radiology of Emergency Medicine.* 3rd ed. Baltimore, MD: Williams & Wilkins; 1993:458:461.

Leggit JC, Meko CJ. Acute finger injuries: Part I. Tendons and ligaments. *Am Fam Physician.* 2006;73:810–816.

Leggit JC, Meko CJ. Acute Finger Injuries: Part II. Fractures, dislocations, and thumb injuries. *Am Fam Physician.* 2006;73:827–839.

Nance EP, Kay JJ, Milek MA. Volar plate fractures. *Radiology.* 1979;133:61–64.

CHAPTER 45

Phalangeal Fractures

George M. Bridgeforth, Jessica Peelman, and Charles Carroll IV

SECTION 9 Hand

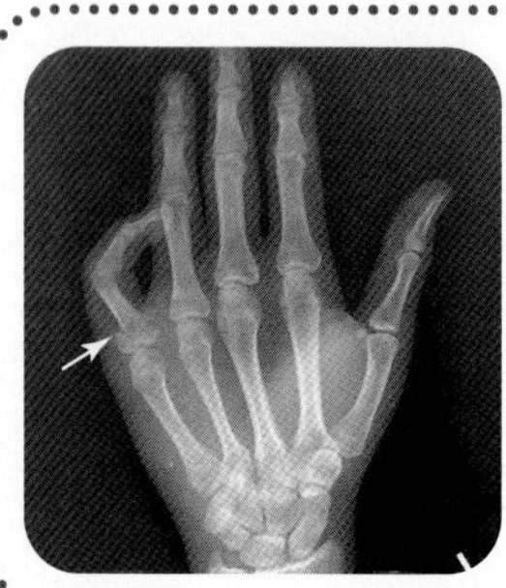

A 21-year-old man presents with laceration and gross deformity of the fifth finger of his left hand after a motor vehicle collision.

Clinical Presentation

Phalangeal fractures may occur in the proximal, middle, or distal phalanx, with the distal phalanx being the most commonly fractured bone in the finger. These fractures may lead to a significant loss of hand function if not properly treated. The mechanism of injury is usually direct trauma to the digit when the finger is hit by an object or during a fall. Crushing injuries, twisting injuries, or axial loads (jamming of the finger) may also lead to phalangeal fractures. These injuries are also frequently sports-related, especially in younger patients.

Clinical examination is essential. An important clinical test is to have the patient clinch his or her fist. Normally, the tips of fingers should all point to the scaphoid. If one of the fingers points away from the scaphoid, the examiner should suspect a fracture with a torsion deformity of the finger. It is also necessary to check for tendon injuries by assessing the patient's ability to independently flex and extend each joint in the finger—the distal and proximal interphalangeal joints as well as the metacarpophalangeal joint. In addition, it is important to check for wounds, nail bed injuries, and open fractures. There may be other associated injuries of the hand or fingers as well. Comparison with fingers of the contralateral hand is crucial. Finally, it is always essential to document the neurovascular status carefully.

CLINICAL POINTS

- Finger fractures often occur in sports activities
- Without proper treatment, loss of hand function can occur

PATIENT ASSESSMENT

1. Marked tenderness, swelling, and deformity at the site of the fractured phalanx
2. Pain-limited range of motion of the digit and grip strength
3. Bruising and ecchymosis

Radiographic Evaluation

Radiographic tests include posteroanterior (PA), lateral (Fig. 45.1), and oblique views. If the injury is isolated to one finger, finger radiographs provide better resolution. If the injury involves multiple fingers or the hand, hand radiographs are more appropriate.

Radiographs should be analyzed for location and pattern of the fracture. Fracture location can typically be divided into the head, neck, shaft, or base of the phalanx. Important fracture characteristics include orientation, comminution (multiple pieces), displacement, angulation, stability, and joint involvement (Fig. 45.2). It is important to evaluate the fracture pattern in both the PA and lateral planes (Fig. 45.3).

NOT TO BE MISSED

- Finger contusion and/or sprain
- Finger dislocation with or without fracture
- Subungual hematoma (a collection of blood under the nail)
- Fingernail avulsion or nail bed injury
- Tenosynovitis
- Mallet finger
- Jersey finger
- Volar plate injury
- Central slip finger injury
- Collateral ligament rupture (varus valgus instability)
- Finger infection (paronychia or felon)
- Cellulitis
- Dysvascular finger
- Oligoarthritis

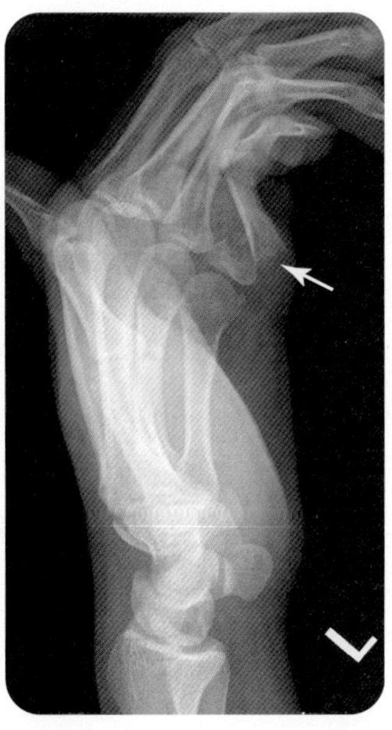

Figure 45.1 Lateral radiograph of the left hand from the patient in the introductory case, demonstrating an acute, volar displaced fracture of the fifth proximal phalanx.

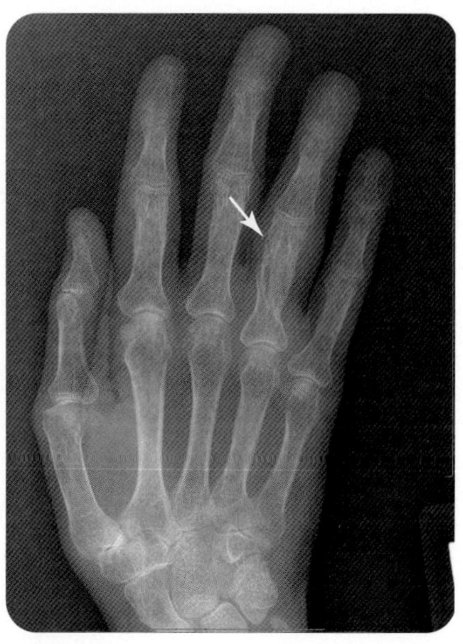

Figure 45.2 AP radiograph of the right hand in a 63-year-old man who fell demonstrates osteopenia and an acute comminuted fracture of the fourth proximal phalanx.

Treatment

Referral for treatment of most phalangeal fractures is warranted, because both overtreatment and undertreatment can lead to significant functional problems, such as chronic pain, stiffness, and deformity. The treatment of phalangeal fractures involves a delicate balance of providing enough immobilization to allow

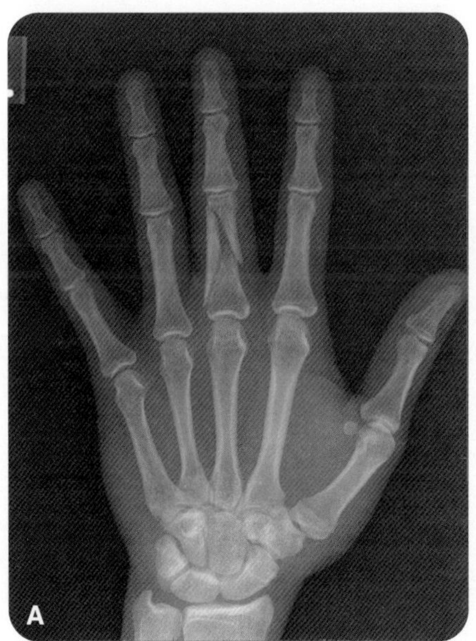

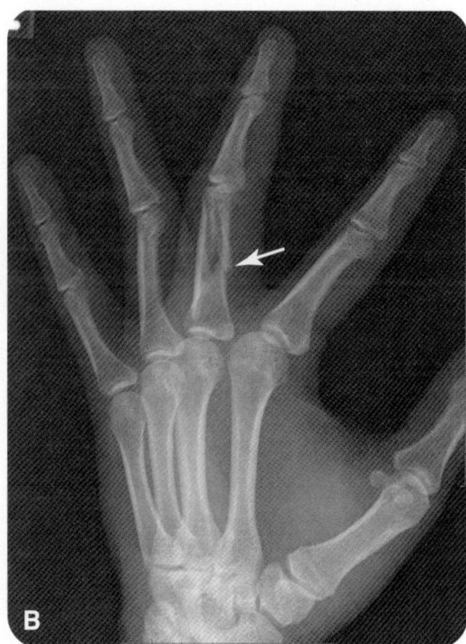

Figure 45.3 A 31-year-old man involved in an altercation. **(A)** The AP radiograph of the left hand demonstrates an acute, comminuted fracture of the left proximal phalanx with distraction of the fracture fragments. **(B)** The oblique projection illustrates the additional volar angulation (*arrow*) not visualized on the AP projection.

WHEN TO REFER

- Fractures with angular or rotational deformity or open fractures require immediate, urgent treatment.
- Unstable fractures and articular fractures require referral for possible surgical treatment.
- Stable fractures may warrant referral to a specialist if the primary physician is not familiar with treating them.

healing while permitting early motion to prevent stiffness. Therapy for most nondisplaced, stable fractures involves splinting in the "safe position" (metacarpophalangeal flexion and proximal interphalangeal extension) along with an adjacent finger for 3 to 4 weeks. Protected mobilization with buddy taping to an adjacent digit until union is achieved should follow.

Reduction and immobilization is necessary for displaced, angulated, or rotated fractures. If the fracture is stable after closed reduction, treatment with splinting followed by protected mobilization is appropriate. Patients with these fractures have a significant risk of recurrent deformity and warrant close follow-up with frequent clinical and radiographic evaluation. Fractures that are irreducible or unstable require operative fixation. Other operative indications include open fractures and fractures involving the articular surface.

Suggested Readings

Eiff MP, Hatch RL, Calbach WL. *Fracture Management for Primary Care*. 2nd ed. Philadelphia, PA: Saunders; 2003:48–65.

Harris JH, Harris WH, Novelline RA. *The Radiology of Emergency Medicine*. 3rd ed. Baltimore, MD: Williams & Wilkins; 1993:458–467.

Hoffman DF, Schaffer TC. Management of common finger injuries. *Am Fam Physician*. 1991;43(5):1594–1607.

Kozin SH, Thoder JJ, Lieberman G. Operative treatment of metacarpal and phalangeal shaft fractures. *J Am Acad Ortho Surg*. 2000;8:111–121.

Leggit JC, Meko CJ. Acute finger injuries: Part II. Fractures, dislocations and thumb injuries. *Am Fam Physician*. 2006;73:827–834.

Leggit JC, Meko CJ. Acute finger injuries: Part I. Tendons and ligaments. *Am Fam Physician*. 2006;73:810–816.

Oetgen ME, Dodds SD. Non-operative treatment of common finger injuries. *Curr Rev Musculoskelet Med*. 2008;1(2):97–102.

Slade JF III, Oetgen ME. Phalangeal injuries. In: Trumble TE, Budoff JE, eds. *Hand Surgery Update IV*. Rosemont, IL: American Society for Surgery of the Hand; 2007:3–7.

Wang QC, Johnson BA. Fingertip injuries. *Am Fam Physician*. 2001;63(10):1961–1966.

CHAPTER 46

Distal Phalanx (Tuft) Fractures

George M. Bridgeforth, David Roberts, and Charles Carroll IV

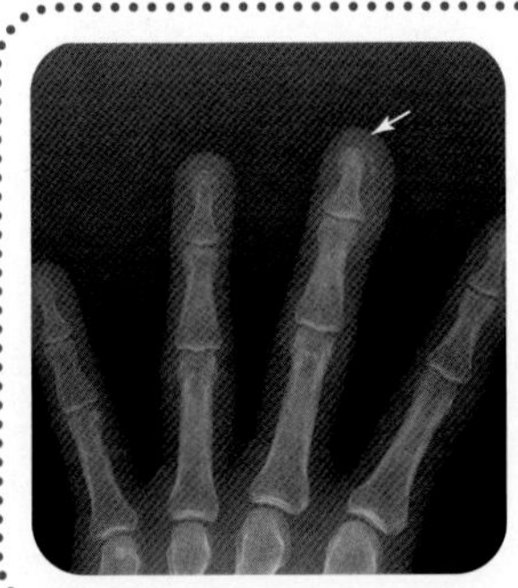

A 48-year-old man has caught his left middle finger in a machine at work. He complains of marked pain, swelling, and tenderness of his fingertip. He denies any coldness, numbness, or discoloration.

Clinical Presentation

Tuft fractures are most commonly comminuted fractures of the distal phalanx. Common sports- and work-related injuries, tuft fractures account for approximately 50% of all hand fractures. The thumb, index, and middle fingers are most frequently involved because they extend the most during usual activities. Crush injuries are the most common cause of tuft fractures—a falling object hitting the finger, catching the finger(s) in a machine or door, or hitting the finger(s) with a hammer. Subungual hematomas, which usually accompany tuft fractures, produce a blue-black, tender bruise, which may elevate the nail. The presence of a hematoma indicates a nail bed laceration, another condition that is commonly associated with tuft fractures.

Pain, swelling, and tenderness are characteristic. Most patients exhibit pain-limited range of motion. It is necessary to evaluate flexor and extensor tendon function by observing ability to actively extend and flex distal interphalangeal (DIP) joint. In addition, it is essential to check neurovascular status carefully:

- Observe skin color, warmth, and capillary refill to assess blood flow.
- Evaluate sensation to light touch and two-point discrimination to assess integrity of the digital nerves.
- Beware of a cold, dusky, cyanotic, numb finger!

A mallet finger, a fingertip injury, is characterized by a flexed posture at the DIP joint and inability to actively extend the finger at the DIP joint. For more information about mallet finger injuries, see Chapter 47.

CLINICAL POINTS

- Tuft fractures are comminuted fractures of the distal phalanx.
- The most common cause of these fractures is a crush injury.
- Dislocations are more common at the proximal interphalangeal joint and relatively rare at the distal interphalangeal joint.

PATIENT ASSESSMENT

1. Marked pain and tenderness of the distal phalanx
2. Swelling, ecchymosis, skin abrasions, and deformity of the distal phalanx
3. Limited range of motion

Radiographic Evaluation

For isolated finger injuries, three radiographic views are necessary: posteroanterior (PA), lateral, and oblique (Fig. 46.1A–C). Hand and/or wrist radiographs may be necessary for fractures of multiple digits or other associated injuries.

Distal phalanx fractures can be classified as simple (a single, clean fracture line) or comminuted (multiple fracture lines and small fragments) (Fig. 46.2). They may be extra-articular (not involving the DIP joint) or intra-articular (extending to the DIP joint). Intra-articular fractures of the dorsal lip of the DIP

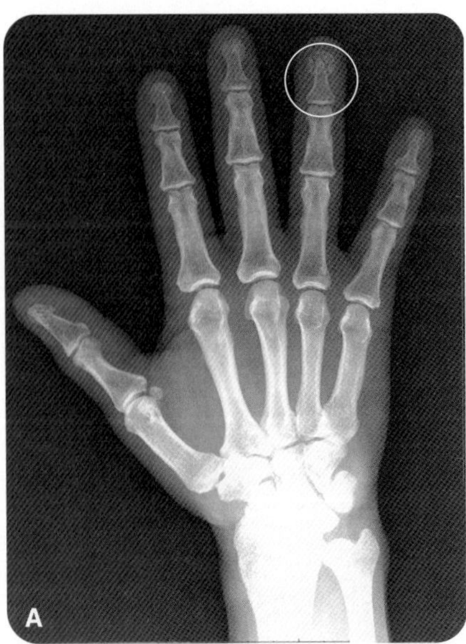

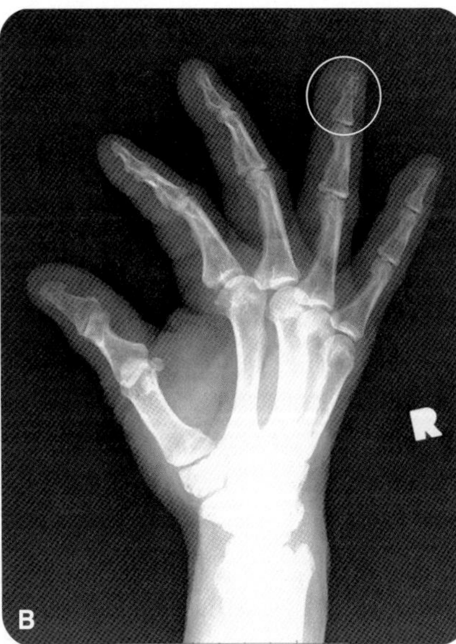

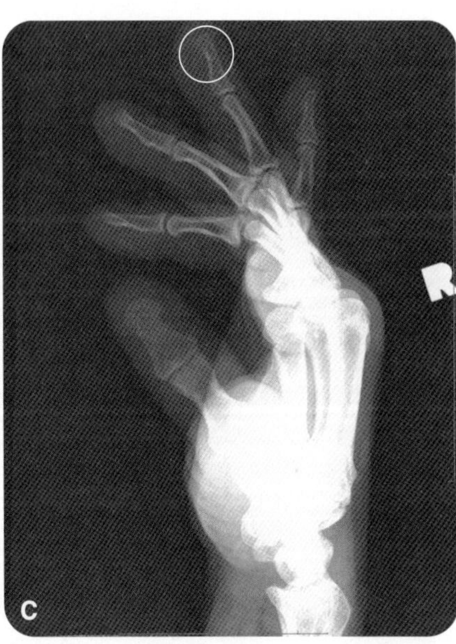

Figure 46.1 A 57-year-old man was lifting a heavy object when the object slipped and crushed his right ring finger. **(A–C)** AP, oblique, and lateral radiographs of the right hand demonstrate an acute fracture of the right fourth phalangeal tuft (*circled*).

joint are associated with mallet finger injuries (see Chapter 47), and fractures of the palmar lip are associated with jersey finger injuries. Displaced oblique and transverse fractures as well as articular fractures warrant discussion with a hand specialist.

Treatment

Treatment for most tuft fractures involves 4 to 6 weeks of immobilization using a short finger splint. Various types of splints are available. A proper splint should immobilize the distal phalanx and DIP joint but leave the proximal

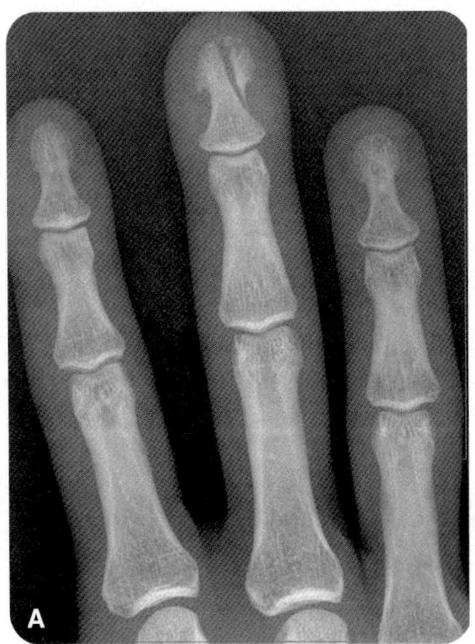

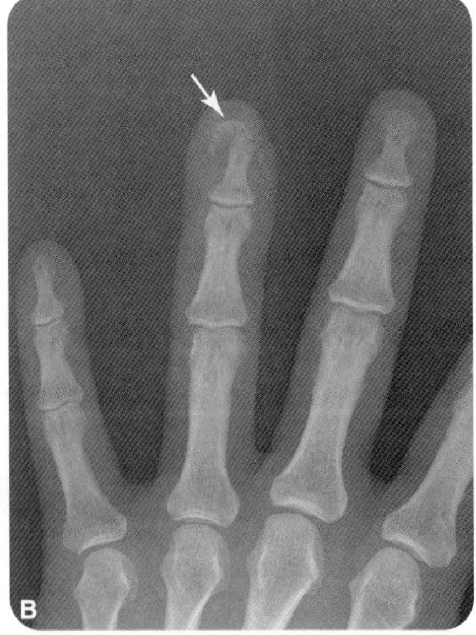

Figure 46.2 **(A)** A 36-year-old man dropped a 40-lb weight on his hand. A magnified AP view of the right middle finger demonstrates an acute fracture through the third phalangeal tuft with a dominant clean fracture line and comminution at the tip. **(B)** A 40-year-old man has caught his ring finger between two dumbbells at a gym. An anteroposterior radiograph of the left hand demonstrates an acute, comminuted fracture of the left distal phalangeal tuft.

NOT TO BE MISSED

- Open fractures
- Neurovascular injuries
- Finger contusions/sprains
- Subungual hematoma
- Nail plate avulsion and injury
- Mallet finger (inability to extend the finger at the DIP joint)
- Jersey finger
- Paronychia
- Felon
- Herpetic whitlow
- Osteoarthritis
- Gout
- Psoriatic arthritis ("sausage digit," "mouse ears" deformity at the DIP joint)

WHEN TO REFER

- Open fractures and neurovascular injuries
- Large subungual hematomas or nail plate avulsions
- Flexor or extensor mechanism injuries

interphalangeal (PIP) joint free, because immobilization of the PIP joint would lead to unnecessary stiffness at an uninjured joint. A hand therapist can provide a custom-fitted splint that can comfortably protect and immobilize the fracture. Although comminuted fractures of the distal phalanx are the most common, monoarticular nondisplaced oblique and transverse fractures of the distal phalanx are usually treated in a similar fashion.

Generally, tuft fractures do not require surgery. However, open fractures, or those associated with partial amputations and neurovascular injuries, may require reconstructive surgery by a hand specialist. Wound irrigation, debridement, and closure, followed by a course of oral antibiotics, are necessary to reduce the risk of deep infection in open fractures. Physicians who are not familiar with treating complicated distal phalanx fractures should refer these patients immediately to minimize the risk of complications such as osteomyelitis or even amputation.

Decompression of subungual hematomas can provide dramatic pain relief and involves trephinating the nail plate with an 18-gauge needle, heated paper clip, or, if no nail polish is on the nail, with an electrocautery device. If trephination is done gently and rapidly, anesthesia is often unnecessary. (Reports of excessive bleeding have occurred in patients who have a concomitant distal phalangeal fracture. The American College of Emergency Physicians cautions against trephination in patients with fractures of the distal phalanges.) Large subungual hematomas can be associated with nail bed injuries, which may require repair and hand surgery referral. Markedly disrupted nail beds are repaired with sutures but are best left alone if the nail is closely adherent to the nail bed. An avulsed nail plate generally grows back over 3 to 6 months, but there is the possibility of residual nail plate deformity. Fortunately, this is generally of no functional significance.

Follow-up of the healing process should involve serial radiographs and clinical examinations. By 4 to 6 weeks, the fracture is usually no longer tender, and the patient may begin to mobilize the injured digit and gradually strengthen the hand. Hand therapy may be necessary under supervision of a trained hand therapist. It is necessary to check carefully for complications, especially in high-risk patients (e.g., those with conditions such as diabetes mellitus).

Most of the recovery occurs in the first 8 to 12 weeks, but the total process may be prolonged in some cases. One study reported that less than one-third of patients had reached full recovery by 6 months, usually due to persistent numbness, cold sensitivity, hyperesthesia, DIP joint stiffness, and nail growth abnormalities. An appropriately trained physician should treat secondary infections, such as paronychia, with incision and drainage.

Suggested Readings

DaCruz DJ, Slade RJ, Malone W. Fractures of the distal phalanges. *J Hand Surg Br.* 1988;13(3):350–352.

Eiff MP, Hatch RL, Calbach WL. *Fracture Management for Primary Care.* 2nd ed. Philadelphia, PA: Saunders; 2003:48–65.

Green DP. *Green's operative hand surgery.* 5th ed. Philadelphia, PA: Elsevier/Churchill Livingstone; 2005:2 v. (xv, 2313, lii).

Harris JH, Harris WH, Novelline RA. *The Radiology of Emergency Medicine.* 3rd ed. Baltimore, MD: Williams & Wilkins; 1993:458–467.

Hoffman DF, Schaffer TC. Management of common finger injuries. *Am Fam Physician.* 1991;43(5):1594–1607.

Leggit JC, Meko CJ. Acute finger injuries: Part I. Tendons and ligaments. *Am Fam Physician.* 2006;73:810–816.

Leggit JC, Meko CJ. Acute finger injuries: Part II. Fractures, dislocations and thumb injuries. *Am Fam Physician.* 2006;73:827–834.

Oetgen ME, Dodds SD. Non-operative treatment of common finger injuries. *Curr Rev Musculoskelet Med.* 2008;1(2):97–102.

Simon RR, Wolgin M. Subungual hematoma: association with occult laceration requiring repair. *Am J Emerg Med.* 1987;5(4):302–304.

Sloan JP, et al. Antibiotics in open fractures of the distal phalanx? *J Hand Surg Br.* 1987;12(1):123–124.

Wang QC, Johnson BA. Fingertip injuries. *Am Fam Physician.* 2001;63(10):1961–1966.

CHAPTER 47

Mallet Finger

George M. Bridgeforth, David Roberts, and Charles Carroll IV

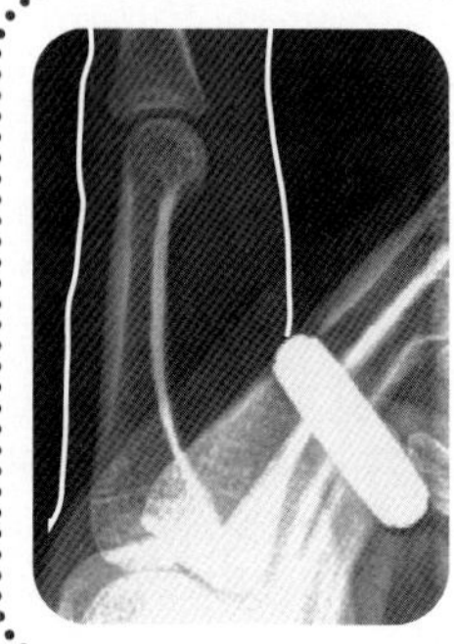

A 49-year-old man jams his left index finger playing softball. He is now unable to extend his finger and reports moderate pain, swelling, and soreness. He denies any coldness or discoloration.

Clinical Presentation

A mallet finger is an injury to the extensor mechanism of the finger. It is characterized by an inability to extend the distal phalanx at the distal interphalangeal (DIP) joint. The joint rests in an abnormally flexed position. The dorsum of the joint may be slightly tender and swollen, although there may be little pain. Patients may continue activities and notice the loss of extension after a day or more. There are two forms of mallet finger. The tendinous form is an extensor tendon rupture, and the bony form is a bony avulsion fracture of the distal phalanx.

In the workplace setting, mallet finger injuries are usually caused by crush injuries or from falling objects. In sports, they are caused by high-velocity balls that strike the dorsal surface of the DIP joint while it is flexed. These injuries result when traumatic forced flexion of the extended fingertip causes disruption of the distal extensor mechanism. Classically, they occur during athletic activities, when an extended finger is struck at the tip by a basketball, volleyball, baseball, or softball. Other mechanisms of injury include crush injuries (e.g., slamming finger in a door) or falling objects. However, mallet finger injuries can also result from seemingly trivial trauma of everyday activities, such as pushing off a sock or tucking in a bed sheet.

It is always important to check the neurovascular status carefully. Mallet injuries may occur with or without an avulsion fracture at the DIP joint.

The opposite of a mallet finger is a jersey finger. A patient with a jersey finger is not able to flex his or her finger at the DIP joint. Causes include getting a finger (usually the fourth, or ring, finger) caught in an opponent's jersey while making a tackle in football or rugby.

The patient with a mallet finger not only has a painful and swollen distal finger but is unable to extend the DIP joint actively. During the examination, it is important to check neurovascular status carefully:

- Observe skin color, warmth, and capillary refill to assess blood flow
- Evaluate sensation to light touch and two-point discrimination to assess integrity of the digital nerves

CLINICAL POINTS

- The mechanism that straightens the DIP joint is disrupted.
- The injury may occur when a person is trying to catch a ball.
- The extensor tendon is damaged (possibly ruptured).

PATIENT ASSESSMENT

1. Flexion deformity of the DIP joint
2. Inability to extend the distal phalanx actively
3. Most tenderness to palpation over the dorsal distal phalanx and DIP joint
4. Possible compensatory swan neck deformity
5. Possible subungual hematoma (blood under the nail plate)

NOT TO BE MISSED

- Open fractures
- Neurovascular injuries
- Finger contusions/sprains
- Subungual hematoma
- Nail plate avulsion and injury
- Jersey finger
- Paronychia
- Felon
- Herpetic whitlow
- Osteoarthritis
- Gout
- Psoriatic arthritis ("sausage digit," "mouse ears" deformity at the DIP joint)

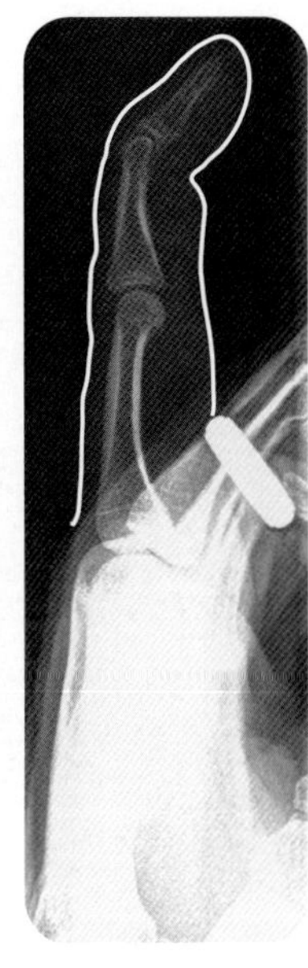

Figure 47.1 Lateral radiograph of the left hand of the patient in the introductory case, demonstrating soft tissue swelling over the left, second distal interphalangeal joint with a flexion deformity at that joint consistent with a mallet finger.

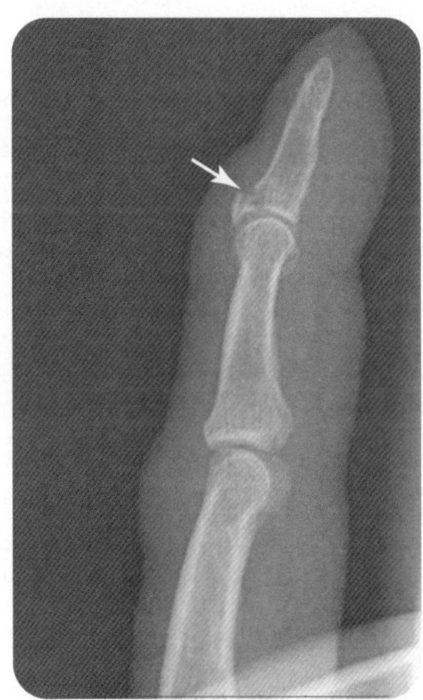

Figure 47.2 A 73-year-old man jammed his left second digit with mallet finger deformity. The lateral radiograph of the affected digit demonstrates an acute avulsion of the dorsal base of the distal phalanx (*arrow*) at the attachment site of the extensor tendon. The examination is windowed so that the soft tissue outline of the finger demonstrates fixed flexion of the DIP joint.

Radiographic Evaluation

A radiograph shows changes of osteoarthritis at the DIP joint with full extension. Finger radiographs to obtain include posteroanterior, lateral (Fig. 47.1), and oblique views. A mallet finger results from injury to the extensor mechanism. On the lateral radiograph, the flexion deformity caused by lack of integrity of the extensor mechanism is clearly evident. The examiner should check this film for a flexion deformity at the DIP joint, with the distal phalanx flexed like a mallet. A tendinous or soft tissue mallet is an avulsion or tear of the distal extensor tendon at the DIP joint (Fig. 47.2). A bony mallet has an associated fracture of the dorsal base of the distal phalanx involving the insertion of the extensor tendon. A pure tendon injury shows no evidence of fracture, only the mallet deformity (Fig. 47.3).

In addition, it is necessary to check for any subluxation of the DIP joint (lack of congruency of the joint surfaces). A fracture at the base of the distal phalanx may be present and attached to the end of the extensor tendon (Fig. 47.4). If the fracture is large (>50% of the articular surface), palmar subluxation of the distal phalanx may occur.

Large Heberden's nodes at the DIP joint sometimes occur if there is an extension injury to the DIP joint. Heberden's nodes, which usually appear in older patients with degenerative osteoarthritis, may appear as a pseudomallet deformity, with a flexion deformity resulting from degeneration of the DIP joint. Distinguishing a dorsal osteophyte from a mallet fracture requires careful evaluation. An osteophyte appears well circumscribed with a circumferential sclerotic rim, whereas a fracture has a clean fracture line. In addition, there may be other evidence of osteoarthritis changes affecting other joints (DIP joints, both knees).

Treatment

Only experienced practitioners or specialists should treatment mallet finger injuries. The initial treatment for most mallet injuries, regardless of the age of injury, presence of a fracture, or even subluxation of the DIP joint, is a splint that immobilizes the DIP joint in extension. Success rates exceed 80%. Various splints are commercially available, including the stack-type splint, palmar or dorsal padded splints, or custom thermoplastic splints made by a hand therapist. The proximal interphalangeal joint does not require immobilization and should be kept free to allow motion and avoid stiffness. (Even with optimal care, a residual dorsal prominence or slight loss of DIP motion (5–10 degrees) may result. A short course of hand therapy to mobilize a stiff digit or weak hand may be necessary.)

It is critical that the splint be worn continuously for the duration of treatment. If the splint is removed, the DIP joint must be kept in the

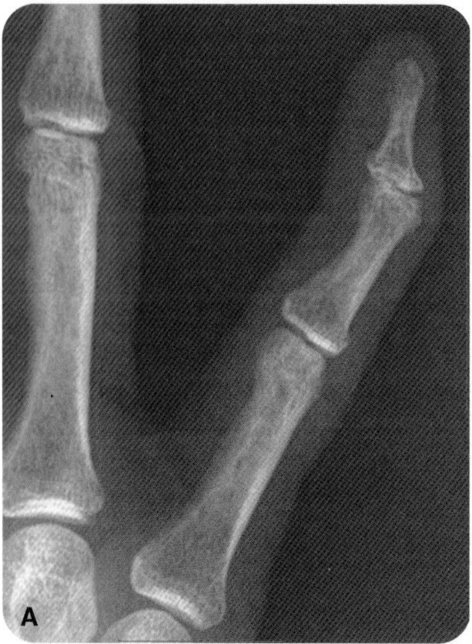

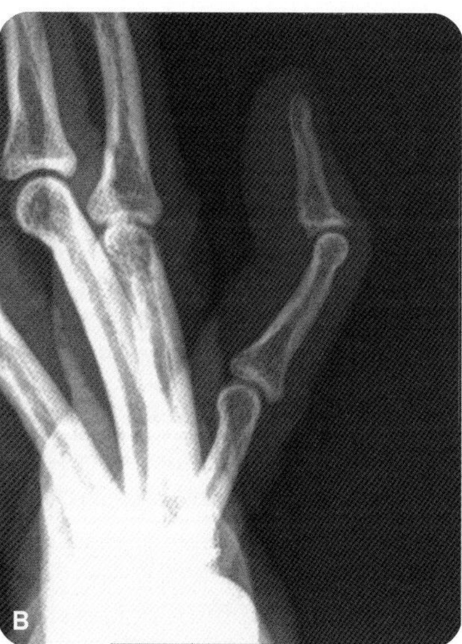

Figure 47.3 A 50-year-old woman complains of right hand pain after being assaulted. **(A)** AP and **(B)** lateral radiographs magnified over the right fifth digit demonstrate fixed flexion of the fifth DIP joint. A fracture is not present in this case.

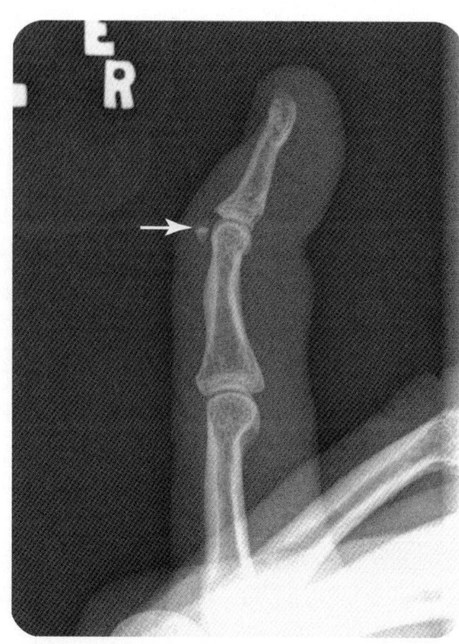

Figure 47.4 A lateral radiograph of the left fifth digit demonstrates a small acute avulsion (*arrow*) of the dorsal base of the fifth distal phalanx with an associated mallet finger deformity.

extended position by supporting it with the thumb or the opposite hand at all times. If the DIP joint is allowed to flex prematurely, reinjury to the partially healing tendon or bone can occur. In this situation, splinting should resume. It is necessary to extend the original treatment period and consider the new splinting as the beginning of the treatment extension. The length of treatment for full-time splinting ranges from 6 weeks for a mallet fracture to 12 weeks for a purely soft tissue injury. This is usually followed by an additional 6 weeks of splinting at night or during strenuous activities.

Careful observation of the skin is important because the constant pressure of a splint can lead to dorsal skin irritation and skin breakdown. Fortunately, this usually responds to adjustment of the size and fit of the splint.

Surgery is appropriate only in selected patients, such as those with open injuries, those whose occupation does not allow continuous use of a splint, and those who have chronic injuries with DIP contracture and associated swan neck deformity.

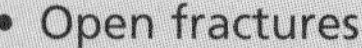

WHEN TO REFER

- Open fractures
- Neurovascular compromise
- Any complex fracture pattern

Suggested Readings

Bendre AA, Hartigan BJ, Kalainov DM. Mallet Finger. *J Am Acad Orthop Surg*. 2005;13(5):336–344.

Brzezienksi MA, Schneider LH. Extensor tendon injuries at the distal interphalangeal joint. *Hand Clin*. 1995;11(3):373–386.

Chan DY. Management of simple finger injuries: the splinting regime. *Hand Surg*. 2002;7(2):223–230.

Eiff MP, Hatch RL, Calbach WL. *Fracture Management for Primary Care*. 2nd ed. Philadelphia, PA: Saunders; 2003:43–47.

Green DP. *Green's operative hand surgery*. 5th ed. Philadelphia, PA: Elsevier/Churchill Livingstone; 2005:2 v. (xv, 2313, lii p.).

Harris JH, Harris WH, Novelline RA. *The Radiology of Emergency Medicine*. 3rd ed. Baltimore, MD: Williams & Wilkins; 1993:458–463.

Kalainov DM, et al. Nonsurgical treatment of closed mallet finger fractures. *J Hand Surg Am*. 2005;30(3):580–586.

McCue FC, Meister K. Common sports hand injuries. An overview of aetiology, management and prevention. *Sports Med*. 1993;15(4):281–289.

Moore KL, Dalley AF. *Clinically Oriented Anatomy*. 4th ed. Philadelphia, PA: Lippincott Williams & Wilkins; 1999:808–809.

Oetgen ME, Dodds SD. Non-operative treatment of common finger injuries. *Curr Rev Musculoskelet Med*. 2008;1(2):97–102.

Rosen P, Doris PE, Barkin SZ, Markovchick VJ. *Diagnostic Radiology in Emergency Medicine*. Saint Louis, MO: Mosby Year Book; 1992:181.

Tuttle HG, Olvey SP, Stern PJ. Tendon avulsion injuries of the distal phalanx. *Clin Orthop Relat Res*. 2006;445:157–168.

CHAPTER 48 Thumb Fractures

George M. Bridgeforth, Brian Weatherford, and Charles Carroll IV

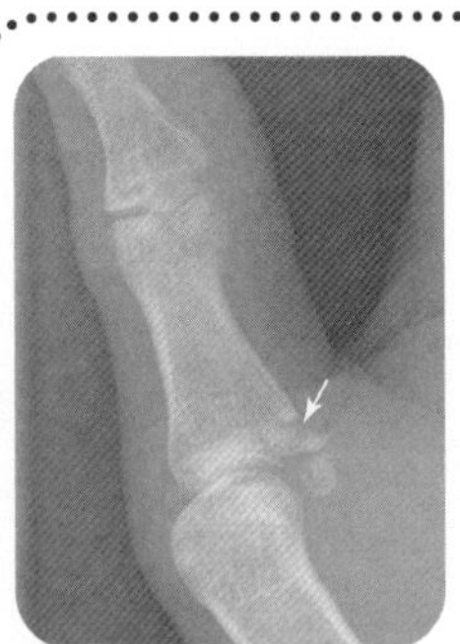

A 24-year-old man injures his right hand while wrestling with his brother. He complains of marked swelling, pain, and tenderness in his thumb, as well as limited range of motion.

CLINICAL POINTS

- A broken thumb affects a person's ability to grasp.
- Sports activities may lead to thumb fractures.
- Using protective taping may reduce the risk of a thumb fracture.

PATIENT ASSESSMENT

1. Marked pain, soreness, and swelling at the fracture site
2. Pain and limited range of motion of the thumb
3. A misshapen thumb
4. Possible numbness or coldness in the thumb

Clinical Presentation

A broken thumb is a serious injury. It is especially critical because the opposable thumb, when working properly, allows humans to grasp and pinch. Thumb function accounts for as much as 50% of overall hand function, which in turn depends on an intact and functional joint at the base of the thumb. The bones in the thumb consist of two phalanges and a metacarpal (actually a primordial phalanx) (Fig. 48.1). The distal phalange runs from the tip of the thumb to the knuckle, and the proximal phalange runs from the knuckle to the base of the thumb. Although a fracture can occur in any of these bones, the most serious breaks occur near the joints. A fracture at the base of the thumb, near the wrist, may be especially problematic. A Bennett fracture is an oblique intra-articular fracture of the base of the first metacarpal bone that extends into the carpometacarpal (CMC) joint (Fig. 48.2). A Rolando fracture also involves a break at the base of the thumb, except that it is a comminuted fracture (Fig. 48.3).

The mechanism of injury in thumb fractures is usually an axial load (downward force), with the thumb in flexion or extension. Direct stress, such as from a fall, is often the cause. Hyperextension, flexion, and rotational injuries also occur. Indirect trauma may also lead to thumb fractures. People with a history of bone disease are also at risk. Victims are most likely to be males between 10 and 30 years of age. Injuries most often result from sports injuries (football, baseball, basketball) on weekends.

The physician should examine the injury carefully and take a medical history. Severe pain and swelling at the site of the break are common in all types of thumb fractures. Characteristic signs of a Bennett or Rolando fracture include pain, swelling, and ecchymosis around the base of the thumb as well as instability of the CMC joint. During the examination, the physician should also check for open fractures (associated wounds). In addition, it is important to check neurologic and vascular status:

- Cold, dusky, cyanotic hand
- Decreased or absent pulses
- Numbness

Dorsal view

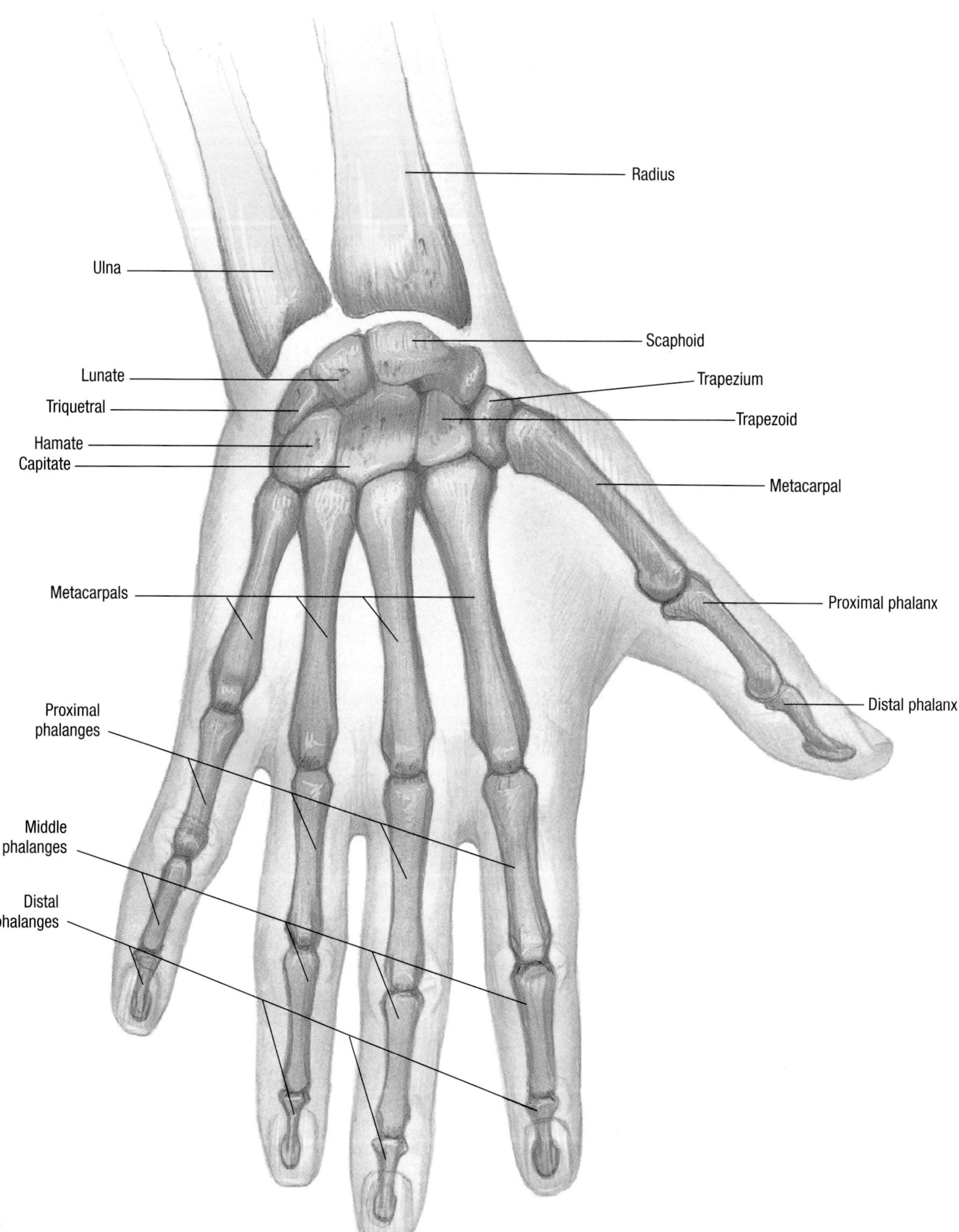

Figure 48.1 Wrist and hand bones. Dorsal view. Asset provided by Anatomical Chart Co.

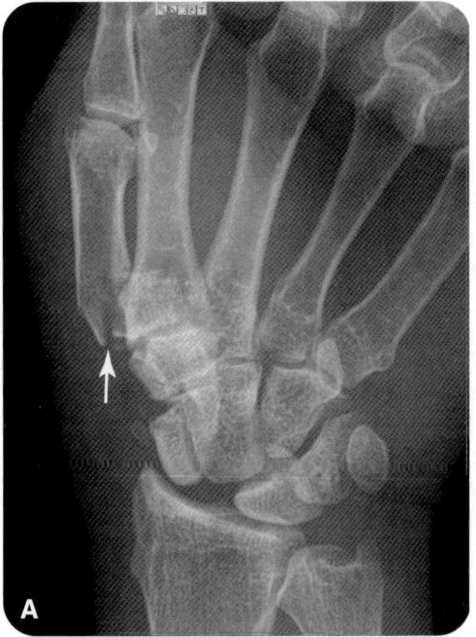

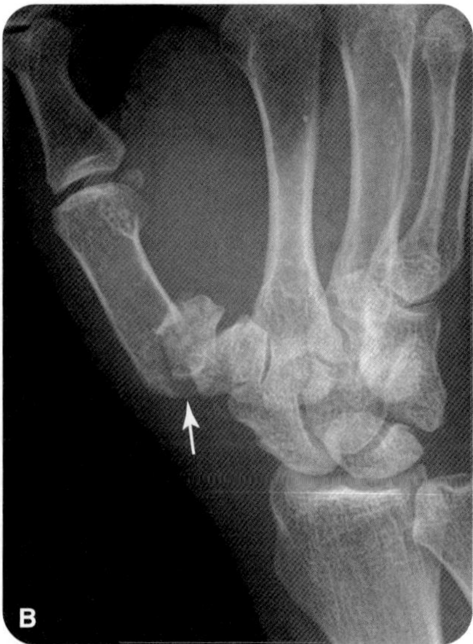

Figure 48.2 **(A)** Anteroposterior and **(B)** oblique radiographs of the right hand in a 55-year-old man involved in a motorcycle collision. These radiographs demonstrate an acute comminuted fracture of the base of the first metacarpal consistent with a Rolando fracture, which has a worse prognosis than the Bennett fracture.

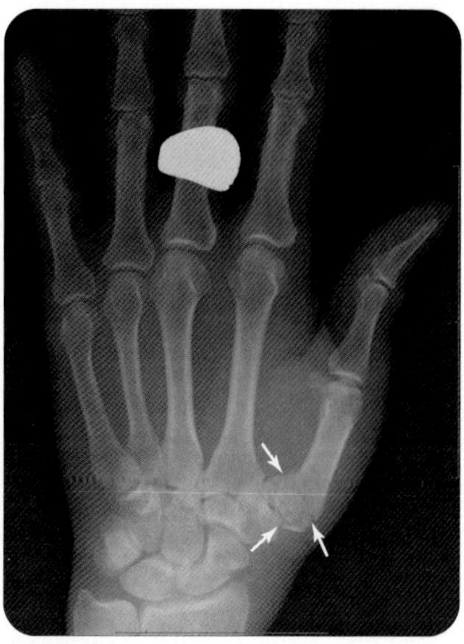

Figure 48.3 A 68-year-old man presents with left thumb pain after falling. The AP radiograph of the left hand demonstrates a T-shaped fracture of the base of the first metacarpal with intra-articular extension compatible with a Rolando fracture.

NOT TO BE MISSED

- Thumb sprain/contusion
- De Quervain's tendonitis
- Tenosynovitis of the thumb
- CMC osteoarthritis
- Osteoarthritis of the saddle joint
- Dislocation of the saddle joint (uncommon)
- Scaphoid fracture
- Subungual hematoma
- Nail avulsion
- Gamekeeper's thumb
- Collateral ligament tear
- Flexor tendon rupture
- Mallet thumb (very rare)
- Herpetic whitlow

Radiographic Evaluation

Three views of the thumb as well the hand are necessary: posteroanterior (PA), lateral, and oblique (Figs. 48.2 and 48.3).

When evaluating a patient for a possible Bennett fracture, it is necessary to first look for a fracture involving the base and the proximal shaft of the first metacarpal. Classically, there are two fragments: a displaced (avulsion) fragment of the radial aspect of the metacarpal in continuity with the remainder of the thumb and a small bone fragment (from the ulnar metacarpal base) that remains attached to the volar ligament at the trapezium or saddle joint of the thumb. In addition, there is dorsal and radial displacement as well as supination of the detached fragment due to the unopposed pull of the abductor pollicis longus and extensor pollicis brevis. The fracture is typically unstable and truly is a fracture subluxation or fracture dislocation of the thumb CMC joint.

When evaluating a patient for a possible Rolando fracture, it is important to remember that radiographs of the thumb may not disclose the full extent of articular comminution. If the fracture at the base of the thumb is a comminuted fracture (i.e., three or more parts) with a Y- or a T-shaped configuration, it is a Rolando fracture.

Treatment

DISTAL PHALANGEAL FRACTURES

These fractures require splinting and care of the nail bed. Wound and nailed care may be necessary. Otherwise, a removable splint for 4 to 6 weeks is appropriate (Fig. 48.4).

THUMB METACARPAL FRACTURES

For thumb fractures of the metacarpal shaft of the thumb that are simple and nondisplaced, treatment with a splint or cast with frequent follow-up is warranted. Typically, closed splint immobilization is necessary. Those fractures

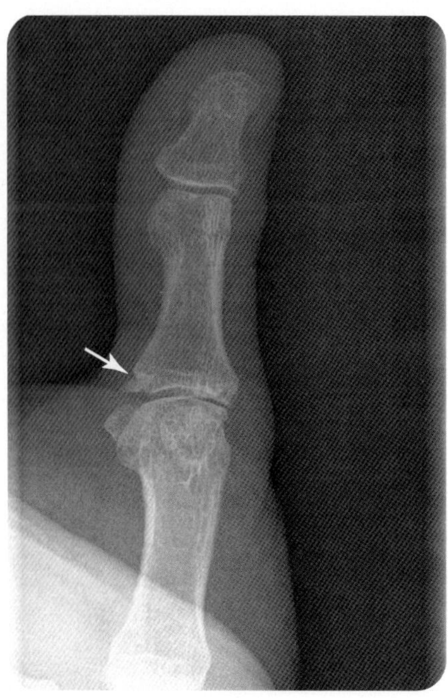

Figure 48.4 A 59-year-old man presents with thumb pain after a bicycle accident. The oblique radiograph of the first digit demonstrates an avulsion fracture of the ulnar base of the first proximal phalanx (*arrow*) known as the "gamekeeper's thumb" or "skier's thumb." The avulsion occurs at the attachment of the ulnar collateral ligament on the proximal phalanx.

that are displaced, angulated, rotated, or unstable require pinning or placement of plates and screws with postsurgical therapy. These fractures typically heal over 6 to 12 weeks with splint treatment.

For thumb fractures of the metacarpal neck that are nondisplaced, treatment with a dorsal blocking splint ("clamdigger" splint) is appropriate, as in other metacarpal neck fractures. To facilitate and maintain reduction of the fracture, it is necessary to flex the metacarpophalangeal joint. Fractures that are unstable or displaced may require pinning or an open reduction and internal fixation.

For fractures involving the articular joint surfaces of the metacarpophalangeal joint and interphalangeal joint, treatment involves a thumb spica splint for 4 to 6 weeks. Displaced articular fractures may require and open reduction on internal fixation.

BENNETT AND ROLANDO FRACTURES

Generally, Bennett fractures require stabilization with pinning. Because the thumb CMC joint is a complex multiplanar joint, any fracture that is either displaced or involves the articular surface (i.e., joint space) of the saddle joint on the trapezium should be evaluated by a specialist. Care should be taken to look for an isolated or concomitant fracture of the trapezium. The trapezium fracture requires anatomic reduction to prevent posttraumatic arthritis of the CMC joint and pain.

Treatment of most Bennett fractures involves outpatient pinning and stabilization of the base of the thumb metacarpal. After obtaining appropriate anesthesia of the thumb, reduction consists of a combination of axial traction, abduction, and pronation while applying pressure over the metacarpal base. The physician should carefully scrutinize radiographs to determine whether the CMC joint is properly located. If the joint appears dislocated or subluxated, it is necessary to attempt reduction. Occasionally, the fracture is not displaced and requires a thumb spica cast or splint for 6 weeks with a reasonable clinical outcome.

However, a Rolando fracture may require open (operative) reduction and fixation.

WHEN TO REFER

- All thumb fractures require immediate referral

Suggested Readings

Carlsen BT, Moran SL. Thumb trauma: Bennett fractures, Rolando fractures, and ulnar collateral ligament injuries. *J Hand Surg Am*. 2009;34(5):945–952.

Freeland AE, Geissler WB, Weiss APC. Operative treatment of common displaced and unstable fractures of the hand. *JBJS*. 2001;83:928–945.

Green DP. *Green's operative hand surgery*. 5th ed. Philadelphia, PA: Elsevier/Churchill Livingstone; 2005:2 v. (xv, 2313, lii p.).

Greenspan A. *Orthopedic Imaging: A Practical Approach*. Philadelphia, PA: Lippincott Williams & Wilkins; 2004:206–208.

Harris JH, Harris WH, Novelline RA. *The Radiology Emergency Medicine*. 3rd ed. Baltimore, MD: Williams & Wilkins; 1993:435–440, 452, 458.

Henry MH. Fractures of the proximal phalanx and metacarpals in the hand: preferred methods of stabilization. *J Am Acad Orthop Surg*. 2008;16(10):586–595.

Lang J, Counselman F. Common orthopedic hand and wrist injuries. *Emedmag*; 2009. query:www.emedmag.com. Accessed July, 2009.

Leggit JC, Meko CJ. Acute finger injuries: Part I. Tendons and ligaments. *Am Fam Physician* 2006;73:810–816.

Leggit JC, Meko CJ. Acute finger injuries: Part II. Fractures, dislocations, and thumb injuries. *Am Fam Physician*. 2006;73:827–839.

Moore KL, Dalley AF. *Clinically Oriented Anatomy*. 4th ed. Philadelphia, PA: Lippincott Williams & Wilkins; 1999:748–767.

Peterson JJ, Bancroft LW. Injuries of the fingers and thumb in the athlete. *Clin Sports Med*. 2006;25(3):527–542.

Ring D, Jupiter JB, Herndon JH. Acute fractures of the scaphoid. *J Am Acad Orthop Surg*. 2000;8(4):225–231.

Rockwood CA, Green DP, Bucholz RW. *Rockwood and Green's fractures in adults*. 6th ed. Philadelphia, PA: Lippincott Williams & Wilkins; 2006.

Soyer AD. Fractures of the base of the first metacarpal: current treatment options. *J Am Acad Orthop Surg*. 1999;7(6):403–412.

Zuidema GD. *The Johns Hopkins Atlas of Human Functional Anatomy*. 4th ed. Baltimore, MD: The John Hopkins University Press; 1997:14.

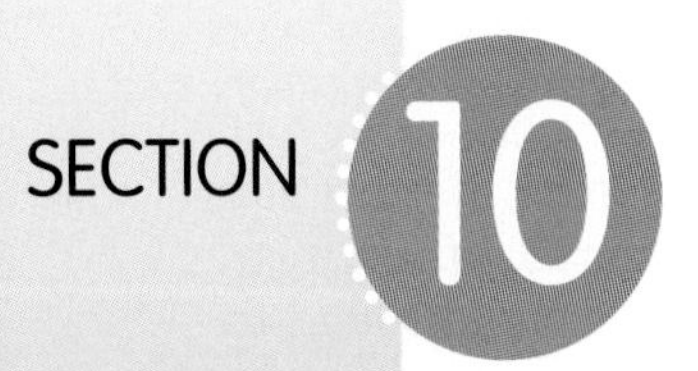

SECTION 10

Other Radiologic Problems

Metastatic bone diseases may not only be disabling but also be life threatening. Unrecognized, spinal metastatic lesions may cause unstable fractures, acute spinal cord compression, and permanent paralysis, as well as lead to premature demise. In addition, inflammatory conditions such as rheumatoid arthritis, gout, psoriatic arthritis, and degenerative osteoarthritis may be seen in patients with acute pain or trauma. It is very important to recognize the early manifestations as well as the natural progression of these disorders. Patients with long-term inflammatory conditions may face daily challenges and disabilities. Understanding the natural progression of these disorders not only helps develop better treatment plans but also helps differentiate pain and discomfort from an inflammatory arthritis as opposed to an acute injury.

With a deeper understanding of these radiologic conditions, the primary care physician is better equipped to recognize and serve the needs of these special populations. Early recognition and intervention may help delay further disease progression, lead to a more favorable long-term outcome, and maintain the patient's quality of life.

CHAPTER 49

Metastatic Cancer in Bones

George M. Bridgeforth and Mark Nolden

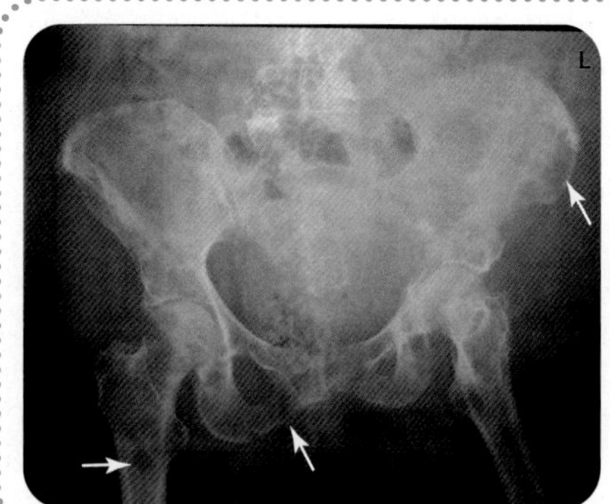

A 64-year-old woman who has had a lump in her right breast for 11 years presents after falling badly and lying on the floor for several days.

Clinical Presentation

Approximately 50% to 80% of all skeletal metastases are caused by breast, prostrate, lung, and prostrate cancers. In addition, renal cancer, gastrointestinal cancer, thyroid cancer, sarcoma, lymphoreticular malignancies, lymphoma, multiple myeloma, and melanoma also metastasize. Metastatic cancer frequently affects bones. The most common site is the spine, although the pelvis, femur, humerus, and skull are often affected.

Patients may complain of pain and soreness in the lower back, pelvis, or hips (cervical metastatic disease is uncommon); limited range of motion; and weakness and weight loss. They may attribute these symptoms to recent strain or trauma. Those with skeletal metastatic lesions may develop pathologic fractures of the spine, femur, and hip.

Physical assessment of patients with metastatic spine disease can be perplexing. It requires a high index of suspicion. Key clues include a patient history of cancer (especially breast, lung, or prostrate), a positive history of smoking (especially in lung or renal cancer), hematuria (renal cancer), or a positive family history of cancer. Other key clues include undiagnosed breast masses, generalized unexplained weakness or weight loss, and sudden onset of severe low back pain with or without the sudden onset of radicular symptoms (e.g., numbness and weakness of the lower extremities).

It is important to note that metastatic cancers may also cause cauda equina injuries to the spinal cord. Affected patients usually present with severe low back pain associated with numbness and weakness of the lower extremities. In addition, they may have new problems with bowel and bladder incontinence and report changes in sexual function, including impotence and loss of libido.

The possibility of a cauda equina injury should be considered, especially if the neurological examination shows saddle anesthesia (S2, S3, S4) at the perianal region. Rectal examination reveals a loss of sphincter tone. Additional neurological findings include new-onset sensory loss, the pattern of which may vary with the type and the location of the spinal core injury. The sensory loss is associated with upper/lower motor signs (e.g., motor weakness with hyperactive or absent reflexes).

CLINICAL POINTS

- Affected patients are usually older than 50 years of age.
- Patients frequently complain of extreme pain.
- A history of associated trauma may be present.

PATIENT ASSESSMENT

1. Patient (or family) history of cancer
2. Pain and soreness
3. Constitutional signs such as malaise, weakness, and weight loss
4. Possible focal tenderness

Radiographic Evaluation

Tests to order include radiographs of the lumbar spine, including anteroposterior, lateral, and oblique views (2). Other recommended imaging tests include a magnetic resonance imaging (MRI) scan if metastatic disease is suspected. A computed tomography (CT) scan (Fig. 49.1) is optional, although if there is a high index of suspicion, a CT with narrow cuts for bone metastasis may be warranted (especially in the hospital setting where the presence of medical equipment may make it difficult to obtain an MRI scan).

It is important to note that not every injury that patients believe is associated with trauma is actually trauma related. When screening back pelvic and hip radiographs (especially in patients with severe pain over fifty years of age), it is always important to check for metastatic cancers. When viewing the anteroposterior lumbar sacral spine, a solitary metastatic lesion may be very subtle. The examiner should always check each pedicle, the ilium, the sacroiliac joints, and the sacrum for lytic or blastic changes. Lytic lesions may be produced by multiple myeloma and by lung, colon, renal, and thyroid cancers. The well-circumscribed punched-out lesions of multiple myeloma are usually apparent on skull films as well. Blastic lesions are caused by metastatic prostrate cancers. Mixed blastic/lytic lesions may be caused by breast and lung tumors as well as by cervical, testicular, and ovarian cancers, although these reproductive cancers are uncommon.

Metastatic lesions should not be confused with osteomyelitis. The following radiological clues may be helpful. Metastatic lesions (whether blastic or lytic) are usually confined to the bony architecture. For example, metastatic lesions involving two adjacent lumbar vertebral bodies shows no evidence of an inflammatory reaction that has spread across the disc space. The lesions are localized to the bony architecture. On the other hand, osteomyelitis has indistinct cortical margins with a white inflammatory reaction that has spread beyond the bones, causing a partial or complete effacement of the disc space. In the absence of widespread disease, metastatic lesions rarely affect the thoracic and cervical spine. The initial metastatic lesions are usually the lower

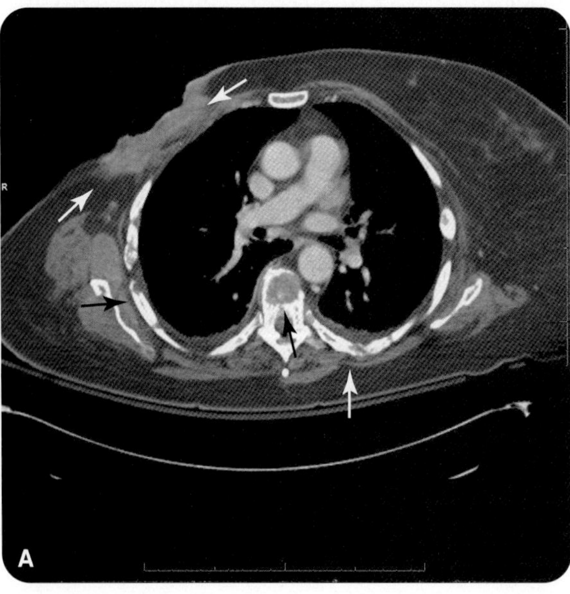

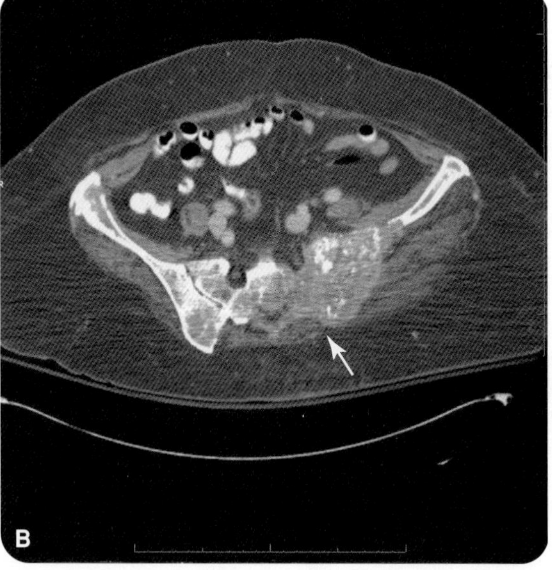

Figure 49.1 (A) An axial computed tomography (CT) image from the patient in the introductory case demonstrating an extensive, infiltrative lesion in the right breast with osseous involvement of the spine and ribs. **(B)** A more inferior CT image through the sacroiliac joints demonstrates multiple lytic soft tissue lesions.

NOT TO BE MISSED

- Low back strain or back contusion
- Acute spinal fracture
- Lumbar radiculopathy
- Osteoarthritis (age usually >50 years)
- Facet arthropathy
- Spinal stenosis
- Spondylosis versus spondylolisthesis
- Spinal cord tumors
- Ankylosing spondylitis (more common in men)
- Pyelonephritis (more common in women) or renal stones
- Abdominal aortic aneurysms
- Osteomyelitis
- Sacroiliitis
- Cauda equina injuries (rare)
- Acute abdomen (e.g., pancreatitis, cholecystitis)
- Vascular malformations (rare)

WHEN TO REFER

- Patients with severe pain, neurological signs, obtunded mental status, or cauda equina injuries should be referred immediately.
- It is recommend that non-emergency referrals should be discussed with a specialist as soon as possible.

thoracic or lumbar spine, hips, and pelvis. Although thoracic osteomyelitis is extremely rare, a patient who presents with this disease, which is characterized by indistinct inflammation and bony destructions, should be evaluated for Pott's disease, or tuberculosis of the spine. Untreated, Pott's disease can lead to marked unstable kyphotic deformity.

Treatment

Treatment may involve any combination of surgery, radiation, and chemotherapy. A multidisciplinary team that respects the wishes of the patient should determine the treatment course. Generally, patients with severe medical problems, severe dementia, or an expected survival time of less than 3 months are not ideal surgical candidates. Indications for surgery include

1. radioresistant tumors (sarcomas, certain lung cancers, colon cancers, and renal cell carcinomas),
2. spinal instability,
3. intractable pain not amenable to conservative measures, and
4. progressive neurological deficit despite radiation/oncology.

Patients with cauda equina injuries should be referred immediately for treatment. These injuries, which may also be caused by herniated discs, are medical emergencies. Usually, cauda equina injuries from metastatic cancers are treated by teams of neurosurgeons (or orthopedic specialists), radiation oncologists, and oncologists. As with metastatic cancer, treatment may consist of a combination of surgery, radiation, and chemotherapy, contingent on the patient's prognosis, tumor type, and level of destruction desired.

Suggested Readings

Ecker RD, Endo T, Wetjen NM, Krauss WE. Diagnosis and treatment of vertebral column metastases. *May Clin Proc.* 2005;80(9):1177–1186.

Georgy BA. Metastatic spinal lesions: state of the art treatment options and future treats. *Am J Neuroradiol.* 2008:29(9):1605–1611.

Jenis LG, Dunn EJ, An HS. Metastatic disease of the cervical spine. *Clin Orthop Relat Res.* 1999;359:89–103.

Klimo P, Schmidt MH. Surgical management of spinal metastases. *Oncologist.* 2004;9(2):188–196.

Loughrey GJ, Collins CD, Todd SM, et al. Magnetic resonance imaging in the management of suspected spinal canal disease in patients with known malignancy. *Clin Radiol.* 2000;55(11):849–855.

Ratliff JK, Coop PR. Metastatic spine tumors. *South Med J.* 2004;97(3):246–253.

Schmidt MH, Klimo P Jr, Vrionis FD. Metastatic spinal cord compression. *J Natl Comr Canc Netw.* 2005;3(5):711–719.

Venkitaraman R, Sohaib SA, Barbachano Y, Parker CC. Detection of occult spinal cord compression with magnetic resonance imaging of the spine. *Clin Oncol (R Coll Radiol).* 2007;19(7):528–531.

Wetzel FT, Phillips FM. Management of metastatic disease of the spine. *Orthop Clin North Am.* 2000;31(4):611–621.

White AP, Kwon BK, Lindskod DM, Friedlaender GE, Grauer JN. Metastatic disease of the spine. *J Am Acad Orthop Surg.* 2006;14(11):587–598.

CHAPTER 50

Rib Fractures

George M. Bridgeforth and Kris Alden

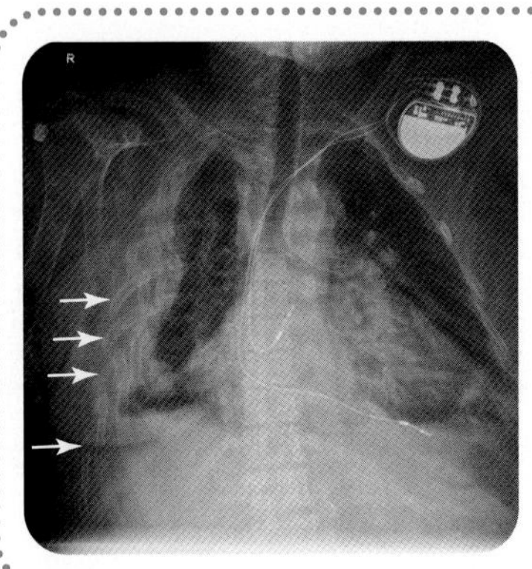

A 63-year-old woman complains of right-sided rib pain after falling on the street. She reports moderate soreness that worsens when she tries to take a deep breath. She notes marked tenderness of the right chest wall as well.

Clinical Presentation

Fracture of one or more ribs is a common chest injury. Generally, rib fractures result from direct trauma or falls sustained in sports activities or motor vehicle accidents. Most often, the middle ribs (4th through the 8th ribs) are fractured (Fig. 50.1). Fractures of the first rib are uncommon but may be associated with serious injuries to the mediastinum (aortic transection), brain, or cervical spinal cord. Although rib fractures occur in both adults and children, children seem to be less vulnerable because their bones are somewhat more flexible. Nontraumatic rib fractures occur more often in older women who have osteoporosis.

Patients with acute rib fractures may present with bruising, swelling, marked focal tenderness of the fractured ribs. There is diminished chest wall expansion due to pain and guarding. Decreased breath sounds (from diminished lung expansion) are a common finding with severe chest wall contusions and rib fractures. Absent breath sounds may be secondary to an associated pneumothorax or a traumatic effusion in the lower lung fields. A pneumothorax may occur with or without a rib fracture. Therefore, it is imperative to order a chest radiograph and rib films (see section, "Radiographic Evaluation"). Although some experts would argue that chest radiographs alone are sufficient.

Decreased breath sounds with dullness to percussion at the base may represent an effusion.

It is necessary to check for respiratory distress (decreased or absent breath sounds, rapid heart rate, rapid respiratory rate with shallow breathing). In addition, the examiner should verify that there are no effusions (dullness at the base with absent breath sounds) or pneumothorax (hyperresonance with percussion, decreased breath sounds). Tension pneumothoraces with flail chests are rare but are serious emergencies. It is also important to check for tension pneumothorax (deviated trachea directed away from the pneumothorax with marked respiratory distress). Patients with displaced rib fractures affecting three or more adjacent ribs may have a flail chest. A flail chest may be accompanied by a sucking or a whistling noise.

CLINICAL POINTS

- The cause of rib fractures is usually direct trauma or falls.
- The middle ribs are the most likely to be fractured.
- Decreased breath sounds with hyperresonance to percussion may be a sign of a pneumothorax.

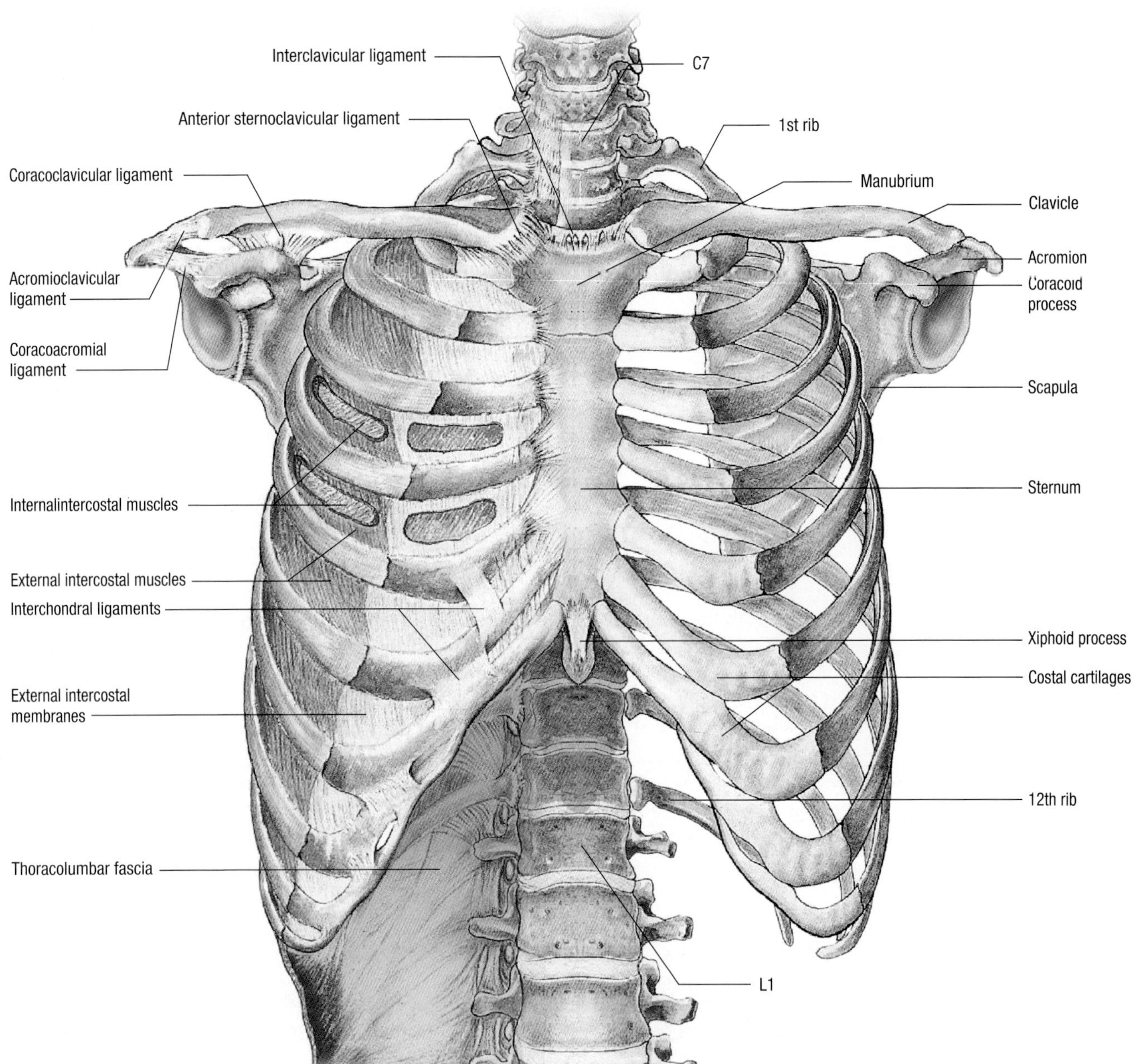

Figure 50.1 Most rib fractures affect the middle ribs (4th to 8th). Fractures involving the upper ribs may be associated with cervical spinal cord or traumatic head injuries. Fractures involving the lower chest wall may be associated with abdominal trauma (lacerations of the liver, acute pancreatitis, or a ruptured spleen). Asset provided by Anatomical Chart Co.

PATIENT ASSESSMENT

1. Pain when breathing or with movement
2. Bruising and focal tenderness of the chest wall
3. Decreased breath sounds on the affected side
4. Possible associated cervical and abdominal injuries

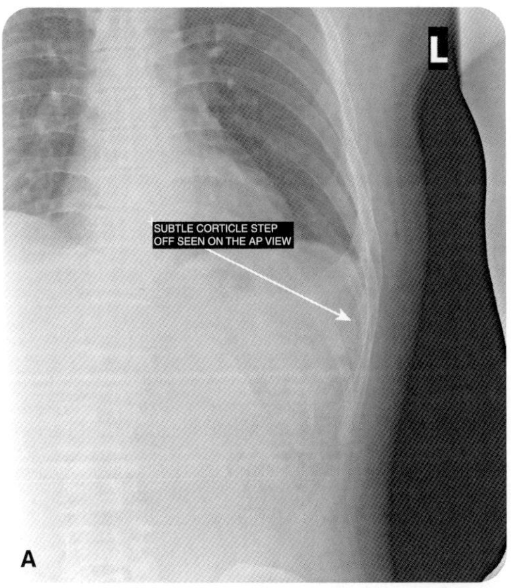
L
SUBTLE CORTICLE STEP OFF SEEN ON THE AP VIEW
A

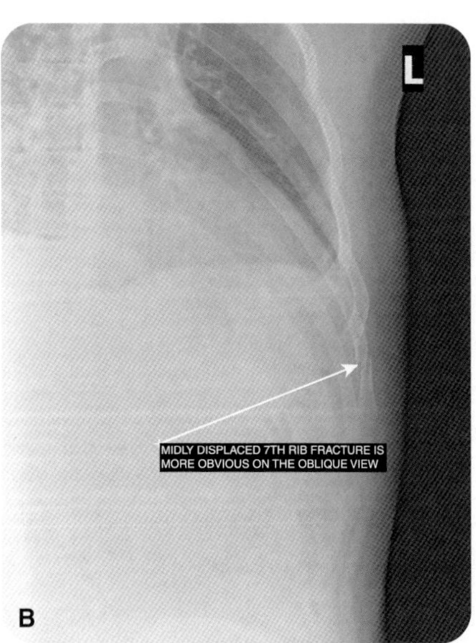
L
MIDLY DISPLACED 7TH RIB FRACTURE IS MORE OBVIOUS ON THE OBLIQUE VIEW
B

Figure 50.2 Mildly displaced left 7th rib fracture is subtle on the anteroposterior view **(A)** but more obvious on the oblique rib view **(B)**. (Courtesy of Richard Kim, MD.)

Radiographic Evaluation

Required images include a chest radiograph (two views: posteroanterior and lateral) rib films may provide additional definition. If digital images are obtained, image enhancement should be considered. In an acute trauma setting, it may not be possible to get a two-view chest radiograph. A portable anteroposterior (AP) view may have to suffice (Fig. 50.2). Although cardiothoracic structures appear larger on an AP view (because the heart and mediastinum are closer to the x-ray machine), an AP view is useful for detecting enlargement of the mediastinum, pneumothorax, or a traumatic effusion. AP views of the chest may also be necessary in bedridden patients (e.g., patients in an intensive care unit). They are useful for checking placement of breathing and nasogastric tubes.

If the patient has serious chest trauma, the physician should strongly consider obtaining a computed tomography (CT) scan. A chest CT scan may be necessary in cases of occult fractures or cardiac or pulmonary effusions. An abdominal CT scan may also yield valuable information.

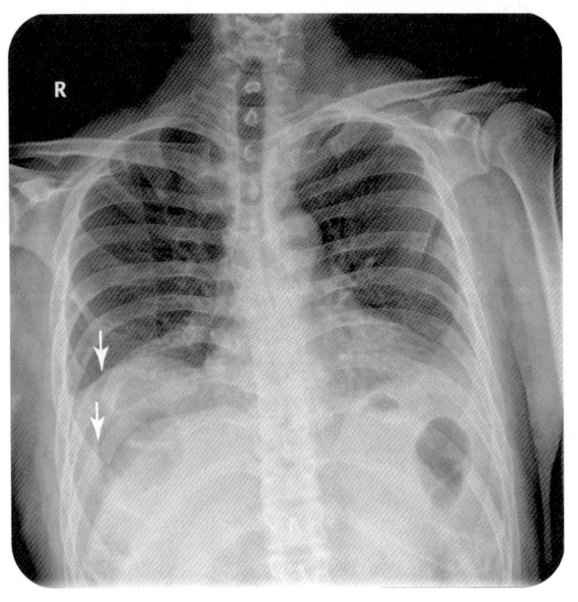
R

Figure 50.3 Acute right rib fractures in a trauma victim.

The examiner should trace the cortical outline of each rib carefully. Obviously, careful attention should be devoted toward any area where there is pain and tenderness. Nondisplaced fractures may appear as thin dark lines that disrupt the cortex. Partially displaced and displaced fractures show an actual break in the cortex and extend into the rib (Fig. 50.3).

Superimposed lung structures, such as small bronchi, can be a pitfall. These structures may be difficult to distinguish from a fractured rib. The following clues may be helpful. Bronchi are usually branched (Y shaped). Generally, bronchi are slightly thicker than fractures. In addition, bronchi may extend outside of the rib to the intercostal space. On the other hand, a rib fracture ends at the cortex. It is important to note that displaced rib fractures with sharp edges can result in a pneumothorax. In addition, the examiner should always check the chest radiographs very carefully for mediastinal enlargement (aortic transaction),

NOT TO BE MISSED

- Pneumothorax
- Hemopneumothorax/ tension pneumothorax (pneumothorax with tracheal deviation to the opposite side)
- Aortic transection
- Cardiac tamponade (hemopericardium)
- Flail chest injury (multiple fractures)
- Associated cervical injuries (cervical fractures, cervical spine injuries, crushed trachea)
- Associated abdominal injuries
- Associated spinal injuries
- Chest contusion
- Myocardial infarctions/angina
- Pneumonia
- Dissecting aortic aneurysm
- Herpes zoster
- Acute pancreatitis
- Acute cholecystitis
- Ulcer
- Kidney stones
- Lung cancer

WHEN TO REFER

- Patients with a flail chest injury from multiple rib fractures, a pneumothorax, a hemopneumothorax, or a widened mediastinum (aortic transaction, cardiac tamponade from a hemo-pericardium)
- Patients with severe cervical or abdominal injuries

pneumothorax, or associated effusion. In addition, it is always necessary to check the thoracic vertebrae on the chest radiograph for fractures or displacement.

It is important to note that rib fractures do not always appear on the initial radiographs. For patients with persistent pain, soreness, and tenderness, repeat films within several days may be warranted. If there are three or more rib fractures (involving two segments of each adjacent rib), the patient may develop a flail chest. The injured segment of the chest wall may be come detached. Clinically, this is apparent as the detached segment is pulled in by the negative intrathoracic pressure (as the intact chest wall expands during inspiration). During expiration, the detached chest wall expands from the positive intrathoracic pressure as the intact chest wall contracts. As previously stated, a pneumothorax (collapsed lung) or hemopneumothorax (bloody effusion with a collapsed lung) may occur with or without associated rib fractures. The examiner should be very suspicious, especially if there is a flail chest or a fracture involving the first rib. In addition, lower chest wall fractures (8th to 12th rib) may be associated with injury to the spleen, liver, or kidneys.

Treatment

Other than supportive care and treatment of the symptoms, there is no specific treatment for rib fractures. The overwhelming majority of these fractures resolve in 6 to 8 weeks with supportive care involving the use of cold packs, rib belts, and pain medications. In general, the pain resolves, and the fractures heal without complications.

Complicated fractures that are associated with large pneumothoraces, large effusions, widened mediastinum, or displaced fractures with sharp edges should be referred immediately. Patients with fractures of the first cervical ribs may have an associated spinal cord trauma. (These cases should be placed in a hard collar and on a spine board. They should be referred for a CT scan.)

Suggested Readings

Bergeron E, Lavoie A, Clas D, et al. Elderly trauma patients with rib fractures are at greater risk of death and pneumonia. *J Trauma*. 2003;54(3):478–485.

Bhavnagri SJ, Mohammed TLH. When and how to image a suspected broken rib. *Cleve Clin J Med*. 2009;76(5):309–314. Query: http://www.ccjm.org/content/76/5/309.full. Accessed October, 2009.

Easter A. Management of patients with multiple rib fractures. *Am J Crit Care*. 2001;10(5):320–327.

Griffith JF, Rainer TH, Ching AS, et al. Sonography compared with radiography in revealing acute rib fractures. *Am J Roentgenol*. 1999;173:1603–1609.

Harris JH, Harris WH, Novelline RA. *The Radiology of Emergency Medicine*. 3rd ed. Baltimore, MD: Williams & Wilkins; 1993:491–498.

Rosen P, Doris PE, Barkin RM, Barkin SZ, Markovchick VJ. *Diagnostic Radiology in Emergency Medicine*. Saint Louis, MO: Mosby Yearbook; 1992:82–83.

Tintinalli JE, Kelen GD, Stapczynsk JS, eds.. *Emergency Medicine: A Comprehensive Study Guide*. 6th ed. New York, NY: McGraw-Hill; 2004:1600–1601.

Vydareny KH, Gover DT, Khan A, et al. ACR *Appropriateness Criteria Rib Fractures*. query: http://www.guideline.gov/summary/summary.aspx?ss=145&doc-id=13680&nbr=7014. Accessed October, 2009.

Ziegler DW, Nikhileshewer N. The morbidity and mortality of rib fractures. *J Trauma*. 1994;37(6):975–979.

CHAPTER 51

Rheumatoid Arthritis

George M. Bridgeforth and Kris Alden

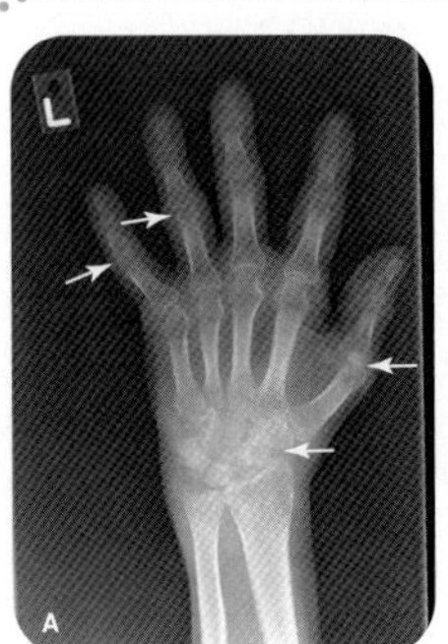

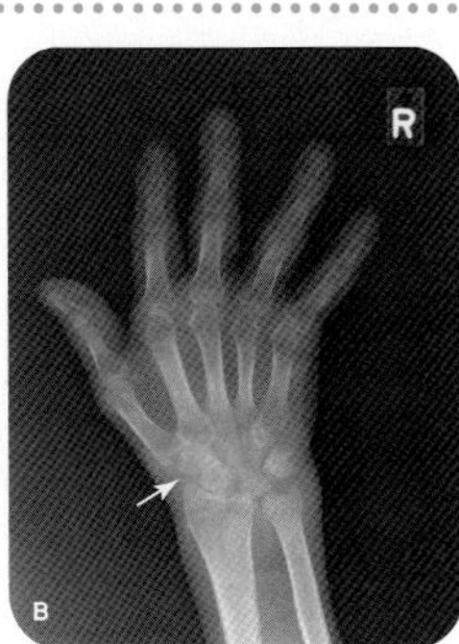

A 63-year-old man has redness, warmth, swelling, and severe pain affecting his wrists and his hands. He complains of pain, swelling, and redness in both knees as well.

Clinical Presentation

More than 2 million Americans have the chronic inflammatory disease rheumatoid arthritis (RA). Women are affected more than men; the female-to-male ratio is approximately 3:1. Although individuals of any age can develop RA, most cases typically occur between the ages of 25 and 55 years. RA is an autoimmune arthritic condition, and its exact cause is unclear. Principally a joint disease, RA also has systemic manifestations, such as weight loss, low-grade fever, and malaise.

Affected joints are swollen, tender, and warm. Patients may complain of morning stiffness, with limited movement. A polyarthritis, RA usually involves the small joints of the hands, feet, and cervical spine but may also affect large joints such as the shoulders and knees. (Patients with RA may be prone to life-threatening cervical subluxations with minor cervical trauma. It is imperative to assume cervical instability until proven otherwise and to use a spine board and a hard cervical collar.) An important feature is the presence of a periarticular osteoporosis that not only involves the metacarpals and the proximal interphalangeal (PIP) joints, but there is some involvement of the distal interphalangeal (DIP) joints as well.

Clinicians use seven criteria to diagnose RA. At least four of the seven criteria must be met (Box 51.1).

Unlike gout and psoriatic arthritis, RA is usually a symmetrical arthritis. It can involve the upper cervical spine, hands, wrists, elbows, knees, ankles, and sacroiliac joints. Unlike osteoarthritis, which involves the DIP joints, RA has predilection for the carpal (wrist), metacarpals, and PIP joints. In the latter stages, there may be involvement of the DIP joints as well. Also, unlike osteoarthritis, RA is not characterized by prominent subchondral sclerosis or osteophyte formation at the joint margins. When these latter two findings are present (especially at the DIP joints of the hands), it indicates a concomitant osteoarthritis.

CLINICAL POINTS

- Rheumatoid arthritis (RA) is a chronic inflammatory disease.
- Women are more likely than men to develop RA.
- Morning stiffness is a common complaint.

Radiographic Evaluation

Usually an examiner would like a minimum of three views of any affected area. Optional tests include a cervical computed tomography scan with contrast (for cervical trauma) to rule out atlantoaxial instability (Fig. 51.1).

PATIENT ASSESSMENT

1. Redness, warmth, and swelling of the wrists, metacarpals, PIP joints, knees, ankles, and elbows
2. Moderate disease: ulnar deviation of the hands; hypertrophy of the metacarpals, PIP joints, and knees
3. Advanced disease: joint erosions with permanent joint deformities (pannus formation), swan neck and boutonniere deformities
4. Deformities of the hands
5. Hypertrophy with severely impaired range of motion of the wrists, hands, and knees

Box 51.1 Diagnostic Criteria for Rheumatoid Arthritis (RA)*

1. Morning stiffness of the joints that lasts for at least 1 hour.
2. Arthritis in three or more joint areas. At least three joints demonstrate soft tissue swelling or fluid accumulation that has been verified by a physician. The possible areas of involvement are the proximal interphalangeal (PIP) joints, metacarpophalangeal (MCP) joints, wrist, elbow, knee, ankle, and metatarsophalangeal joints.
3. Arthritis affecting the joints of the hand, with at least one swollen area affecting the wrist, MCP, or PIP joint.
4. Symmetric arthritis. Bilateral arthritis affecting the same joints listed in item 2—the inflammatory changes do not have to be identical. (Although it is uncommon, there is an asymmetric form of RA.)
5. Rheumatoid nodules. The presence of subcutaneous nodules over bony prominences, extensor surfaces, or juxta-articular regions, verified by a physician.
6. Positive (serum) rheumatoid factor.
7. Radiographic changes secondary to RA identified on the posteroanterior hand and wrist radiographs.

*The first four criteria must be present for at least 6 weeks.

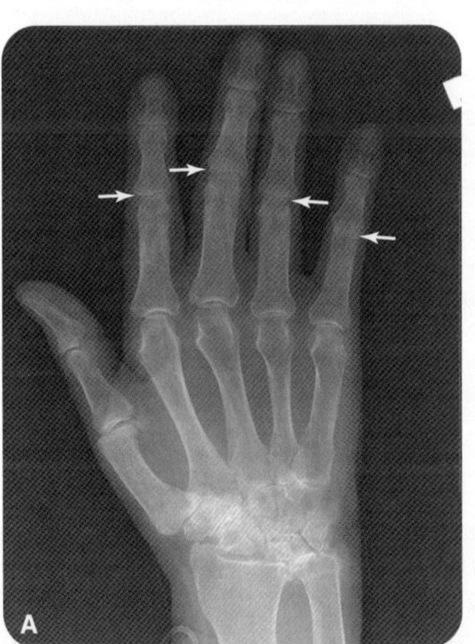

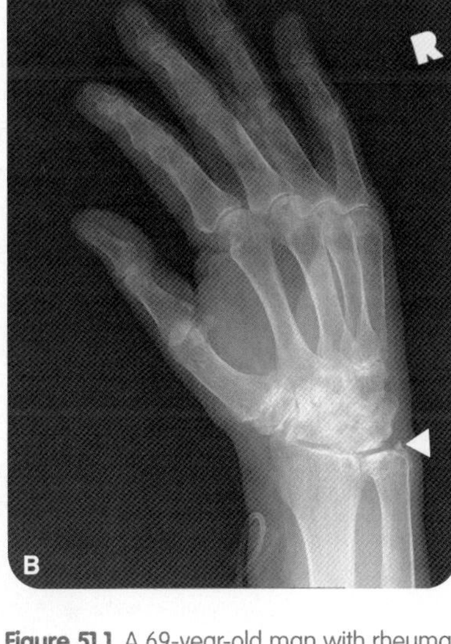

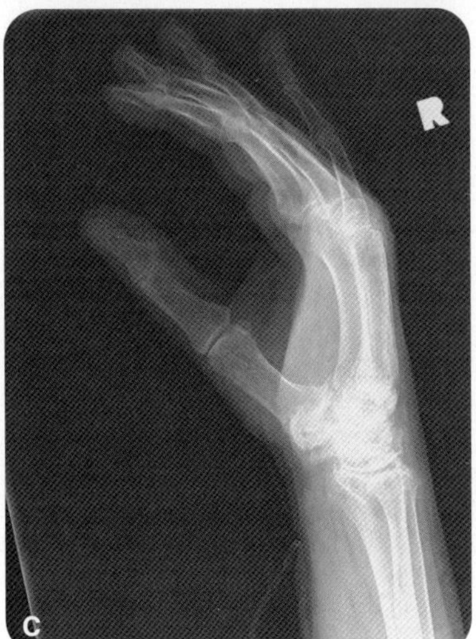

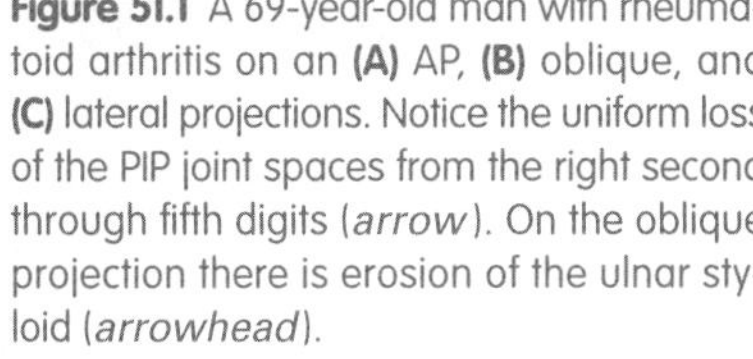
Figure 51.1 A 69-year-old man with rheumatoid arthritis on an **(A)** AP, **(B)** oblique, and **(C)** lateral projections. Notice the uniform loss of the PIP joint spaces from the right second through fifth digits (*arrow*). On the oblique projection there is erosion of the ulnar styloid (*arrowhead*).

NOT TO BE MISSED

- Osteoarthritis
- Psoriatic arthritis
- Gout
- Fractures/contusions
- Septic joint
- Collagen vascular disease (systemic lupus erythematosus, scleroderma)

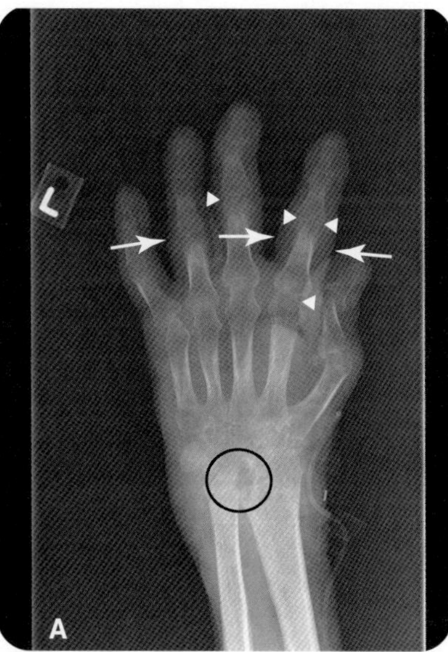

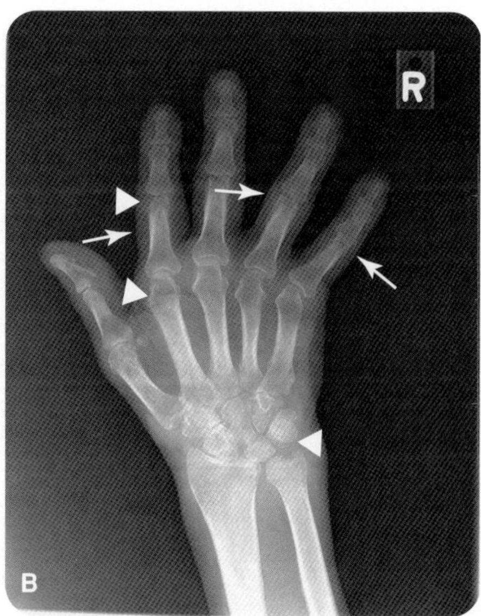

Figure 51.2 A 66-year-old man with advanced rheumatoid arthritis. Anteroposterior radiographs of the **(A)** left and **(B)** right hands demonstrate diffuse osteopenia, proximal periarticular soft tissue swelling (*arrows*), marginal erosions (*arrowheads*), and ulnar deviation of the right fourth and fifth MCP joints. Also note widening of the scapholunate interval and proximal migration of the capitate in the left hand (*circled*) compatible with scapholunate advance collapse (SLAC).

With early RA, there is an ulnar deviation of the wrists associated with a nonspecific soft tissue swelling (Fig. 51.2). With advanced RA, there is extensive erosive destruction of the carpal bones. Commonly associated findings include boutonniere and swan neck deformities of the fingers. Moreover, there is joint space narrowing with marginal erosions of the PIP joint. Hallmarks of early RA include soft tissue swelling with periarticular osteoporosis (Fig. 51.3). With joint space narrowing there are marginal erosions (i.e., erosions at the corners of the joints). More advanced involvement can lead subluxations of the metacarpals; these subluxations result in the ulnar deviation of the hand seen on clinical

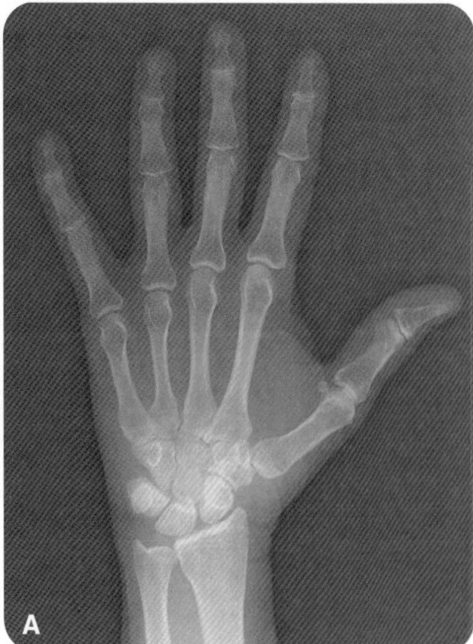

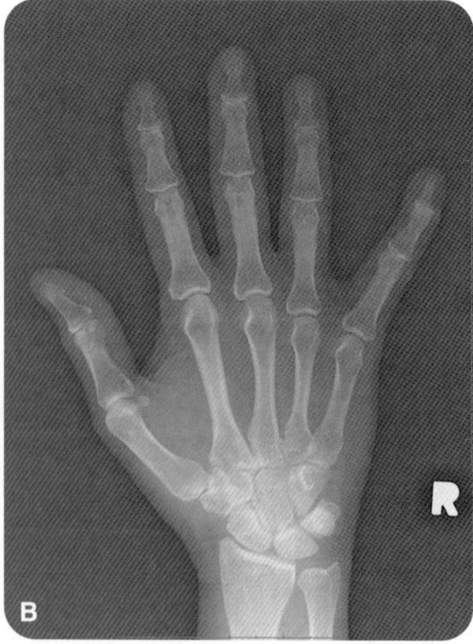

Figure 51.3 A 49-year-old female with rheumatoid arthritis demonstrating periarticular osteopenia, an early phase of the disease process.

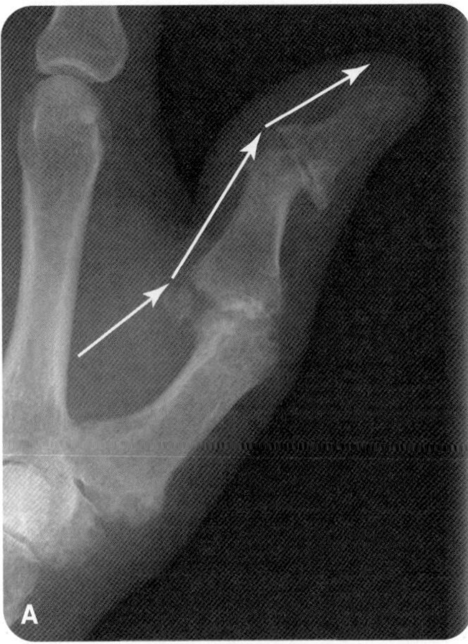

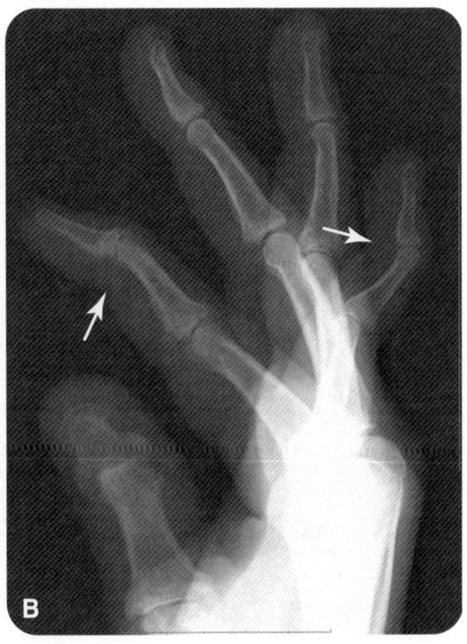

Figure 51.4 A 51-year-old man with rheumatoid arthritis demonstrating **(A)** boutonniere deformity of the left first digit and **(B)** swan neck deformities of the second and fifth DIP joints (*arrows*).

and radiological examinations. Boutonnière and swan neck deformities are classic findings in advanced RA. With a boutonnière deformity, there is prominent flexion at the PIP joint and extension of the DIP joint. Inflammation of the PIP joint results in a synovitis with elongation of the lateral bands. The resulting inflammation leads to attenuation and volar subluxation of the lateral bands (and triangular ligaments). The volar subluxation of the lateral bands exerts a downward force on the PIP joint; the end result is a characteristic flexion deformity of the PIP joint. With a swan neck deformity, the opposite configuration is characteristic. There is hyperextension of the PIP joint with flexion of the DIP joint. There is damage to the extensor mechanism at the DIP joint. Moreover, stretching and inflammatory damage to the volar plate (with an associated tendon imbalance) produces a hyperextension deformity at the PIP joint (Fig. 51.4).

In addition, the radiographic features of osteoarthritis demonstrate joint space narrowing, osteophytic formation, and subchondral cyst formation. The radiographic features of psoriasis include pencil-in-cup deformities of the joints or acroosteolysis (bony resorption of the distal phalanges, which has a classic candle-on-a-flame appearance).

Patients with RA can develop premature degeneration of the odontoid process. This premature degeneration causes atlantoaxial instability at the first and second cervical level (C1–C2) (Fig. 51.5). In patients with RA, flexion–extension films may accentuate an atlantoaxial (C1–C2) subluxation. Instability at this level can lead to ventilator dependent quadriplegia or death.

Treatment

The successful treatment of RA requires a team approach. A primary care physician and a rheumatologist may successfully managed mild-to-moderate cases may be managed by. A surgeon may be necessary in advanced cases, where operative treatment may be warranted to help restore joint mobility and function as well physical and occupational therapy to preserve independence. Because advanced RA may be disabling, early recognition, treatment, and patient education are the keys to a successful outcome. To preserve existing joint function, clinicians should encourage patients to participate in a regular

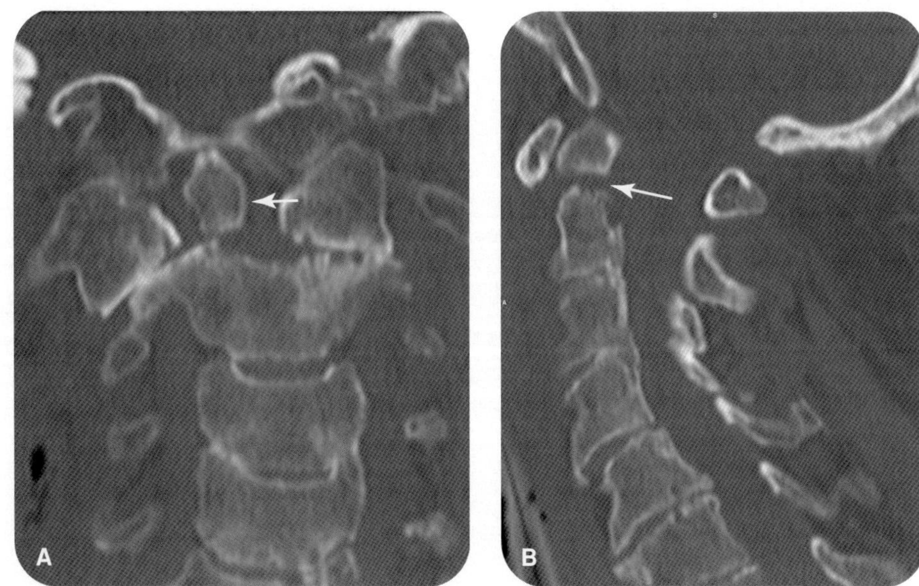

Figure 51.5 **(A)** Coronal and **(B)** sagittal reformatted computed tomography images of the cervical spine of the patient in the introductory case are focused over the atlantoaxial joint, demonstrating chronic nonunion of a type 2 dens fracture and ligamentous instability as evidenced by lateral subluxation of the right lateral mass of C1 on C2.

exercise program. To reduce joint stress in obese patients, clinicians should also encourage a healthy diet and weight loss.

Pharmacological treatment of RA with several different classes of drugs used in combination may be successful. For patients who can tolerate nonsteroidal anti-inflammatory drugs (NSAIDs), such medications may reduce pain and inflammation. However, they can cause gastric irritation, gastritis, and ulcers by blocking cyclooxygenase 1 (COX-1); this enzyme generates prostaglandins that have a protective effect on the gastric mucosa. Patients who are at high risk for gastric irritation may take NSAIDs with food or combined with a proton pump inhibitor or a prostaglandin E1 analog (misoprostol).

A subclass of NSAIDs known as COX-2 inhibitors do not offer increased analgesic effects over standard NSAIDs, but they may provide some protection against gastric irritation. Nevertheless, patients require monitoring for signs of gastrointestinal irritation, including nausea, vomiting, abdominal pain or discomfort, dizziness, and dark tarry stools. Other major side effects of NSAIDs include skin rashes, renal impairment, liver dysfunction, fluid retention, and elevated blood pressure, as well as the precipitation of asthma in aspirin-sensitive patients. NSAIDs may be contraindicated in patients with bleeding diatheses, ulcers, congestive heart failure, and renal insufficiency. Acetaminophen is useful in patients who cannot tolerate NSAIDs. Unlike the NSAIDs, acetaminophen provides some pain relief but does not block the inflammatory cascade. Short-term, but not long-term, use of narcotics may be used in selected cases.

Corticosteroids have been a mainstay in the treatment for RA for decades. Maintenance dosages are usually 5 to 10 mg/day. Traditionally, higher dosages were be used for flare-ups, but this practice is no longer as common. The side effects of corticosteroid limit their usefulness. Long-term steroid use may lead to osteoporosis. A combination of corticosteroids with calcium supplementation (one to one and one-half grams per day) and bisphosphonates may limit bone loss. Other major side effects of corticosteroids include cushingoid features (moon-shaped facies), weight gain, acute gastritis and ulcers, avascular necrosis of the hip (rare), hyperglycemia, hypokalemia, cataract formation, and adrenal suppression. With the introduction of newer agents known as disease-modifying antirheumatic drugs (DMARDs) to combat RA, some clinicians are using a regimen of DMARDs and low-dose corticosteroids for 1 or 2 months until the DMARD medications begin to work.

Although both NSAIDs and DMARDs alleviate the symptoms of RA, research has shown that only DMARDs alter the disease course and improve radiographic outcomes. Several different classes of DMARDs are available. They are described below.

CYTOTOXIC AGENTS

Methotrexate is a first-line medication that is effective against RA. In most cases, it is well tolerated in low dosages. The anti-inflammatory mechanism is not well understood, but it probably involves both immunosuppressive and toxic effects on several different enzymes in the inflammatory cascade. It may be used in combination with other DMARDs. Contraindications include liver disease, alcohol dependency, leukopenia (low white blood cell count), thrombocytopenia, renal insufficiency, and folate deficiency. Common side effects include nausea, vomiting, stomatitis, oral ulcers, and alopecia, as well as headache and fatigue. Administering folate supplements may diminish some side effects.

Cyclosporine is a reserve medication for the treatment of RA. It is usually used for patients who cannot tolerate "biologic" DMARDs—the newer classes of monoclonal antibodies or fusion proteins. Cyclosporine is an immunosuppressive medication that works by impairing the transcription of interleukin-2, a key cytokine that generates inflammation, in T cells. Main side effects include elevations in blood pressure, opportunistic infections, and renal insufficiency. Cyclosporine has been linked to the development of lymphoproliferative disorders. Combined with methotrexate may make the drug more effective.

Cyclophosphamide is a reserve agent, which is used to treat more serious cases of RA that do not respond to other agents. Major side effects of this alkylating agent include nausea, vomiting, diarrhea, oral ulcers, bone marrow, suppression, ovarian toxicity, and hemorrhagic cystitis. The medication has been linked to the development of secondary malignant cancers, including bladder cancer.

Azathioprine is an immunosuppressant that works as a purine analog (substitute). Major side effects include myelosuppression (lowering white blood cell, red blood cell, and platelet counts). Other side effects are secondary opportunistic infections, skin rash, alopecia, pancreatitis, and hepatotoxicity. The toxicity of azathioprine may increase in patients with renal insufficiency or those who are taking angiotensin-converting enzyme (ACE) inhibitors. In addition, patients receiving gold therapy, penicillamine, or antimalarials for RA should not take this drug.

AURAL AGENT

In the treatment of RA, this toxic metal may be administered orally or by injection. Following an injection, patients may complain of dizziness and weakness. It was more commonly used in the past, but it has been largely replaced by the biologic DMARDs. The side effects of gold, which limit its usefulness, include bone marrow suppression and proteinuria. Moreover, skin rashes are common and may vary from a mild itching to a major exfoliative dermatitis. Other side effects include ulcerations of the mouth and oral mucosa. Joint pain may increase for a few days.

CHELATING AGENTS (SEE SECTION, "PENICILLAMINE")

Antimalarial Agent

Hydroxychloroquine is reserved for patients who cannot tolerate biologic DMARDs. Major side effects include retinopathy, corneal deposits, itching, skin pigmentation and skin rashes, blood dyscrasias, nausea, and weakness. Irreversible retinopathy is rare, but baseline and annual eye examinations are recommended.

Tumor Necrosis Factor Blockers

Tumor necrosis factor (TNF) blockers may be effective in the treatment of RA. These agents are contraindicated in patients with active tuberculosis, opportunistic infections, pregnancy, multiple sclerosis, hepatitis (acute or chronic), congestive heart failure, chronic cutaneous ulcerations, catheters, septic arthritis within the past year, or an infected prosthesis. Side effects may include influenza-like illnesses, development of antinuclear antibodies (although the development of full systemic lupus erythematosus is rare), and injection site reactions.

Infliximab, a murine (hamster) chimera monoclonal antibody, is a TNF-α blocker. The drug limits the ability of the TNF-α to generate inflammatory mediators that produce joint damage and destruction. Infliximab is administered intravenously every 2 weeks for the first 6 weeks and then every 8 weeks. To reduce its side effects, infliximab may be administered after diphenhydramine, corticosteroids, and acetaminophen.

Etanercept is a fusion protein composed of a human immunoglobulin G and two p75 TNF receptor blockers. The drug binds to p75 receptors on TNF-α, thereby rendering it ineffective. It is given subcutaneously once to twice per week.

Adalimumab is a human immunoglobulin G monoclonal antibody. It also binds to TNF-α, thus limiting its effectiveness. It is given subcutaneously every 2 weeks.

Newer monoclonal antibodies such as golimumab require monthly administration.

T-Cell Costimulatory Blocker

Abatacept is a Y-shaped fusion protein that binds to the CD28 receptor on T lymphocytes, thus downregulating the T cell and preventing it from producing inflammatory cytokines. Abatacept is administered by intravenous infusion at baseline, 2 weeks, 4 weeks, and then monthly. Major side effects of abatacept include infusion reactions and opportunistic infections. The drug may be associated with a higher risk of secondary lymphomas and lung cancers. It should not be used concomitantly with tumor necrosis factor blockers.

B-Cell Depleting Agent

Rituximab is a B-cell depleting chimeric murine monoclonal immunoglobulin G antibody that works by binding to the CD20 receptor on B cells. Research has shown that deleting B cells help reduce the signs and symptoms of RA and slow disease progression. Major side effects include opportunistic infections and infusion reactions such as fever, chills, nausea, vomiting, dizziness, and headache, which may be reduced by administering oral acetaminophen as well as intravenous glucocorticoids and diphenhydramine prior to the infusion. Other reported side effects include pruritus (itching), lupus antibodies, polyarticular arthritis, and vasculitis. During the infusion of rituximab, monitoring of patients for chest pain, chest tightness, and shortness of breath is necessary. Cardiovascular events and fatal bronchiolitis obliterans are uncommon but have been reported.

Rituximab is a reserve-line biologic DMARD for patients who do not respond to tumor necrosis factor blockers or other biologic DMARDs. If rituximab is administered with tumor necrosis factor blockers or biologic DMARDs, there is an increased risk of opportunistic infections.

WHEN TO REFER

- Patients with RA who have sustained acute spinal cord injuries may be prone to cervical atlantoaxial dislocations, which can be life-threatening
- Patients with advanced disease

Interleukin-1 Receptor Antagonist

By binding to its receptor, anakinra blocks the actions of interleukin-1, a major cytokine that generates inflammation. Daily administration by subcutaneous injection is necessary. Because of a higher risk of neutropenia and opportunistic infections, anakinra should not be given concomitantly with other biologic DMARDs. It is necessary to monitor the neutrophil count at baseline and then every 3 months. Other common side effects include injection site erythema, weakness, influenza-like illnesses, and gastrointestinal disturbances.

Penicillamine

Penicillamine, a chelating agent, is useful for refractory cases of RA that do not respond to other DMARDs. It binds metals such as copper and iron. Its anti-inflammatory action in RA is not well understood. Major side effects include systemic lupus erythematosus, skin rashes (that may vary in scope from minor to serious), and impaired renal function.

Suggested Readings

Brown JH, Deluca SA. The radiology of rheumatoid arthritis. *Am Fam Physician.* 1995;52(5):1372–1380.

Greenspan A. *Orthopedic Imaging: A Practical Approach.* 4th ed. Philadelphia, PA: Lippincott Williams & Wilkins; 2004:474–490.

Harris JH, Harris WH, Novelline RA. *The Radiology of Emergency Medicine.* 3rd ed. Baltimore, MD: Williams & Wilkins; 1993:465.

Jacobson JA, Girish G, Jiang Y, Resnick D. Radiographic evaluation of arthritis: inflammatory conditions. *Radiology.* 2008;248:378–379.

Matusmoto AK, Bathon J, Bingham CO. *Rheumatoid Arthritis Treatment.* Query: http://www.hopkins-arhthritis.org/arthritis-info/rheumatoid-arthritis/rheum_treat.html. Accessed October, 2009.

Nash PT, Florin TH. Tumor necrosis factor inhibitors. *Med J Aust.* 2005;183(4):205–308.

O'Dell JR. Therapeutic strategies for rheumatoid arthritis. N Eng J Med. 2004;350:2591–2602.

Olsen NJ, Stein M. New drugs for rheumatoid arthritis. *N Eng J Med.* 2004;350:2167–2179.

Rindfleisch JA, Muller D. Diagnosis and management of rheumatoid arthritis. *Am Fam Physician.* 2005;72:1037–1047, 1049–1050.

Scott DL, Kingsley MB. Tumor necrosis factor inhibitors for rheumatoid arthritis. *N Eng J Med.* 2006;355: 704–712.

Smith MR. Rituximab (monoclonal anti-CD20 antibody): mechanism of action and resistance. *Oncogene.* 2003;22:7359–7268.

CHAPTER 52

Psoriatic Arthritis

George M. Bridgeforth and Kris Alden

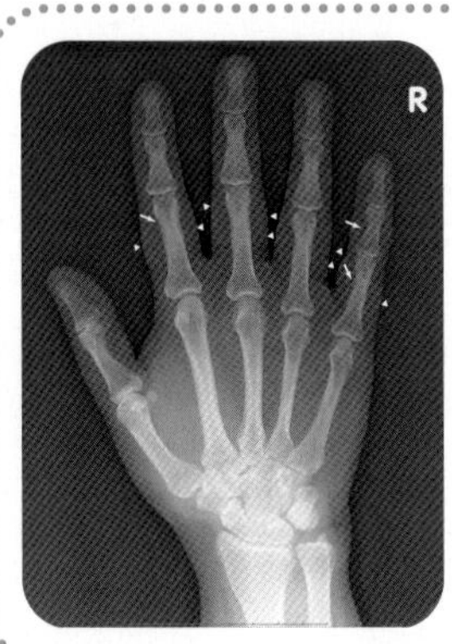

A 35-year-old woman with psoriasis complains about bilateral hand pain and back pain.

Clinical Presentation

Psoriatic arthritis is an oligoarticular, asymmetric arthritis. It may affect the distal interphalangeal (DIP) joints of the fingers, the spine, the sacroiliac joints, the hips, the knees, and the ankles. The diagnosis should be suspected in any patient with an acute joint inflammation and a history of psoriasis, an immune skin disorder. Psoriasis is characterized by salmon-colored plaques with fine silver reticular striae. Common sites of psoriasis include the knees, the tips of the elbows, the gluteal folds, the shins, as well as the soles and palms of the hands.

Psoriatic arthritis affects between 2% and 3% of the general population. It is has an equal distribution among males and females and is more common in Caucasians. The arthritic condition occurs in approximately 5% to 8% of the patients with psoriasis.

In psoriatic arthritis, nail changes, including discoloration, fungal infections (onycholysis of the nail), and small pinpoint depressions (nail pitting) may occur in up to 50% of cases. Yellow–pink and yellow–brown discolorations of the nails (oil-drop sign) may also occur. Tendinitis may be present, and patients may complain of swollen fingers. Such sausage-like swelling of the digits is referred to as dactylitis.

There are five types of psoriatic arthritis, as described below.

1. Asymmetric: typically involves three joints or less on different sides of the body and is generally mild.
2. Symmetric: usually affects the same joints, in multiple matching pairs, on both sides of the body. This form of disease, which is somewhat similar to rheumatic fever (see Chapter 51, "Rheumatoid Arthritis"), is more severe than the asymmetric type and may be disabling.
3. Spondylitis: involves the spine and neck, leading to inflammation and stiffness. It may also affect the joints of the arms, hips, legs, and feet.
4. DIP predominant: generally involves the most distal joints in the fingers and toes, resulting in inflammation, stiffness, and nail changes.
5. Arthritis mutilans: predominantly affects the small joints in the fingers and toes closest to the nail but often is associated with back and neck pain. This severe form of psoriatic arthritis is deforming and destructive.

CLINICAL POINTS

- The large majority of cases of this oligoarticular arthritis are asymmetric.
- Psoriatic sacroiliitis may lead to complaints of low back pain.
- Tendinitis may occur.

PATIENT ASSESSMENT

1. May be associated with pitting of the nails (up to 50% of the cases)
2. Early involvement: sausage digits and swollen DIP joints and involvement of the fingers
3. Late involvement: pencil-in-cup deformities and acro-osteolysis (flame-shaped erosions of the distal tufts of the hands and feet)

NOT TO BE MISSED

- Contusion
- Fracture
- Cellulitis
- Septic joint
- Osteoarthritis
- Osteomyelitis
- Rheumatoid arthritis
- Gout

Radiographic Evaluation

Psoriatic arthritis may affect several different joints, including the hands, the feet, and the sacroiliac joints. Radiographic evaluation depends on the affected area. If the sacroiliac joint is affected, radiographs of this joint may be helpful, as well as advanced imaging modalities including computed tomography and/or magnetic resonance imaging.

The examiner should look for oligoarticular involvement of the DIP joints of the hands. Early psoriatic involvement of the hands or feet can result in sausage digits. On the radiograph, look for a sausage-like pattern of soft swelling around a digit (Fig. 52.1). In addition, the examiner should observe radiographs for bone erosions at the joint margins of the joints (second and third phalanges) associated with new bone formation at the proximal border. These changes result in a characteristic mouse ear deformity ("Mickey mouse" sign) of the DIP joints (Fig. 52.2). The mouse ear configuration associated with erosive changes is a common feature of advanced psoriatic arthritis. Other advanced changes include the development of tuft erosions of the distal phalanx. This type of terminal erosion, which may appear as a small flame on a candle, is called an acro-osteolysis. Moreover, advanced cases may manifest as an asymmetric ankylosis of the proximal interphalangeal joints and the DIP joints. Other advanced findings of psoriatic arthritis include the development of pencil-in-cup deformities (Fig. 52.3). With this classic deformity, there is a marked erosion of the distal portion of the proximal joint so that it appears like a pencil that is surrounded by a cup.

In addition, psoriatic arthritis may produce a sacroiliitis (inflammation of the sacroiliac joint). Patients may complain of lower back pain (Fig. 52.4). Most sacroiliac joint deformities may be identified as a sclerotic thickening of the joint on standard radiographs.

Treatment

Patients with psoriasis may receive treatment with topical steroids, psoralen (a light-sensitive medication) combined with ultraviolet light A (PUVA) phototherapy,

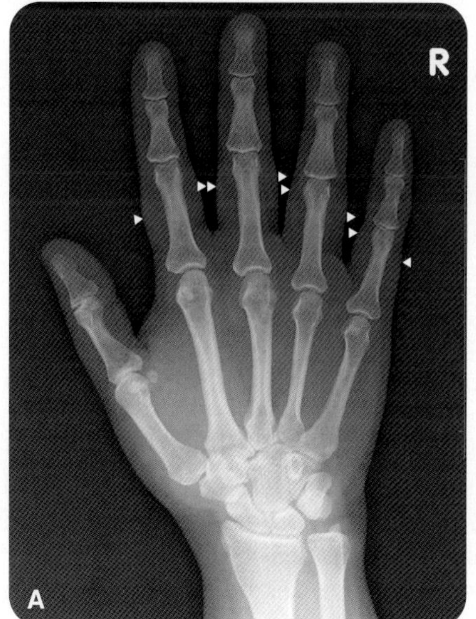

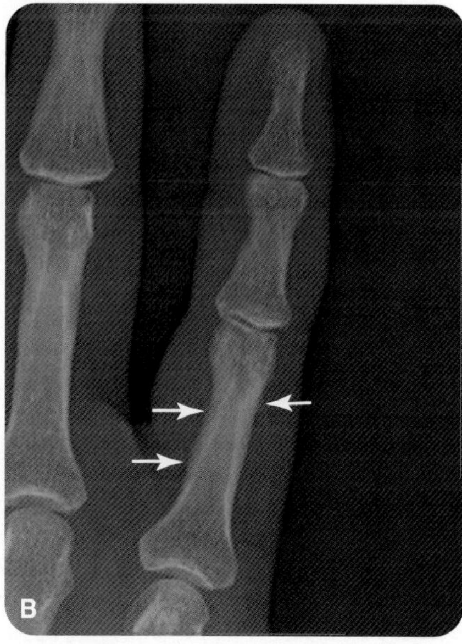

Figure 52.1 (A) Anteroposterior radiograph of the right hand of the patient in the introductory case demonstrates soft tissue swelling seen as a sausage digit (*arrowheads*). **(B)** A magnified view of the right fifth proximal phalanx demonstrates subtle periosteal reaction (*arrows*), a classic finding in psoriatic arthritis when the appropriate history is present.

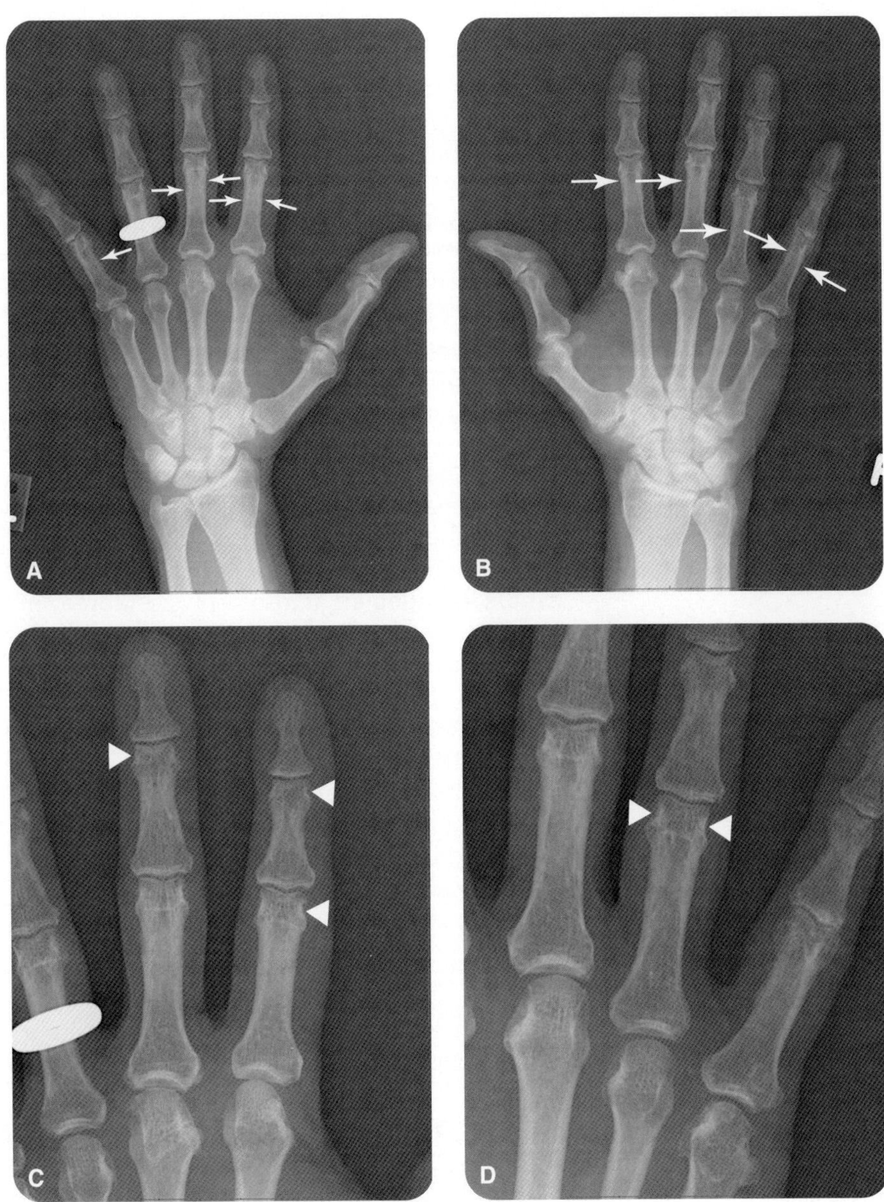

Figure 52.2 A 75-year-old man with documented psoriatic arthritis presents with bilateral hand pain. Anterior posterior radiographs of the **(A)** left and **(B)** right hands demonstrate subtle enlargement of the digits and periosteal reaction of the proximal phalanges (*arrows*). Magnified views of the **(C)** left second and third digits and **(D)** right fourth proximal interphalangeal joint demonstrate marginal erosions (*arrowheads*), which can simulate the appearance of "Mickey Mouse."

oral retinoids for desquamation, methotrexate, or cyclosporine. The retinoids include acitretin and sulfasalazine. Cyclosporine and methotrexate, as well as azathioprine, are orally administered immunosuppressive agents. Each medication has a host of side effects, including kidney or liver damage, which must be monitored carefully. Cyclosporine and methotrexate do have some secondary effects that may help combat psoriatic arthritis. Treatment of more severe cases of psoriasis requires monoclonal antibodies known as biologics or tumor necrosis factor (TNF) inhibitors.

Ideally, patients with psoriatic arthritis should have their treatment coordinated by a dermatologist and a rheumatologist. Early recognition and intervention results in a more favorable long-term outcome. Therapy for arthritic pain may include nonsteroidal anti-inflammatory drugs (NSAIDs). Patients

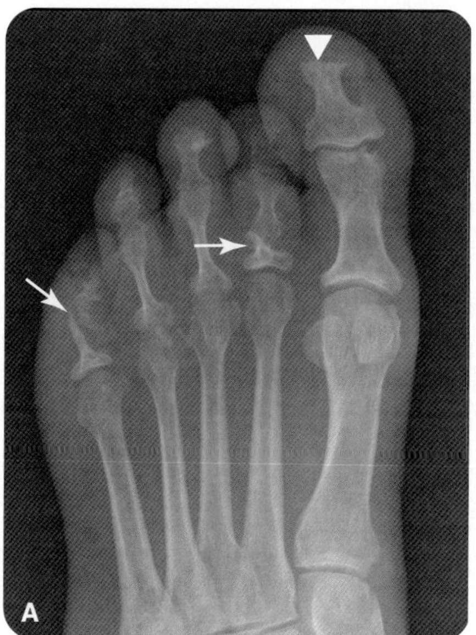

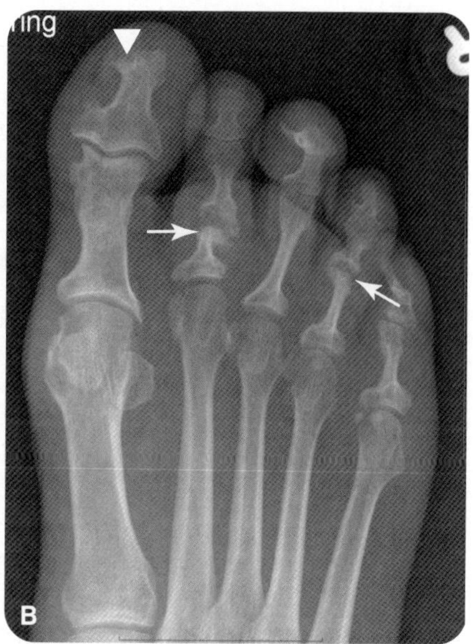

Figure 52.3 Anteroposterior radiographs of the **(A)** left and **(B)** right feet demonstrating acroosteolysis (*arrowheads*) of the first distal phalanges. In addition, there are pencil-in-cup deformities (*arrows*) of the left second and fifth proximal phalanges and right second and fourth proximal phalanges.

who cannot tolerate NSAIDs may take acetaminophen. Clinicians should discourage the long-term use of narcotics or oral steroids.

TNF blockers such as adalimumab, etanercept, or infliximab, which are sometimes referred to as fusion proteins, work by binding to the receptors of TNF. They may be effective in limiting inflammation. Infliximab is administered intravenously at baseline and then every 2 weeks for 6 weeks. Maintenance infusions are administered every 8 weeks. Etanercept is usually administered twice weekly subcutaneously. Adalimumab is administered subcutaneously every 2 weeks.

Longer acting TNF blockers such as golimumab are now on the market. Golimumab requires once-monthly administration via subcutaneous injection.

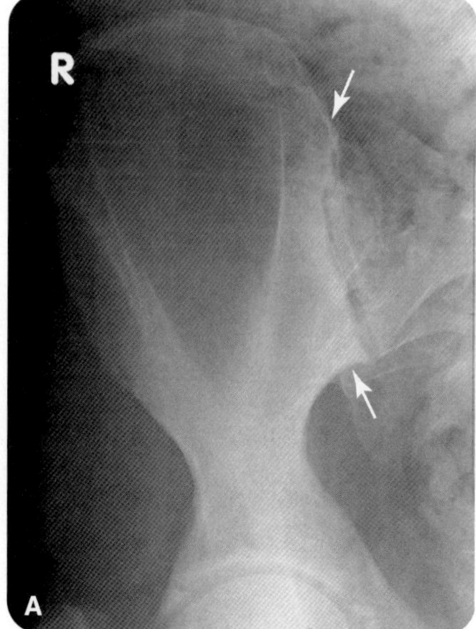

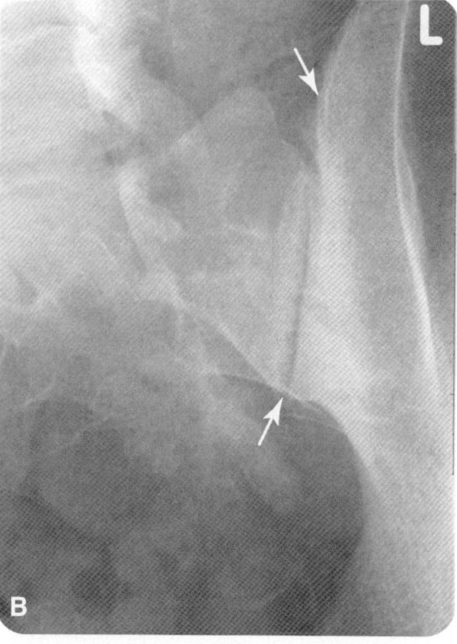

Figure 52.4 Frontal radiographs of the **(A)** right and **(B)** left sacroiliac joints in the patient from the opening case demonstrates asymmetrically increased sclerosis of the left more than right sacroiliac joint (*arrows*).

WHEN TO REFER

- For moderate and advanced cases, a dermatological and rheumatological referral should be considered.
- Patients with advanced disease should be referred to an orthopedic surgeon or a physician specialized in physical medicine and rehabilitation.

Often, clinicians prescribe TNF blockers together with methotrexate when combating psoriatic arthritis. However, it is important not to combine TNF blockers, although another TNF blocker may be substituted if a different TNF blocker is ineffective. Combining TNF blockers does not offer any greater efficacy but runs the risk of higher complications such as opportunistic infections.

Although the TNF blockers may be useful, they may result in immunosuppression and serious infections, including tuberculosis. Moreover, there may be an increased risk of lymphoproliferative disorders (lymphomas), but more long-term data are needed. These medications block TNF-α, which is a cytokine, a chemical mediator that can lead to damage and destruction of cartilage and bone. These medications may worsen chronic hepatitis and multiple sclerosis. Moreover, patients may develop antinuclear antibodies; however, the actual development of systemic lupus erythematous is rare.

Suggested Readings

Barton AC. Genetic epidemiology: psoriatic arthritis. *Arthritis Res.* 2002;4:247–251.

Callen JP, Jorizzo JL, Bolognia JL, et al. *Dermatological Signs of Internal Disease.* 3rd ed. Philadelphia, PA: Saunders; 2003:35–37, 328.

FitzpatrickTB, Polano MK, Surrmond D. *Color Atlas and Synopsis of Clinical Dermatology.* New York, NY: McGraw-Hill; 1983:46–63.

Gottlieb A, Korman NJ, Gordon KB, et al. Guidelines of Care for the Management of Psoriasis and Psoriatic Arthritis: Section 2. Psoriatic Arthritis: Overview and Guidelines of Care for Treatment with an Emphasis on the Biologics. *J Am Acad Dermatol.* 2008;58(5):851–864.

Greenspan A. *Orthopedic Imaging.* 4th ed. Philadelphia, PA: Lippincott Williams & Wilkins; 1994:493–499.

Habif T, Campbell JL, Quitadamo M, Zug K. *Skin Disease Diagnosis and Treatment.* Saint Louis, MO: Mosby; 2001:84–93.

Jacobson JA, Girish G, Jiang Y, Resnick D. Radiographic evaluation of arthritis: inflammatory conditions. *Radiology.* 2008;248:378–389.

Jones J, Brenner C, Chin N, Bunker CB. Radiological associations with dermatological disease. *Br J Radiol.* 2005;78:662–671.

Mease DJ, Goffe BS, Netz J, et al. Etanercept in the treatment of psoriatic arthritis and psoriasis: a randomized trial. *Lance.* 2000;356:385–390.

National Psoriasis Foundation. *Treating Psoriatic Arthritis: Biologic Drugs.* Query: http:www.psoriasis.org/netcommunity?sublearn02-treat-bio. Accessed October, 2009.

National Psoriasis Foundation. *Treating Psoriatic Arthritis: Traditional Systemic Drugs.* Query:nttp://www.psoriasis.org/netcommunity/sublearn02-treat-system. Accessed October, 2009.

Schoellnast H, Deutschmann HA, Hermann J, et al. Psoriatic arthritis and rheumatoid arthritis: findings in contrast enhanced MRI. *Am J Radiol.* 2006;187:351–357.

White GM, Cox NH. *Diseases of the Skin: A Color Atlas and Text.* Saint Louis, MO: Mosby; 2000:47–61.

CHAPTER 53 Gout

George M. Bridgeforth and Kris Alden

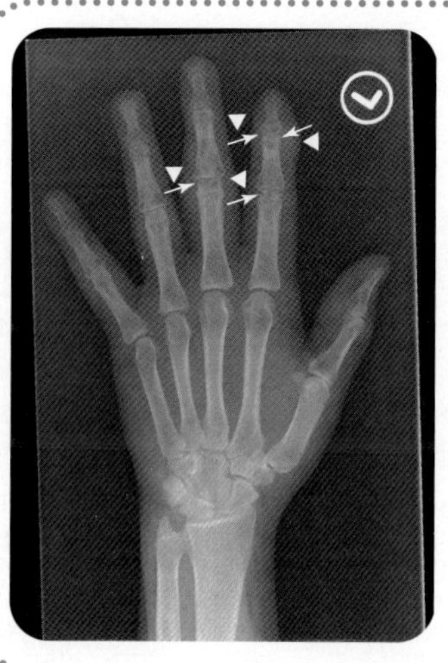

A 57-year-old postmenopausal woman presents with acute bilateral hand pain, swelling, and erythema. She has had intermittent attacks characterized by redness swelling of the great toe, the knee, and the ankle for several days.

Clinical Presentation

Gout is a condition that affects approximately 2% of the population. In younger age groups, it affects men more than women 9:1. However, the ratio declines with advancing age with a male to female ratio of 3:1 following menopause. Moreover, the age distribution is different as well. It commonly begins in males between 30 and 45 years of age and in postmenopausal females. The incidence of gout continues to increase with advancing age.

Gout usually presents as an oligoarthritis; it is caused by the deposition of monosodium urate crystals in the joint space. The disease is manifested by either an overproduction or an underexcretion of uric acid.

Gout is characterized by a history of acute attacks and remissions. Acute attacks usually last for several (5–10) days and are characterized by marked redness, warmth, swelling, and tenderness. Sixty percent of patients with gout have a second attack within 1 year, and 78% have a second attack within 2 years. The most commonly affected joint is the great toe. However, other joints such as the knees, ankles, fingers, and elbows may be affected. Most flare-ups affect a single joint. However, severe cases may affect multiple joints. Widespread, disabling joint destruction is uncommon, except in severe cases.

Tophi, which are permanent collections of uric acid crystals, may be seen in severe cases. They may be seen on the metacarpal heads (i.e., the knuckles), lower ear lobes, olecranon (tips of the elbows), and the Achilles tendons. In addition, tophi may appear over the distal interphalangeal or proximal interphalangeal joints in patients with concomitant osteoarthritis. Generally, it takes more than 10 years to develop gouty tophi. However, tophi have a higher risk of developing in untreated or poorly treated patients. Kidney stones occur in approximately 15% of patients with gout.

CLINICAL POINTS

- Gout is more common in men.
- Periodic attacks and remissions characterize gout. Au2 noted and appreciated.
- The most commonly affected joints are in the feet or hands, as well as the knee, ankle, elbow, or wrist.

Radiographic Evaluation

Usually standard radiographs are sufficient. CT or MRI scans are usually not required. Necessary tests depend on the area of involvement. It is not uncommon for patients with nontraumatic medical conditions to relate them to injuries.

PATIENT ASSESSMENT

1. Marked redness, warmth, and swelling of virtually any joint
2. Usually oligoarticular and asymmetric arthritis characterized by flare-ups followed by periods of remission
3. Severe pain; complaint of painful weight bearing when pain affects the lower extremities

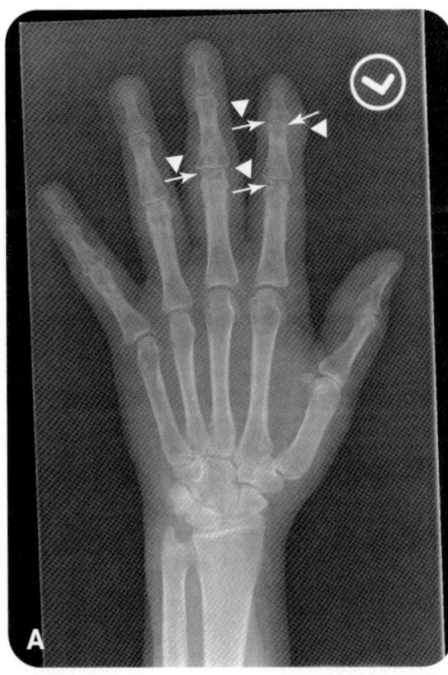

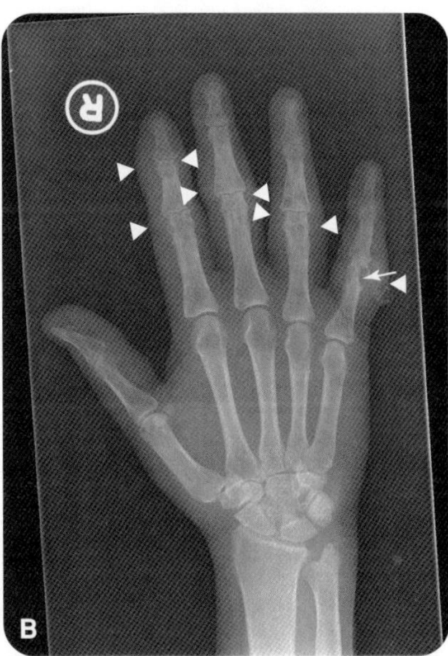

Figure 53.1 AP radiographs of the **(A)** left and **(B)** right hands from the patient in the opening case demonstrating periarticular soft tissue swelling (*arrowheads*), marginal erosions (*arrows*), and preservation of the joint space and bone mineralization compatible with gouty arthritis.

Gout can often manifest as periarticular erosions with predominant soft tissue swelling involving the affected joint. One of the pathognomonic features of gout are the hourglass-shaped periarticular erosions with a characteristic appearance, resembling bites out an apple with sharp rounded edges (Fig. 53.1). Greenspan describes these erosions as having a characteristic "overhanging edge" (Fig. 53.2). If the examiner looks closely (especially if the patient has had a history of a prior attack affecting the particular joint), there may be radiographic evidence of early periarticular involvement. The periarticular bone may appear less dense in that region.

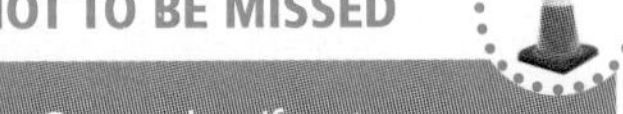

NOT TO BE MISSED

- Contusion/fracture
- Cellulitis
- Septic joint
- Osteoarthritis
- Osteomyelitis
- Rheumatoid arthritis
- Psoriatic arthritis

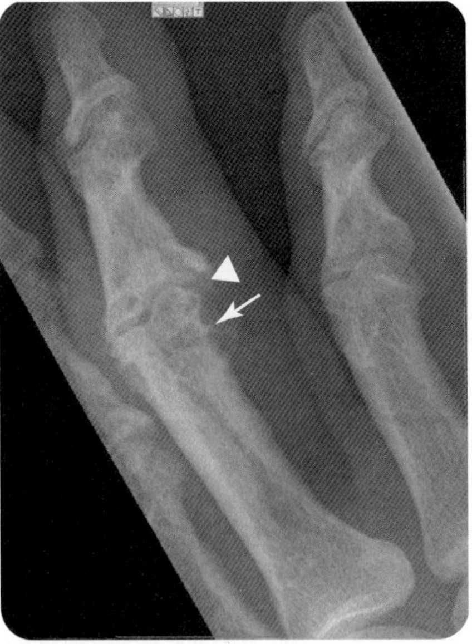

Figure 53.2 Oblique radiograph of the left hand in a patient with gout demonstrating the typical "rat bite" erosions (*arrow*) of the third proximal interphalangeal joint and overhanging edge (*arrowhead*).

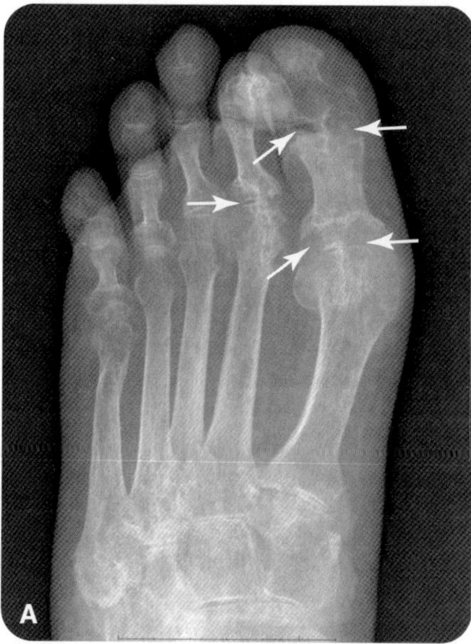

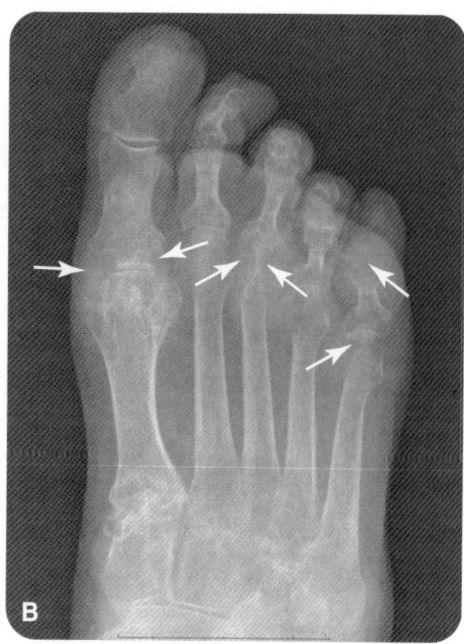

Figure 53.3 AP radiographs of the **(A)** left and **(B)** right feet demonstrating advanced gouty arthritis in a 71-year-old man. Advanced marginal erosions are demonstrated affecting the proximal and distal aspects of the joint spaces (*arrows*). Pencil-in-cup appearance is present at the right third metatarsal distally. Notice, however, that the central joint spaces are preserved particularly evident at the first MTP joints bilaterally.

In addition, the examiner should note the preservation of the joint space, which is an important finding with gout (Fig. 53.3). The joint space is usually preserved because gouty attacks (unlike many other inflammatory rheumatological conditions) are sporadic. Usually, even in advanced gout, there is some preservation of the joint space. (In rheumatoid arthritis, usually the presentation is usually more symmetrical and not oligoarticular. Moreover, one of the hallmarks of rheumatoid arthritis is a disuse osteopenia. This finding is associated with progressive joint destruction (Fig. 53.4). Because most gouty attacks

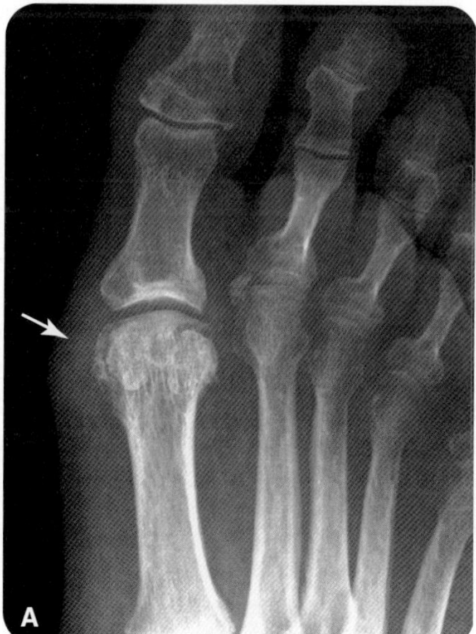

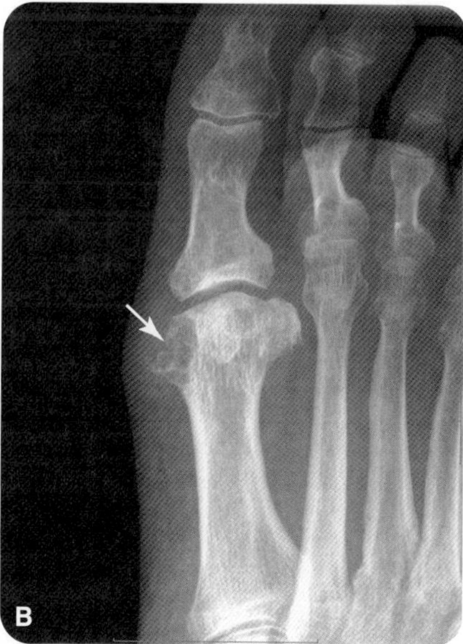

Figure 53.4 A 80-year-old intoxicated man present with acute first metatarsal pain. **(A)** Initial AP radiograph of the right first MTP joint demonstrates a soft tissue calcification (*arrow*) and marginal erosions compatible with tophaceous gout. **(B)** Repeat radiograph after 4 months demonstrates progression of the marginal erosion of the medial first MTP joint.

are of short duration, a long-term disuse osteopenia does not have time to develop.)

Treatment

Treatment for acute flare-ups involves a combination of pain medications (nonsteroidal anti-inflammatory drugs [NSAIDs] if tolerated), short-term corticosteroids, and cold packs. Patients who are elderly; who have chronic renal disease, severe congestive heart failure, or peptic ulcers, or aspirin-sensitive asthma; or who are taking warfarin may not be able to tolerate oral steroids and NSAIDs. Acetaminophen may be substituted. Also, oral colchicine may be used as a second-tier medication. Common side effects with colchicine include transient diarrhea. Thiazides, which can lead to hyperuricemia, should be avoided if possible. Clinicians should discourage the long-term use of narcotics.

One of the main goals of effective treatment is to decrease the serum urate level to equal to or less than 6.0 mg/dL. It is necessary to monitor urate levels every 4 to 6 weeks until patients reach target levels and then every 6 to 12 months. Clinicians use allopurinol, a xanthine oxidate inhibitor, to treat hyperuricemia. Allopurinol may be taken daily and in combination with probenecid, a uricosuric (promotes the excretion of uric acid) medication. However, probenecid may not be used in patients with compromised renal function (glomerular filtration rate <50%). The dosage of allopurinol should be reduced in patients with renal impairment as well. Side effects of allopurinol include skin rashes and a rare but fatal hypersensitivity syndrome. Moreover, allopurinol and probenecid have many common drug interactions, which may limit their use.

Newer medications, including febuxostat, have recently challenged the efficacy of allopurinol. Like allopurinol, febuxostat is an uricostatic drug that inhibits xanthine oxidase. However, unlike allopurinol, febuxostat has fewer reported side effects, and patients who are allergic to allopurinol may use febuxostat. Furthermore, the dose of febuxostat needs no adjustment in elderly patients or patients with mild-to-moderate renal impairment. Major side effects of febuxostat include headaches, liver function abnormalities, and gastrointestinal disturbances. Other newer medications include uricolytic drugs that degrade uric acid, which are formulated by combining the porcine enzyme urate oxidase with chains of polyethylene glycol (PEG). Uricase-PEG 20 and pegloticase, which is given intravenously every 2 to 4 weeks, decreases the level of immunological reactions. In addition, the PEG component prolongs the half-life of the medication. These medications may be useful in decreasing or eradicating gouty tophi as well. They may be used for treating advanced cases or gout or for patients who cannot tolerate standard uricostatic and uricosuric medications.

Finally, dietary education and weight reduction (in obese patients) can help reduce the incidence of future attacks. Foods and beverages rich in purines such as meat, seafood, and alcohol should be limited. They should be replaced by healthy portions of chicken, ham, pork, and vegetables. Blood pressure and renal function should be monitored.

WHEN TO REFER

- Patients with recurrent flare-ups that are not controlled by a regimen of diet and medications should be followed by a rheumatologist as well as a primary care practitioner.
- It may be difficult to differentiate a septic arthritis from a gout flare up. In these cases, the joint fluid should be apirated analyzed under a microscope for crystals vs. bacteria and sent for cultures.

Suggested Readings

Bloch C, Hermann G, Yu TF. A radiologic reevaluation of gout: a study of 2,000 patients. *Am J Roentgenol.* 1980;134(4):781–787.

Choi HK, Atkinson K, Karlson EW, Willett W, Curhan G. Purine-rich foods, dairy and protein intake and the risk of gout in men. *N Eng J Med.* 2004;350:1093–1103.

Dore RK. Gout: what primary care physicians want to know. *J Clin Rheumatology.* 2008;14(S):547–554.

Edwards LN. Clinical manifestations of gout in seniors: causes, co-morbidities, and complications of long-standing hyperuricemia. *Suppl Clin Geriat*. September 2009:5–14.

Eggebeen A. Gout: an update. *Am Fam Physician*. 2007;76:801–808, 811–812.

Greenspan A. *Orthopedic Imaging: A Practical Approach*. 4th ed. Baltimore, MD: Lippincott Williams & Wilkins; 2004:509–514.

Harris JH, Harris WH, Novelline RA. *The Radiology of Emergency Medicine*. 3rd ed. Baltimore, MD: Williams & Wilkins; 1993:432.

Mandell BF. Clinical manifestations of hyperuricemia and gout. *Cleve Clin J Med*. 2008;75(S):55–58.

National Institute of Health. Pegylated Recombinant Mammalian Uricase (PEG- Uricase) as Treatment for Refractory Gout. http://clinicaltrials,gov/ct1/show/NCT001111657. Updated July 10, 2009. Accessed October, 2009.

Rosen P, Doris PE, Barkin RM, Barkin SZ, Markovchick VJ. *Diagnostic Radiology in Emergency Medicine*. Saint Louis, MO: Mosby Year Book; 1992:520–522.

Tintinalli JE, Kelen GD, Stapczynski JS. *Emergency Medicine: A Comprehensive Study Guide*. 6th ed. New York, NY: McGraw-Hill; 2004:909–910.

Index

Page numbers in *italics* denote Figures (*f*) and Tables (*t*).